MOUNT SINAI
EXPERT GUIDES

Neurology

MOUNT SINAI EXPERT GUIDES

Neurology

EDITED BY

Stuart C. Sealfon, MD
Glickenhaus Professor and Chairman Emeritus, Department of Neurology
Professor of Neurobiology, Pharmacology and Systems Therapeutics
Director, Center for Advanced Research on Diagnostic Assays
Icahn School of Medicine at Mount Sinai
New York, NY, USA

Rajeev Motiwala, MD
Associate Professor of Neurology
Director, Neurology Clerkship
Icahn School of Medicine at Mount Sinai
New York, NY, USA

Charles B. Stacy, MD
Assistant Professor of Neurology
Director of General Neurology
Icahn School of Medicine at Mount Sinai
New York, NY, USA

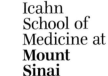

Icahn
School of
Medicine at
**Mount
Sinai**

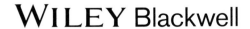

WILEY Blackwell

Contents

PART 3: NEUROLOGIC DISEASES AND THERAPEUTICS

Contributors

Kenneth W. Altman MD, PhD, FACS
Professor and Vice Chair for Clinical Affairs
Department of Otolaryngology – HNS
Director, The Institute for Voice and
Swallowing at BCM
Baylor College of Medicine
Houston, TX, USA

Shannon E. Babineau MD
Division of Child Neurology
Goryeb Children's Hospital
Morristown, NJ, USA

Joshua Bederson MD
Professor and System Chair
Department of Neurosurgery
Icahn School of Medicine at Mount Sinai
New York, NY, USA

Florence Ching-Fen Chang MBBS
Robert and John M. Bendheim Parkinson and
Movement Disorders Center at Mount Sinai
Department of Neurology
Icahn School of Medicine at Mount Sinai
New York, NY, USA

Barbara Kelly Changizi MD
Assistant Professor
Departments of Neurology and Psychiatry
The Ohio State University Wexner Medical Center
Columbus, OH, USA

Catherine Cho MD, MSCR
Associate Professor
Departments of Neurology and Otolaryngology
New York University Langone Medical Center
New York, NY, USA

Bernard Cohen MD
Morris B. Bender Professor
Department of Neurology
Icahn School of Medicine at Mount Sinai
New York, NY, USA

Reade De Leacy MD, MBBS
Assistant Professor
Department of Radiology
Icahn School of Medicine at
Mount Sinai
New York, NY, USA

Mandip S. Dhamoon MD, MPH
Assistant Professor
Department of Neurology
Vascular Neurology Fellowship Director
Icahn School of Medicine at Mount Sinai
New York, NY, USA

Michelle T. Fabian MD
Assistant Professor
Department of Neurology
Corinne Goldsmith Dickinson Center
for Multiple Sclerosis
Icahn School of Medicine at Mount Sinai
New York, NY, USA

Steven H. Feinsilver MD
Professor
Department of Medicine
Division of Pulmonary, Critical Care and
Sleep Medicine
Director, Center for Sleep Medicine
Icahn School of Medicine at
Mount Sinai
New York, NY, USA

Madeline C. Fields MD
Assistant Professor
Department of Neurology
Co-Director of the Mount Sinai Epilepsy
Center
Clinical Neurophysiology Fellowship
Director
Icahn School of Medicine at Mount Sinai
New York, NY, USA

Steven J. Frucht MD
Professor
Department of Neurology
Director, Movement Disorders Division
Robert and John M. Bendheim Parkinson
and Movement Disorders Center
Icahn School of Medicine at Mount Sinai
New York, NY, USA

Sam Gandy MD, PhD
Mount Sinai Professor of Alzheimer's Disease
    Research
Departments of Neurology and Psychiatry
Director, Mount Sinai Center for Cognitive
Health
Director, NFL Neurological Center
Associate Director, Mount Sinai Alzheimer's
Disease Research Center
Icahn School of Medicine at Mount Sinai
and James J. Peters Veterans Association
Medical Center
New York, NY, USA

Isabelle M. Germano MD, FACS
Professor
Departments of Neurosurgery, Neurology,
Oncological Sciences
Director, Comprehensive Brain Tumor
    Program
Co-Director, Radiosurgery Program
Icahn School of Medicine at Mount Sinai
New York, NY, USA

Martin Goldstein MD
Associate Professor
Department of Neurology
Medical Director, Mount Sinai Center for
    Cognitive Health
Icahn School of Medicine at Mount Sinai
New York, NY, USA

Errol L. Gordon MD
Assistant Professor
Departments of Neurosurgery and
    Neurology
Neurocritical Care
Icahn School of Medicine at Mount Sinai
New York, NY, USA

Mark W. Green MD, FAAN
Professor
Departments of Neurology, Anesthesiology,
and Rehabilitation Medicine
Director, Headache and Pain Medicine
Icahn School of Medicine at Mount Sinai
New York, NY, USA

Deborah R. Horowitz MD
Associate Professor
Department of Neurology
Icahn School of Medicine at Mount Sinai
New York, NY, USA

Asha Iyer MD, PhD
Resident
Department of Neurosurgery
Icahn School of Medicine at Mount Sinai
New York, NY, USA

Stephen Krieger MD
Associate Professor
Department of Neurology
Corinne Goldsmith Dickinson Center for MS
Director, Neurology Residency Program
Icahn School of Medicine at Mount Sinai
New York, NY, USA

Ruby J. Lien MD
Attending Radiologist
Neuroradiology and Emergency/
Trauma Radiology
Winthrop Radiology Associates
Mineola, NY, USA

Fred D. Lublin MD, FAAN, FANA
Saunders Family Professor
Department of Neurology
Director, The Corinne Goldsmith Dickinson
Center for Multiple Sclerosis
Icahn School of Medicine at Mount Sinai
New York, NY, USA

Lara V. Marcuse MD
Assistant Professor
Department of Neurology
Co-Director, Mount Sinai Epilepsy Center
Icahn School of Medicine at Mount Sinai
New York, NY, USA

Justin Mascitelli MD
Resident
Department of Neurosurgery
Icahn School of Medicine at Mount Sinai
New York, NY, USA

Aaron Miller MD, FAAN, FANA
Professor
Department of Neurology
Director, Clinical Affairs, Corinne Goldsmith
Dickson Center for Multiple Sclerosis
Icahn School of Medicine at Mount Sinai
New York, NY, USA

Rajeev Motiwala MD
Associate Professor
Department of Neurology
Director, Neurology Clerkship
Icahn School of Medicine at Mount Sinai
New York, NY, USA

Michael P. Mullen MD
Professor
Departments of Medicine and Infectious Diseases
Director, Institute for Advanced Medicine
Icahn School of Medicine at Mount Sinai
New York, NY, USA

Thomas P. Naidich MD
Vice-Chair of Radiology for Academic Affairs
Irving and Dorothy Regenstreif
Research Professor of Neurosciences
  (Neuroimaging)
Professor of Radiology, Neurosurgery,
and Pediatrics
Icahn School of Medicine at Mount Sinai
New York, NY, USA

Margaret Pain MD
Resident
Department of Neurosurgery
Icahn School of Medicine at Mount Sinai
New York, NY, USA

Ritesh A. Ramdhani MD
Assistant Professor
Department of Neurology and Neurosurgery
Robert and John M. Bendheim Parkinson
and Movement Disorders Center
Icahn School of Medicine at Mount Sinai
New York, NY, USA

Jessica Robinson-Papp MD, MS
Assistant Professor
Departments of Neurology and Pathology
Icahn School of Medicine at Mount Sinai
New York, NY, USA

Janet C. Rucker MD
Bernard A. and Charlotte Marden
Associate Professor of Neurology
NYU Langone Medical Center
New York, NY, USA

Stuart C. Sealfon MD
Glickenhaus Professor and Chairman Emeritus
Department of Neurology
Professor of Neurobiology, Pharmacology and
Systems Therapeutics
Director, Center for Advanced Research
on Diagnostic Assays
Icahn School of Medicine at Mount Sinai
New York, NY, USA

Susan Shin MD
Assistant Professor
Department of Neurology
Icahn School of Medicine at Mount Sinai
New York, NY, USA

David M. Simpson MD, FAAN
Professor
Department of Neurology
Director, Clinical Neurophysiology Laboratories
Director, Neuromuscular Division
Director, Neuro-AIDS Program
Icahn School of Medicine at Mount Sinai
New York, NY, USA

Mark A. Sivak MD
Assistant Professor
Department of Neurology
Icahn School of Medicine at Mount Sinai
New York, NY, USA

Eric Smouha MD
Associate Professor
Department of Otolaryngology
Director of Otology-Neurotology
Icahn School of Medicine at Mount Sinai
New York, NY, USA

Charles B. Stacy MD
Assistant Professor
Department of Neurology
Director, General Neurology
Icahn School of Medicine at Mount Sinai
New York, NY, USA

Jeremy M. Steinberger MD
Resident
Department of Neurosurgery
Icahn School of Medicine at Mount Sinai
New York, NY, USA

Winona Tse MD
Assistant Professor
Department of Neurology
Movement Disorders Division
Icahn School of Medicine at Mount Sinai
New York, NY, USA

Stanley Tuhrim MD
Professor and Vice Chair for Clinical Affairs,
Department of Neurology
Professor, Geriatrics and
Palliative Medicine
Director, Mount Sinai Stroke Center
Icahn School of Medicine at Mount Sinai
New York, NY, USA

Jamie S. Ullman MD, FACS
Associate Professor
Department of Neurosurgery
Hoftstra Northwell School of Medicine
Hempstead, NY, USA

Jonathan M. Vapnek MD
Associate Professor
Department of Urology
Icahn School of Medicine at Mount Sinai
New York, NY, USA

Geena Varghese DO
Attending Physician
Infectious Disease and Internal Medicine
Westmed Medical Group
West Harrison, NY, USA

Ruth H. Walker MD
Associate Professor
Department of Neurology
Icahn School of Medicine at Mount Sinai and
James J. Peters Veterans Affairs Medical
  Center
Bronx, NY, USA

Hailun Wang MD
Resident
Department of Otolaryngology
Icahn School of Medicine at Mount Sinai
New York, NY, USA

Steven J. Weissbart, MD
Resident
Department of Urology
Icahn School of Medicine at Mount Sinai
New York, NY, USA

Lan Zhou MD, PhD
Associate Professor
Departments of Neurology, Pathology,
and Neurosurgery
Director, Mount Sinai Neuromuscular
Pathology Laboratory
Icahn School of Medicine at Mount Sinai
New York, NY, USA

Sarah Zubkov MD
Assistant Professor
Epilepsy and Neurophysiology
Temple University Hospital
Philadelphia, PA, USA

Series Foreword

Now more than ever, immediacy in obtaining accurate and practical information is the coin of the realm in providing high quality patient care. The Mount Sinai Expert Guides series addresses this vital need by providing accurate, up-to-date guidance, written by experts in formats that are accessible in the patient care setting: websites, smartphone apps, and portable books. The Icahn School of Medicine, which was chartered in 1963, embodies a deep tradition of pre-eminence in clinical care and scholarship that was first shaped by the founding of the Mount Sinai Hospital in 1855. Today, the Mount Sinai Health System, comprised of seven hospitals anchored by the Icahn School of Medicine, is one of the largest healthcare systems in the United States, and is revolutionizing medicine through its embracing of transformative technologies for clinical diagnosis and treatment. The Mount Sinai Expert Guides series builds upon both this historical renown and contemporary excellence. Leading experts across a range of disciplines provide practical yet sage advice in a digestible format that is ideal for trainees, mid-level providers, and practicing physicians. Few medical centers in the USA could offer this type of breadth while relying exclusively on its own physicians, yet here no compromises were required in offering a truly unique series that is sure to become embedded within the key resources of busy providers. In producing this series, the editors and authors are fortunate to have an equally dynamic and forward-viewing partner in Wiley Blackwell, which together ensures that healthcare professionals will benefit from a unique, first-class effort that will advance the care of their patients.

Scott L. Friedman, MD
Series Editor
Fishberg Professor of Medicine
Dean for Therapeutic Discovery
Chief, Division of Liver Diseases
Icahn School of Medicine at Mount Sinai
New York, NY, USA

Preface

Our goal in creating this volume along with the associated App and dedicated website is to provide a resource that is readily available to assist students, young neurologists, and physicians in other specialties in their approach to diagnosis and treatment of patients with diseases of the nervous system. In favor of accessibility, which implies rapid orientation and practical guidance, we have chosen simplicity and clarity over comprehensiveness.

It was not long ago that the practice of neurology consisted largely of descriptive phenomenology in the absence of effective therapeutics. But presently the field has been transformed by tremendous growth in the understanding of neurologic diseases so that vastly increased diagnostic precision is joined to a complex armamentarium of highly effective therapies. Skilled neurologic practice currently demands an extraordinary fund of knowledge, one that continues to change rapidly. Many disorders that now figure prominently in differential diagnosis of patients encountered on a daily basis in the hospital or the clinic were considered arcane or simply not recognized a decade or so ago, and in other cases diagnosis did not need to be precise since there were no treatments. A very abbreviated list of examples includes: anti-NMDA receptor encephalitis presenting as seizures or psychosis and effectively treated through immunomodulation; poorly controlled seizures arising from an epileptogenic focus that can be mapped and resected; dystonia responsive to botulinum toxin; multiple sclerosis variants treated by different immune modulators; acute ischemic stroke etiologies treated by thrombolytics or intravascular retraction; and various severe movement disorders controlled by site-specific deep brain stimulation. As the complexity of patients encountered in the hospital and clinic increases, neurologists must interact with other medical and surgical specialties in all aspects of care. The assiduous application of our particular knowledge is required to establish accurate diagnosis and enact effective therapy in this context. The contributions of the neurologist can dramatically and decisively improve the lives of patients with hundreds of different neurologic conditions. Diseases of the nervous system are generally a high-stakes issue for patients, so starting the process on the right track is crucial. We endeavor to provide a guide to help the reader to approach these patients.

We acknowledge our gratitude for all those who helped with this project. We thank the Wiley team and the respective editors along the way. We thank all of the experts who dedicated themselves to writing the various sections. We thank the superb neurology housestaff at Mount Sinai for so often asking the right questions. Especially we thank our families: our wives, Celia Gelernter Sealfon, Sunghui Stacy, and Neeta Motiwala, and our children Rebecca, Rachel, and Adam Sealfon, Anna and Charles Stacy, and Shweta and Tej Motiwala, who were so endlessly giving and supportive of us while we pursued this project.

Stuart C. Sealfon
Rajeev Motiwala
Charles B. Stacy

List of Abbreviations

ABR	auditory brainstem responses
ACE	angiotensin-converting enzyme
ACHR	acetylcholine receptor
ACTH	adrenocorticotrophic hormone
AD	Alzheimer's disease
ADAS-COG	cognitive subscale of the Alzheimer's disease assessment scale
ADC	average diffusion coefficient
ADEM	acute disseminated encephalomyelitis
ADHD	attention deficit hyperactivity disorder
ADL	activities of daily living
AED	antiepileptic drug
AFP	alphafetoprotein
AHI	Apnea Hypopnea Index
AIDP	acute inflammatory demyelinating polyneuropathy
ANA	antinuclear antibody
ApoE	apolipoprotein E
APP	amyloid precursor protein
APS	antiphospholipid antibody syndrome
aPTT	activated partial thromboplastin time
ARDS	adult respiratory distress syndrome
ASL	arterial spin labeling
ASO	anti-streptolysin O
BA	basilar artery
BAEP	brainstem auditory evoked potential
BAER	brainstem auditory evoked response
BiPAP	bilevel positive airway pressure (ventilation)
BMD	Becker muscular dystrophy
BMP	basic metabolic panel
BMT	bone marrow transplant
BP	blood pressure
BPH	benign prostatic hyperplasia
BPPV	benign paroxysmal positional vertigo
BUN	blood urea nitrogen
bvFTD	behavioral variant frontotemporal dementia
CAS	carotid artery stenting
CASPR2	contactin-associated protein-like 2
CBD	corticobasal degeneration
CBF	cerebral blood flow
CBGD	corticobasal ganglionic degeneration
CBT	cognitive behavioral therapy
CDC	Centers for Disease Control and Prevention

CDR	Clinical Dementia Rating
CEA	carotid endarterectomy
CHD	coronary heart disease
ChEI	cholinesterase inhibitor
CIC	clean intermittent catheterization
CIDP	chronic inflammatory demyelinating polyradiculoneuropathy
CIS	clinically isolated syndrome
CJD	Creutzfeldt–Jakob disease
CK	creatine kinase
CLIPPERS	chronic lymphocytic inflammation with pontine perivascular enhancement responsive to steroids
CM	centromedian nucleus
CMAP	compound muscle action potential
CMD	congenital muscular dystrophy
CMT	Charcot–Marie–Tooth (disease)
CN	cranial nerve
CNS	central nervous system
COMT	catechol-*O*-methyl transferase
COPD	chronic obstructive pulmonary disease
CPAP	continuous positive airway pressure
CPK	creatine phosphokinase
CPM	central pontine myelinolysis
CPP	cerebral perfusion pressure
CRMP	collapsing response mediator protein
CRP	C-reactive protein
CRPS	complex regional pain syndrome
CSW	cerebral salt wasting
CTA	CT angiography
CTE	chronic traumatic encephalopathy
CVE	cerebrovascular event
DAI	diffuse axonal injury
DAT	dopamine transporter
DBS	deep brain stimulation
DEXA	dual-energy X-ray absorptiometry
DLB	dementia with Lewy bodies
DM	dermatomyositis
DMD	Duchenne muscular dystrophy
DO	detrusor overactivity
DSA	digital subtraction angiogram
DSD	detrusor-sphincter dyssynergia
DSS	double simultaneous stimulation
DTI	diffusion tensor imaging
DTT	diffusion tensor tractography
DVT	deep vein thrombosis
DWI	diffusion-weighted imaging
ECHO	enteric cytopathic human orphan (virus)
ECoG	electrocochleography
EDSS	expanded disability status scale

ENoG	electroneuronography
ENG	electronystagmography
EOM	1. extraocular movements; 2. extraocular muscle
ESI	epidural steroid injection
ESR	erythrocyte sedimentation rate
ET	essential tremor
EV7	echovirus 7
EVD	external ventricular drain
FA	fractional anisotropy
FDG-PET	fludeoxyglucose positron emission tomography
FEES	functional endoscopic evaluation of swallow
FIRDA	frontal intermittent rhythmic delta activity
FLAIR	fluid-attenuated inversion recovery
fMRI	functional magnetic resonance imaging
FSHMD	facioscapulohumeral muscular dystrophy
FTD	frontotemporal dementia
FTD-MND	frontotemporal dementia-motor neuron multiplex disease
FTLD	frontotemporal lobar degeneration
FXTAS	fragile X-associated tremor/ataxia syndrome
GAD	glutamic acid decarboxylase
GBM	glioblastoma multiforme
GBS	Guillain–Barré syndrome
GCS	Glasgow Coma Scale
GDS	global depression scale
GERD	gastro-esophageal reflux disease
GFR	glomerular filtration rate
GI	gastrointestinal
GM-1	ganglioside monosialic acid 1
GPED	generalized periodic epileptiform discharge
GPi	globus pallidus interna
GTCC	generalized tonic clonic convulsion
GU	genitourinary
HA	headache
HCV	hepatitis C virus
HHV	human herpesvirus
HITs	high intensity transients
HLA	human leukocyte antigen
HNPP	hereditary neuropathy with tendency for pressure palsies
HR	heart rate
HSP	hereditary spastic paraplegia
HSV	herpes simplex virus
5-HT	5-hydroxytryptophan
Hx	history
IBM	inclusion body myositis
ICD	impulse control disorder
ICH	intracerebral hemorrhage
ICP	intracranial pressure
ICU	intensive care unit

IDDM	insulin-dependent diabetes mellitus
IEM	inborn error of metabolism
IIM	idiopathic inflammatory myopathy
ILD	interstitial lung disease
IMNM	immune-mediated necrotizing myopathy
IMRT	intensity modulated radiation therapy
INO	internuclear ophthalmoplegia
INR	international normalized ratio
IS	ischemic stroke
IVH	intraventricular hemorrhage
IVIG	intravenous immunoglobulin
JCV	John Cunningham virus
JME	juvenile myoclonic epilepsy
KPS	Karnofsky Performance Status
KSS	Kearns–Sayre syndrome
LEMS	Lambert–Eaton myasthenic syndrome
LGMD	limb-girdle muscular dystrophy
LHON	Leber's hereditary optic neuropathy
LMN	lower motor neuron
LOC	loss of consciousness
LP	lumbar puncture
LPA	logopenic aphasia
LPDs	lateralized periodic discharges
MAG	myelin-associated glycoprotein antibody
MAO-B	monoamine oxidase-B
MAP	mean arterial pressure
MBS	modified barium swallow
MCA	middle cerebral artery
MCI	mild cognitive impairment
MdDS	mal de debarquement syndrome
MDS-UPDRS	Movement Disorder Society Unified Parkinson Disease Rating Scale
MEF	maximum expiratory force
MELAS	mitochondrial encephalopathy, lactic acidosis, and stroke-like episodes
MERRF	myoclonic epilepsy with ragged-red fibers
MG	myasthenia gravis
MIBG	[131]m-iodobenzylguanidine
MMSE	mini mental status examination
MND	motor neuron disease
MoCA	Montreal Cognitive Assessment
MPS	mucopolysaccharidosis
MRS	magnetic resonance spectroscopy
MRSA	methicillin-resistant *Staphylococcus aureus*
MS	1. mental status; 2. multiple sclerosis
MSA	multiple system atrophy
MSLT	multiple sleep latency testing
MTT	mean transit time
MUAP	motor unit action potential
MuSK	muscle specific tyrosine receptor kinase

NAION	non-arteritic anterior ischemic optic neuropathy
NARP	neurogenic weakness, ataxia, and retinitis pigmentosa
NBI	neuronal brain iron accumulation
NBIA	neurodegeneration with brain iron accumulation
NCS	nerve conduction study
NCT	non-contrast CT
NCV	nerve conduction velocity
NF1	neurofibromatosis type 1
NIDDM	non-insulin-dependent diabetes mellitus
NIF	negative inspiratory force
NIHSS	NIH Stroke Scale
NIV	non-invasive ventilation
NMDA	N-methyl-D-aspartate
NMJ	neuromuscular junction
NMO	neuromyelitis optica
NPH	normal pressure hydrocephalus
NSC	neural stem cells
NTD	neural tube disease
OCB	oligoclonal bands
OCD	obsessive compulsive disorder
OH	orthostatic hypotension
ONSM	optic nerve sheath meningioma
OSA	obstructive sleep apnea
OT	occupational therapy
OTC	over-the-counter
PCA	patient-controlled analgesia
PCA	posterior cerebral artery
PCC	prothrombin complex concentrate
PCNSL	primary CNS lymphoma
PCR	polymerase chain reaction
PCV	polycythemia vera
PD	Parkinson's disease
PDE-5	phosphodiesterase type 5
PE	pulmonary embolism
PEG	percutaneous endoscopic gastrostomy
PHACE syndrome	Posterior fossa brain malformations, Hemangioma, Arterial lesions, Cardiac abnormalities, Eye abnormalities
PHS	parkinsonism-hyperpyrexia syndrome
PKAN	pantothenate kinase-associated neurodegeneration
PKU	phenylketonuria
PLEDs	periodic lateralized epileptiform discharges
PLS	primary lateral sclerosis
PM	polymyositis
PMA	progressive muscular atrophy
PMC	pontine micturition center
PML	progressive multifocal leukoencephalopathy
PNET	primitive neuroectodermal tumor
PNFA	progressive non-fluent aphasia

PNS	peripheral nervous system
POSTS	positive occipital sharp transients of sleep
POTS	postural orthostatic tachycardia syndrome
PPA	primary progressive aphasia
PPI	proton pump inhibitor
PPMS	primary progressive MS
PRES	posterior reversible encephalopathy syndrome
PRLES	posterior reversible leukoencephalopathy syndrome
PRMS	progressive relapsing MS
PS-1	presenilin 1
PSP	progressive supranuclear palsy
PT	physiotherapy
PVE	periventricular edema
PVR	post-void residual volume
PVS	persistent vegetative state
RA	rheumatoid arthritis
RAS	reticular activating system
rCBF	regional cerebral blood flow
RCT	randomized controlled trial
REM	rapid eye movement
RIS	radiologic isolated syndrome
RNS	responsive neurostimulation
ROM	range of movement
RPR	rapid plasma reagin
RR	respiration rate
RRMS	relapsing-remitting multiple sclerosis
SAH	subarachnoid hemorrhage
SBP	systolic blood pressure
SCA	spinocerebellar ataxia
SCI	spinal cord injury
SCIWORA	spinal cord injury without radiologic abnormalities
SD	semantic dementia
SEGA	subependymal giant cell astrocytoma
SI	signal intensity
SIADH	syndrome of inappropriate antidiuretic hormone secretion
SLE	systemic lupus erythematosus
SLR	straight leg raising
SMA	spinal muscular atrophy
SNAP	sensory nerve action potential
SNHL	sensorineural hearing loss
SNRI	serotonin norepinephrine reuptake inhibitor
SPECT	single photon emission computed tomography
SPMS	secondary progressive MS
SRP	signal recognition particle
SRS	stereotactic radiosurgery
SRT	stereotactic radiotherapy
SSPE	subacute sclerosing panencephalitis
SSRI	selective serotonin reuptake inhibitor

STN	subthalamic nucleus
SUDEP	sudden unexplained death in epilepsy
SVZ	subventricular zone
SW	Sturge–Weber (syndrome)
SWI	susceptibility-weighted imaging
T4	thyroxine
TBI	traumatic brain injury
TCA	tricyclic antidepressant
TCD	transcranial Doppler
TFT	thyroid function test
TIA	transient ischemic attack
TMVL	transient monocular vision loss
tPA	tissue plasminogen activator
Trop.	troponin
TS	Tourette's syndrome
TS	tuberous sclerosis
TSH	thyroid-stimulating hormone
TTG	tissue transglutaminase
TTP	thrombotic thrombocytopenic purpura
TVO	transient visual obscuration
UA	urine analysis
UMN	upper motor neuron
UPDRS	Unified Parkinson Disease Rating Scale
UPPP	uvulopalatopharyngoplasty
UTI	urinary tract infection
UTR	untranslated region
VaD	vascular dementia
Vc	vital capacity
VDRL	venereal disease research laboratory
VEMP	vestibular evoked myogenic potential
VGCC	voltage-gated calcium channel
VIM	nucleus ventralis intermedius
VNS	vagal nerve stimulation
VOG	video-oculography
VOR	vestibulo-ocular reflex
VP	ventriculoperitoneal
VS	vital signs
VZV	varicella zoster virus
wnl	within normal limits
WBC	white blood cell
XLDC	X-linked dilated cardiomyopathy

About the Companion Website

This series is accompanied by a companion website:

www.mountsinaiexpertguides.com

The website includes:
- Case studies
- Figures and Tables:
  - Where a figure or table is on the companion website only, the citation will notify the reader of this: see the citation for Figure 3.1, for example.
  - Where a figure or table is in this printed book, the citation will include the figure number only: see the citation for Figure 3.2, for example.
- Interactive MCQs
- Patient advice
- Reading lists
- Video clips

PART 1

INTRODUCTION

CHAPTER 1

Neurologic History and Examination

Stuart C. Sealfon
Icahn School of Medicine at Mount Sinai, New York, NY, USA

Overview

The goal of the history and examination is to guide the diagnosis, workup, and treatment strategy and to provide a simple and clear record, so any subsequent changes can be easily determined.

- Avoid forcing the history and examination results into categories (e.g. cerebellar tremor) – just describe what you hear and observe precisely and quantitatively.
- Customize the history and examination for each patient.
- Do not substitute imaging studies and other tests for bedside clinical localization – for many neurologic diseases, such as headache syndromes, myasthenia, myopathies, Parkinson disease, and dystonias, imaging studies are not typically useful.
- Establish the neuroanatomic localization first, then consider the differential diagnosis.
- Try to formulate a specific hypothesis about localization and etiology as you obtain the history and then devise a strategy for critically testing this by follow-up questions and during the examination.
- Be definitive and precise about examination findings – avoid "equivocal," "+/–," "possible."

Approach to history taking for the neurologic patient

- Ask open-ended questions and try to avoid listing choices.
- Beware of asking questions that merely confirm your preconceptions as patients may tend to tell you what they think you expect to hear.
- Focus on onset, recovery, timing, and pace of events.
- Characterize the nature and distribution of symptoms (e.g. is pain sharp, dull, aching, shooting, burning, tingling?), distribution, and comparators (e.g. like a toothache, hitting finger with hammer, etc.).
- Determine how witnesses describe the symptoms, especially for disorders of cognition or consciousness.
- Inquire about other medical conditions, review medical and neurologic history and systems, prescription drug use, drugs of abuse, HIV status, and family history, especially for similar conditions.

Approach to the neurologic examination

- The examination is tailored to the complaint, history, and initial findings.
- Not every bedside test is performed for each patient. *Always* tell the patient what you will be doing and what to expect throughout the examination.
- When useful, demonstrate what you want the patient to do.

Mount Sinai Expert Guides: Neurology, First Edition. Edited by Stuart C. Sealfon, Rajeev Motiwala, and Charles B. Stacy.
© 2016 John Wiley & Sons, Ltd. Published 2016 by John Wiley & Sons, Ltd.
Companion website: www.mountsinaiexpertguides.com

Screening neurologic examination

- Mental status:
  - Assess language and cognition during the patient interview.
- Cranial nerves:
  - Confrontation visual fields. Visual acuity on Snellen card, eye movements in all six directions, funduscopy, pupillary reflex while focusing at distance, facial pinprick sensation, facial movement (close eyes tightly, smile), hearing to finger rub, whispered numbers, vocal clarity, movement of palate and uvula, shoulder shrug and neck turning, tongue protrusion.
- Motor:
  - Inspect bulk, tone, assess posture and movements.
  - Assess strength of shoulder shrug, elbow flexion and extension, wrist flexion and extension, grip, pronator drift with eyes closed, foot dorsiflexion and plantarflexion.
- Sensory:
  - Pinprick sensation in all four extremities.
  - Joint position sense, vibratory sensation in toes.
  - Detection of double simultaneous touch stimuli.
- Coordination:
  - Assess finger-nose-finger, coordination and speed of fine finger and rapid alternating movements.
  - Assess gait, tandem gait, Romberg test.
- Reflexes:
  - Biceps, triceps, brachioradialis, patellar, ankle, and plantar reflexes.

Mental status

- Carry out a formal mental status examination if there is any suggestion of abnormality during the history taking.
- Describe the deficits observed as simply as possible and give examples in your records.
- Memory and cognition cannot be fully evaluated in patients with aphasia or impaired alertness.
- See Chapter 6 for discussion of the examination of cognitive function, and Chapter 7 for other cognitive deficits and standardized screening tests – such as the mini mental status examination (MMSE) and Montreal Cognitive Assessment (MoCA).
- The Glasgow Coma Scale (see Chapter 41) is a screen developed for rapid assessment of head trauma and should not substitute for a full examination.

Principal components of the mental status examination

- Orientation and alertness:
  - Level of alertness.
  - Orientation to time, place, person.
  - Ability to spell "world" backwards.
- Memory and calculations:
  - Ability to retain three words at 5 minutes.
  - Ability to recall recent verifiable events or remote history.
  - Subtract 7 from 100 and continue subtracting.
- Language: Dysphasia or aphasia refer to acquired impairments of expressive or receptive language function. Dysphasia is impaired language; aphasia is a more complete disruption of

language production or understanding. In testing language, avoid providing non-verbal clues by pointing or facial expressions.
  - Oral expression: evaluated for tempo, errors.
  - Understanding spoken words: avoiding visual cues such as gestures, test spoken commands (close your eyes, lift your left hand).
  - Written expression: open-ended and to dictation.
  - Reading: commands such as open your mouth, point to your right ear, and read aloud.
  - Naming objects: fingers, coins.
  - Repeating phrases.
- Apraxia: This is an acquired inability to perform a task despite having the motor ability and comprehension needed.
  - Ask the patient to draw a clock with the current time (constructional apraxia).
  - Ask the patient to show how they would use a comb, scissors, or toothbrush.
- Agnosia: This is an impairment of perception of sensory stimuli in the presence of intact primary sensory or visual modalities.
  - Is the patient unable to recognize faces of famous people (prosopagnosia)?
  - Does the patient not recognize their body parts, especially on the left (asomatognosia)?
  - Is the patient unaware of limitations such as paresis caused by their illness (anosognosia)?
  - When testing visual fields, see if finger movement is detected in each quadrant when presented simultaneously bilaterally. Test light touch similarly on the backs of both hands. Does the patient detect visual or sensory stimuli on both sides, but neglects one if they are presented simultaneously (visual or sensory hemi-neglect)?
  - Visual neglect can also be detected by asking a patient to draw a line across the middle of a horizontal line or by placing short lines at different angles all across a page and asking the patient to cross each line.
  - Does the patient have difficult recognizing coins or a safety pin (astereognosis) or numbers traced on the palm (agraphesthesia)?

Elements of examination of the comatose patient (see also Chapter 4)
- Coma scale rating is not a substitute for performing and recording a careful examination.
- Begin with airway, breathing pattern, circulation, and vital sign assessment.
- Examine for bruises and lacerations, jaundice, cyanosis, needle marks.
- Assess consciousness:
  - Does the patient open his eyes to voice and look at examiner?
  - If unarousable to gentle stimuli, what response is seen to painful stimuli? Be humane and avoid bruising and skin damage. Try repeated pinprick before stronger stimuli such as controlled pressure using the stem of a reflex hammer on the nailbed.
- Test pupillary symmetry and reactivity, funduscopic examination, corneal reflex. After excluding neck injury, test oculocephalic reflex (doll's eyes): rotate head to left then right and observe full eye movement to other side. Cold caloric testing is performed by ice water instillation in the ears with the neck at 30 degrees (initially 1 mL after visualizing an intact eardrum, then up to 50 mL). The expected response in coma (with preserved brainstem function) is full conjugate deviation to the side of irrigation. Test facial movement elicited by pinprick or supraorbital pressure and gag reflex.
- In patients not following commands, movements and sensory level are tested by response to painful stimuli. Are the responses purposeful (moves away from pain in non-stereotyped manner or reaches toward stimulus with other hand) or stereotyped (triple flexion, decorticate, decerebrate responses)?
- Evaluate reflexes and extensor-plantar responses.

Cranial nerves

- I. Olfactory
  - Test each nostril with a fruit slice or cup of juice at bedside, or better with identical vials of peppermint or orange extract.
  - Ammonia detection, a noxious stimulus, does not discern deficits of olfaction.
- II. Optic
  - Test pupillary light responses in reduced lighting. Pupils constrict bilaterally with unilateral stimulus. Paradoxical enlargement of the pupil when moving the light from one pupil to the other indicates a relative afferent defect (swinging flashlight test).
  - Test pupillary accommodation to fixation on a finger moving slowly towards the bridge of the nose.
  - Sitting opposite the patient, test visual fields using fingers or, more accurately, using red and white hatpins (obtainable at a craft store). Unilateral reduction of red intensity (red desaturation) is sensitive for detecting optic nerve dysfunction such as optic neuritis.
  - Test acuity in each eye with correction using Snellen card. Refractive errors can be partly compensated using a pinhole for testing.
  - Examine optic disk, vessels, and eyegrounds using an ophthalmoscope.
- III, IV, VI. Ocular motor (oculomotor, trochlear, abducens)
  - Have the patient follow your finger to all positions as well as look from one hand to the other held at opposite extremes. Note diplopia and inquire about double vision; note nystagmus, smoothness of pursuit. Note lid retraction or ptosis.
- V. Trigeminal
  - Corneal reflex: have the patient look up and away. Moving slowly to avoid eliciting eye closure to a visual threat, touch the cornea edge with twisted cotton wool. Both eyes fail to close with a sensory V deficit; unilateral failure to close occurs with motor (facial) weakness.
  - Compare light touch and pinprick on forehead (V1), upper cheeks (V2), and lower lip (V3).
  - Jaw jerk: when you place your index finger firmly above the chin and tap sharply downward on your finger with the reflex hammer you will feel and see the jaw close slightly.
  - Ask the patient to clasp their teeth (while applying opposing pressure outside the mouth) and to open their jaw against resistance, ask the patient to move the jaw from side to side.
- VII. Facial
  - Observe for asymmetry of palpebral fissures and nasolabial folds. Look for weakness of forehead wrinkling on upward gaze. Have patients close their eyes tightly and squeeze their lips together tightly while testing resistance to opening. Lower motor neuron facial weakness involves entire hemi-face, whereas central upper motor neuron facial weakness usually spares the forehead.
- VIII. Acoustic (vestibulocochlear)
  - Test detection of finger rub and comprehension to whispering numbers in each ear.
  - Rinne test for non-neural conduction defect: compare 516 Hz tuning fork base on mastoid process (bone conduction) to tunes held outside ear (air conduction). Normal: air louder than bone. Bone conduction is increased in a conduction defect.
  - Weber test: hold fork at center top of forehead. Louder in bad ear with conduction defect, in good ear with sensorineural defect.
  - Vestibular tests: evaluate eye movements for nystagmus and gait as described below. Special tests for dizziness include the head thrust test, Fukuda stepping test and Dix–Hallpike test.
    - Head thrust test identifies unilateral hypofunction of the peripheral vestibular system. The examiner sits in front of the patient and asks them to look at the examiner's nose while the examiner abruptly rotates the head through a small arc (10–20 degrees) left and right.

Normally, the gaze is held relatively stable. If the vestibular ocular reflex is abnormal, a corrective saccade is seen on the side of reduced vestibular function back toward the examiner's nose. This corrective saccade supports peripheral vestibular hypofunction on the side toward which the head rotation occurred.

  - Stepping test: the patient steps in place for 1 minute with their eyes closed. The normal response is to continue facing in the same direction. A patient with an acute vestibular deficit slowly rotates toward the side of the deficit.
  - Dix–Hallpike test: reposition the patient from a sitting position to reclining with their head hanging and chin 45° to the left; get them to hold the position for at least a minute while inquiring about symptoms and observing for nystagmus. Repeat with chin to the right. In benign paroxysmal positional vertigo, vertigo and rotatory nystagmus begin after a latency of about 5 to 20 seconds, usually improving within 1 minute and decreasing with repeat of the process.

- IX, X: Glossopharyngeal and vagus
  - Evaluate symmetry of palate elevation while the patient says "ah" in a deep voice and while eliciting the gag reflex with stimulation on each side.
- XI: Spinal accessory
  - Get the patient to shrug their shoulder against resistance – the contracting trapezius can be seen and palpated. Rotate the patient's head to each side against resistance – the contracting sternocleidomastoid muscle can be seen and palpated.
- XII: Hypoglossal
  - Evaluate the symmetry of tongue protrusion by having the patient push their tongue against the inside of their cheek on each side against the examiner's hand held outside the cheek.

Motor examination
Overview
- Note tremor, abnormalities of posture, wasting, fasciculations, and tone (see below).
- A comprehensive motor examination is indicated for symptoms of weakness.
- Have the patient maintain arms outstretched in front with palms up and evaluate for drift or rotation suggestive of mild corticospinal deficit (pronator drift).
- Evaluate fine finger movements: demonstrate and ask the patient to play the piano in midair or to drum on a table rapidly using individual fingers. Rapid foot taps can also be evaluated.
- Firmly support the limb proximal to each joint to be tested.
- Evaluate pattern of weakness: hemiparesis, paraparesis, distal, proximal.
- Determine consistency of weakness and fatigability.
- Quantify strength of individual muscles according to the MRC scale (Box 1.1).

BOX 1.1 MRC SCALE FOR MUSCLE STRENGTH

0 No contraction
1 Trace contraction
2 Active movement with gravity
3 Active movement against gravity
4– Active movement against slight resistance
4 Active movement against moderate resistance
4+ Active movement against strong resistance
5 Full strength

- Tests for individual muscles are described in *Aids to the Examination of the Peripheral Nervous System* (see Reading list).

Abnormalities of tone

- Hypotonia: usually associated with muscle weakness and has diverse causes.
- Cogwheel rigidity: cogwheel-like catching with slow pronation-supination movements of forearm or extension and flexion of elbow by examiner. Characteristic of Parkinsonism.
- Paratonia (gegenhalten): irregular "gumby-like" resistance to limb movement. Varies with the resistance or effort put forth by the examiner. Associated with diffuse cortical disease.
- Spasticity: increased tone with sudden passive flexion of limb, such as extending the elbow or lifting the knee joint off the examining table. Stiffness depends on speed of passive movement. Associated with upper motor neuron deficits and clasp knife phenomenon, in which resistance suddenly decreases when the joint is passively moved.
- Myotonia: slow relaxation of muscle contraction. Percussion myotonia is elicited by tapping on the muscle.

CLINICAL PEARLS

- Cerebral upper motor neuron weakness preferentially affects the upper extremity: shoulder abduction > elbow extension = wrist and finger extension; lower extremity: hip flexion, knee flexion, and ankle dorsiflexion > extensors.
- In fine motor movements, corticospinal deficit shows slowing and reduced excursions. Cerebellar deficit shows variable amplitude and speed.
- Radial nerve palsy and a hand area stroke can both cause extensor weakness in the arm. The former can be distinguished by involvement of the brachioradialis, which can be felt to contract during elbow flexion against resistance with the thumb towards the ceiling.
- Non-organic motor weakness: variable; apparent strength on moving greater than when testing; normal tone and reflexes. Resistance tends to vary with the force used to test. Can be overcome with weak force, but shows more strength that is similarly overcome when testing with more force. Hoover sign may be present: place hand under opposite heel while the reclining patient lifts leg against resistance. A physiologic response is when the opposite leg pushes downwards when one leg lifted.

Sensory examination
Overview

- The most difficult part of the neurologic examination is to assess accurately and reproducibly due to physiologic differences in sensation, and individual patients tend either to exaggerate physiologically normal perceptual variation or underreport sensory deficits.
- Start from area of deficit, if present, and delineate transition to normal sensation.
- It is neither practical nor necessary to test the entire skin for every sensory modality.
- For a routine examination, test the face for pinprick and touch, and four extremities for pinprick, light touch, and joint position sense.
- Compare proximal to distal and right to left.
- Light touch: use a cotton wisp and avoid skin hairs.
- Pain sensation: test with new safety pin (disposed after use) using slow, light touches.
- If abnormal pinprick sensation is detected, test temperature sensation in that area. Temperature can be screened by comparing sides of a cool tuning fork warmed with your hand on one side, or with tubes filled with hot and cold water.

- Joint position sense: grasp sides of distal joint with one hand and sides of distal phalanx with the other. Move gently up and down, first assuring that there is no resistance to movement by the patient. Ask about the change in position in an unpredictable pattern – e.g. up, up, down, up, down. Determine size of movement reliably sensed. If absent, proceed to more proximal joint.
- Vibration sense: test over bony prominences with large 128 Hz tuning fork.
- Two-point discrimination can be quantified as the minimum distance the backs of two cotton swabs can be perceived.
- For findings with common cervical, lumbar, and sacral root syndromes, see Chapter 17.

CLINICAL PEARLS
- Sensory deficits are very suggestible. Confirm reliability by returning to area of deficit to retest.
- Test sacral sensation if urinary, bowel symptoms, bilateral leg weakness, or sensory loss to evaluate possible conus medullaris or cauda equina lesion.
- Non-organic sensory loss fails to follow anatomic distribution. Non-anatomic decreased facial sensation may stop at hairline and angle of jaw or on the trunk may proceed exactly to the midline. For hemisensory deficit try the crossed hand test: have the patient interweave their fingers with arms hyperpronated and rotate and fold in the arms so that pinkies of the clasped hands are held against the chest. With random testing of sensation of different fingers, a patient with non-organic hemisensory decrease will tend to confuse the fingers involved.
- Positive "functional" signs do not show that the patient does not have disease of the nervous system. Many patients with serious disease embellish their deficits or provide unreliable responses to examination.

Reflexes
Overview
- Tendon reflexes are a crucial and objective component of the examination.
- It is important to explain what you will do to get the patient to relax before hitting them with a reflex hammer. Gently move the joint to be tested to ascertain that the patient is relaxed.
- The tendon should be struck once in the correct spot with a short, free movement of the hammer.
- If the patient is tense, distract by asking to count backwards from 100.
- If reflexes are absent, try reinforcement: the patient links both hands with the fingers flexed and curved and just before the tendon is struck pulls the hands strongly in opposite directions. Clenching the opposite fist can be used to reinforce upper extremity reflexes. The timing of reinforcement is crucial as the effect is very brief.
- The standard reflexes are listed in Box 1.2.
- Grade reflexes from 0 to 4+, with 0 absent, 1+ trace, 2+ average, 3+ increased, and 4+ abnormally increased.
- Note the presence of clonus.
- Test for the presence or absence of the extensor-plantar reflex (Babinski sign) by slowly and firmly scraping the lateral edge of the sole with a tongue depressor or similar object. In a positive response the large toe moves upward.
- Other reflexes are listed in Table 1.1.

CLINICAL PEARLS

- Avoid confusing a pathologic withdrawal reflex (triple flexion) in a patient with upper motor paralysis of the lower extremities with voluntary withdrawal. The reflex can be identified by its stereotyped form and usually confirmed by stimulating with taps of a safety pin on the dorsum of the foot or top of the large toe. Unlike voluntary movement, which moves away from the painful stimulus, the flexion reflex will move the foot toward the pin stimulating the top of the foot.
- Symmetrically hyperactive or absent reflexes can be normal physiologic variants.

BOX 1.2 STANDARD DEEP TENDON REFLEXES

Biceps:	C5,6	Musculocutaneous nerve
Triceps:	C7,8	Radial nerve
Brachioradialis:	C5,6	Radial nerve
Patellar	L3,4	Femoral nerve
Achilles	S1	Sciatic nerve

Table 1.1 Reflex responses.

Name	Response	Significance
Babinski sign	Stimulate lateral sole → large toe moves upward	Corticospinal (upper motor neuron) dysfunction
Triple flexion	Stimulate lateral sole or foot → flexion of hip, knee, dorsiflexion of foot	Corticospinal (upper motor neuron) dysfunction
Hoffmann reflex	Flick distal phalanx of middle finger → flexion of thumb and fingers	Suggests hyperactive reflexes, but may be normal
Glabellar reflex	Repeated tapping with finger on forehead over eyes → normal: eyes blink a few times then stop; abnormal: eyes continue to blink	Frontal release sign suggesting diffuse bilateral frontal lobe or cortical dysfunction as in dementia; also seen in Parkinsonism
Grasp reflex	Stroking the palm → involuntary grasp	Frontal release sign, similar to above
Palmomental reflex	Stroking the palm → wrinkling of chin mentalis muscle	Frontal release sign, similar to above
Decerebrate response	In coma, sternal pressure → rigid extension of neck and all four extremities	Severe dysfunction of brainstem superior colliculi and vestibular nuclei
Decorticate response	In coma, sternal pressure → flexion of arms and extension of legs	Brainstem dysfunction at a level higher than that causing decerebrate response involving both hemispheres, thalamus, or internal capsule

Gait and coordination (Box 1.3)
Overview
- Examine posture (station) and walking. Pay attention to the width of the base and the symmetry of movements. Test heel-toe walking (tandem walk).

- Romberg sign: have the patient stand steadily feet together with their eyes open, then test if balance is maintained with the eyes closed.
- Finger-to-nose and finger-nose-finger tests: with their hands outstretched, have the patient touch their nose with each index finger, then move it back and forth from the examiner's finger to the patient's nose. Perform this with the patient's eyes open and closed. Evaluate for accuracy, smoothness, and tremor.
- Past pointing test: get the patient to extend their arm with their index finger touching the examiner's finger. The patient then raises their arm over their head with their eyes closed and brings the arm back to touch the examiner's finger.
- Heel-shin test of coordination: have the patient slowly rub the heel of one leg from the ankle to the knee of their other leg on the shin.
- Rapid alternating movements: this involves alternate tapping of the palm and back of hand on a flat surface. Examine and listen for speed and regularity.
- Note involuntary movements at rest and with movement (see further on).

Involuntary movements
- Tremor: constant, steady oscillation
  - Parkinsonian tremor: pill rolling, most prominent at rest, decreases with purposeful movement.
  - Essential tremor: head and voice often involved. Worsens with precise movement. Decreases at rest.
- Chorea: sudden, rapid, purposeless movements. Causes include Huntington disease, Sydenham chorea (post-rheumatic fever), polycythemia vera.
- Athetosis: slow writhing movements of arms and legs. Causes include cerebral palsy, Wilson disease, neurodegeneration with brain iron accumulation (NBIA), ataxia telangiectasia.
- Dystonia: sustained involuntary muscle contractions causing unnatural postures. Includes writer's cramp, blepharospasm, and generalized dystonia. Many genetic forms have been identified.
- Ballismus: wild, uncontrolled flinging movements with any attempt at movement. Caused by damage in the vicinity of the subthalamic red nucleus.
- Myoclonus: sudden, brief shock-like jerks of a group of muscles.

CLINICAL PEARLS
- Decrease in arm swing on one side is a sensitive sign for hemiparesis.
- Slow or magnetic gait associated with urinary incontinence may be normal pressure hydrocephalus.
- Parkinsonism may show retropulsion – difficulty in regaining center of gravity when gently pulled backwards while standing.

Reading list

Key reading sources for this chapter can be found online at www.mountsinaiexpertguides.com

---

Additional material for this chapter can be found online at:
www.mountsinaiexpertguides.com

This includes a reading list.

CHAPTER 2

Neuroradiology

Thomas P. Naidich[1], Reade De Leacy[1], and Ruby J. Lien[2]
[1]Icahn School of Medicine at Mount Sinai, New York, NY, USA
[2]Winthrop Radiology Associates, Mineola, NY, USA

Introduction

Neuroimaging is *in vivo* gross pathology. It demonstrates the anatomy and pathology within the patient to help confirm or exclude a differential diagnosis, or to uncover unsuspected disease. At present, imaging analysis typically begins with computed (axial) tomography (CT, CAT scan) or magnetic resonance imaging (MRI). Other imaging modalities and applications will not be discussed in this chapter.

Imaging terminology

Most neuroimages are displayed as shades of gray where the brightness or darkness of a structure gives information about its state (Figure 2.1; see also Table 2.1 on the companion website).
- "Hyper" – structures and regions that appear bright (i.e. whiter).
- "Hypo" – structures and regions that appear dark (i.e. blacker).
- "Iso" – structures and regions with a brightness co-equal to a specific reference tissue or region.
- FLAIR (fluid-attenuated inversion recovery) imaging is an MRI sequence/imaging technique that suppresses the signal from large pools of water, such as ventricles and cavities, in order to reveal either gliosis or edema in the adjacent parenchyma.

Assessment of mineralization

Mineral deposition within the brain and meninges alters the density and signal intensity of the images in predictable, often age-dependent, ways. Interpretation of the imaging studies requires familiarity with these patterns of deposition (see Table 2.2 on the companion website; see also Figure 2.2 on the companion website).

Analysis of parenchymal volume

CT and MRI both assess the presence of mass and atrophy.
- *Mass* – occupies space, compresses and displaces adjacent structures, and often induces edema, increasing the total mass effect. The net mass effect may be focal, regional, hemispheric, or diffuse. Marked mass effect leads to midline shift, transincisural and tonsillar herniations (Figure 2.3; see also Table 2.3 on the companion website).
- *Volume loss* – aging, post-surgical changes, and sequelae of trauma may cause loss of neural tissue with reduced parenchymal volume and secondary expansion of the ventricles, sulci, and fissures. Such atrophic expansion of cerebrospinal fluid (CSF) (*ex vacuo*) spaces must be distinguished from high-pressure hydrostatic distension of these spaces (hydrocephalus) (Figure 2.4; see also Table 2.4 on the companion website).

Mount Sinai Expert Guides: Neurology, First Edition. Edited by Stuart C. Sealfon, Rajeev Motiwala, and Charles B. Stacy.
© 2016 John Wiley & Sons, Ltd. Published 2016 by John Wiley & Sons, Ltd.
Companion website: www.mountsinaiexpertguides.com

Contrast enhancement in CT and MRI

Lesions are often detected and characterized more completely by administering a chemical compound that passes into the lesion and increases its conspicuity (see Tables 2.5 and 2.6 on the companion website).

- *CT* – Contrast agents used in CT are based on iodinated compounds (I) given as diverse non-ionic iodinated molecules.
  - Administration – intravenous, intra-arterial, and intrathecal.
  - Mode of excretion – primarily via the kidneys and secondarily via the liver.
- *MRI* – Contrast agents used in MRI are diverse chelates of gadolinium (Gd).
  - Administration – intravenous, intra-arterial, and intrathecal.
  - Mode of excretion: the gadolinium chelates presently used in neuroimaging are eliminated primarily by the renal system. There is a small amount of secondary hepatic excretion.
- Both CT and MRI contrast agents must be used cautiously or avoided in patients with impaired renal function (see Table 2.7 on the companion website) and in those who have had prior contrast-related allergic reactions. Up-to-date premedication regimens can be found through the American College of Radiology website (www.acr.org) with these being divided into elective or emergency premedication strategies. Both forms employ oral or intravenous steroids and antihistamines at differing time intervals.

Clinico-radiologic usefulness and basic pharmacodynamics/kinetics of contrast agents

- Increased conspicuity:
  - Presence within the blood vessels (intravascular contrast enhancement).
  - Extravasation of opacified blood through a defect in the vessel wall.
  - Leakage of contrast into the brain or spinal cord wherever a lesion reduces the integrity of the blood–brain barrier (BBB) (Figure 2.5; see also Figure 2.6 on the companion website).
- Basic pharmacodynamics/kinetics:
  - Following intravenous administration, blood contrast levels peak immediately and then fall as the contrast dilutes in the plasma and equilibrates with the extracranial extracellular space.
  - Peak contrast levels within a lesion depend on the dose administered, the size of the vascular compartment within the lesion, and the extent of damage to the BBB.
  - Typically, peak lesion contrast occurs from 5 to 40 minutes following contrast administration.
  - *Static contrast techniques* demonstrate the site and extent of contrast entry into the lesion at one specific point in time (see Table 2.5 on the companion website).
  - *Dynamic contrast techniques* demonstrate the time course of the passage of contrast into, through, and out of the lesion to quantitate the kinetics of enhancement within the lesion (see Table 2.6 on the companion website).

As with all medications, iodine- and Gd-containing contrast agents must be used cautiously with attention to risk-benefit balances, attention to appropriate dosage, and special attention to those populations of patients especially vulnerable to these agents (see Table 2.7 on the companion website).

In a recent article (see Reading list), McDonald et al. determined that neuronal tissue deposition of gadolinium is likely cumulative over a patient's lifetime and occurs despite the absence of either renal or hepatobiliary dysfunction. They found that this deposition might be seen in all patients exposed to gadolinium, in a dose-dependent fashion. Whilst the clinical significance of these findings remains incompletely understood at this time, further research into the *in vivo* safety and stability of gadolinium chelates is needed and forthcoming.

The principle of diffusion as it refers to MRI

Diffusion weighted imaging (DWI) sequences and their corresponding average diffusion coefficient (ADC) maps can be useful in increasing both the sensitivity and specificity of an imaging study.

- *Diffusion* – the random movement of water molecules through the brain.
- *Isotropic diffusion* – diffusion of water is equal in all directions, which is normal in certain brain locations.
- *Anisotropic diffusion* – diffusion of water is unequal with preferential movement in specific directions, which is normal in certain brain locations (see Table 2.8 on the companion website).

In the intact brain, the asymmetric orientation of the white matter fibers, their myelin sheaths, cell membranes, and intracellular microtubules is detectable as a physiologic pattern of anisotropic diffusion. MR techniques can quantitate the diffusion of water as fractional anisotropy (FA). The FA helps to identify and characterize the coherence and integrity of white matter fibers.

Diffusion tensor MR

- Used to assess the principal direction of diffusion within each individual volume element (voxel) of the brain. Those data may then be used to follow white matter fibers from voxel to voxel across the brain (diffusion tensor tractography) (see Table 2.8 on the companion website). These techniques enable display of the orientation of fiber tracts throughout the brain (see Figure 2.7 on the companion website).

Imaging of cerebral ischemia

CT and MRI may both be used to assess the presence and extent of cerebral ischemia-infarction. The initial goal of imaging is to rule out hemorrhage and to help determine the age and extent of infarction (see Table 2.9 on the companion website).

CT assessment of cerebral ischemia

Focal ischemia may not be detectable for hours until secondary consequences such as mass effect and alteration in gray-white density renders it appreciable. Specific imaging signs may help in early identification:

- *"Loss of gray-white distinction sign"* – blurring or loss of the normal difference in the radiodensity between gray matter and white matter.
- *"Dense MCA" or "dense BA" (basilar artery) sign* – thrombosis of the middle cerebral artery (MCA) or basilar artery (BA) resulting in hyperdensity of either vessel, providing an early clue to the site of occlusion and infarction (see Figure 2.8 on the companion website).
  - Increased hemoglobin (Hb) or hematocrit from dehydration, polycythemia, and other causes can falsely increase vessel density and should be kept in mind when assessing imaging.
- *"Insular ribbon" sign* – infarction of the insular cortex causes blurring or loss of gray-white distinction between the insular cortex and the underlying extreme capsule (see Figure 2.8C).
- *Post cerebral or cardiac catheterization* – infarct zones may be displayed more rapidly when residual contrast administered during the catheterization causes a density difference between the infarcted and ischemic tissue.

CT perfusion and angiography

Multiparametric CT perfusion imaging of the brain with reconstructed or dedicated CT angiograms of the neck and cerebral vessels is now forming the standard of care for assessment of infarct core, penumbra and assessment of large vessel occlusion that may be amenable to endovascular intervention within the treatment window. Parameters assessed include:

- *Mean transit time* (MTT) – the average time it takes blood to pass through a given region of brain tissue (commonly measured in seconds).
- *Time to peak* (TTP) – the time from the start of the scan until the maximum attenuation/ enhancement occurs (seconds).
- *Cerebral blood flow* (CBF) – the volume of blood per unit time passing through a given region of brain tissue (milliliters per minute per 100 g of brain tissue).
- *Cerebral blood volume* (CBV) – the volume of blood in a given region of brain tissue (milliliters per 100 g of brain tissue).

CTP (CT perfusion) assessment

- Acute ischemic stroke:
  - Decreased CBF and CBV
  - Increased MTT
- Infarct core:
  - Matched abnormalities on CBV (decreased) and MTT (increased).
- Penumbra:
  - Mismatched abnormalities with increased MTT and decreased CBF with either normal or increased CBV due to compensatory measures.
  - CBF may also be decreased to a lesser extent within the penumbra.

MRI assessment of cerebral ischemia

- On MRI, ischemic lesions are often detected very rapidly due to the cytotoxic (intracellular) edema, consequent narrowing of the extracellular space, and restriction of diffusion (see Table 2.9 on the companion website, and Figure 2.9 on the companion website).

As with CTP, dynamic contrast enhancement may be used to characterize the site of infarction, the infarct core, and any penumbra of ischemic but salvageable tissue using the same parameters (see Tables 2.10 and 2.11 on the companion website, and also Figure 2.10 on the companion website).

Imaging of parenchymal hemorrhage

CT assessment of parenchymal hemorrhage

- Density of blood depends on the concentration of hemoglobin (Hb). At normal adult hemato-crits, intravascular and parenchymal blood will appear bright white (hyperdense).
- *Early (<1 week)* – Clot density first increases over the short term as clot retraction concentrates the Hb and expresses serum.
- *Subacute (1–3 weeks)* – Progressive degradation of the Hb molecule then leads to reduced CT density. The clot "fades" over the ensuing weeks. At some point it becomes isodense to brain.
- *Chronic (>3 weeks)* – Later the clot appears lucent and hypodense compared to the adjacent brain. Note, CT may fail to distinguish between a chronic parenchymal hemorrhage and a chronic parenchymal infarction.

MRI assessment of parenchymal hemorrhage

MRI allows us to "age" intracranial hemorrhages by noting the characteristic alterations of their T1 and T2 signal intensities (see Figure 2.11 on the companion website). These changes evolve from the periphery toward the center of the hematoma, so rate of change depends on initial size of hemorrhage (see Table 2.12 on the companion website).

In general *five stages* of hematoma evolution are recognized:
- *Hyperacute* (first few hours):
  - intracellular *oxyhemoglobin*
  - T1 – isointense
  - T2 – isointense to slightly hyperintense.
- *Acute* (1 to 2 days):
  - intracellular *deoxyhemoglobin*
  - T1 – hyperintense
  - T2 – very hypointense.
- *Early subacute* (2 to 7 days):
  - intracellular *methemoglobin*
  - T1 – progressively increases in intensity to become hyperintense
  - T2 – remains very hypointense.
- *Late subacute* (7 to 14–28 days):
  - *extracellular methemoglobin* – over the next few weeks – as cells break down releasing methemoglobin
  - T1 – remains hyperintense
  - T2 – now also hyperintense.
- *Chronic* (>14–28 days):
  - Periphery:
    - intracellular hemosiderin
    - T1 hypointense
    - T2 hypointense.
  - Center:
    - extracellular hemichromes
    - T1 – isointense
    - T2 – hyperintense.

Assessing potential for an underlying lesion in intracranial hemorrhage
- Patient age, known risk factors, and hematoma location help to assess the likelihood that a hemorrhage reflects an underlying lesion rather than a spontaneous primary bleed.
- The *secondary intracranial hemorrhage (SICH) score* – this score codifies an approach in patients with parenchymal hematomas but no concurrent subarachnoid hemorrhage (see Table 2.13 on the companion website).
- "*The spot sign*" – Table 2.14 (on the companion website) reviews the use of the "spot sign" to assess the likelihood that a hematoma will enlarge, cause in-hospital mortality, or lead to poor outcome in the survivors (see also Figure 2.6 on the companion website).
- Multidetector CT angiography (CTA) shows an overall sensitivity of 89–96%, a specificity of 92–100%, and an accuracy of 91–99% for the detection of vascular etiologies of hemorrhagic stroke when compared with catheter angiography.

Overview of intracranial vasculature
The intracranial circulation is now displayed routinely on CT and MR angiograms.

Analysis of stroke then requires familiarity with the major arteries, veins, and dural venous sinuses of the intracranial circulation (see Tables 2.15, 2.16 on the companion website and Figure 2.11 on the companion website).
- Systematic analysis of arterial stenoses, occlusions, segmental arteritides, aneurysms, arteriovenous malformations, or venous thromboses depends upon careful review of all these vessels, *in order as the blood flows,* lest a significant lesion be overlooked.

Safety concerns with MRI

MRI requires special attention to safety issues unique to the magnetic environment. The general considerations are presented in Table 2.17 (on the companion website) and in the American College of Radiology (ACR) Guidance Document on MR Safe Practice (2013). However, the recommendations reviewed here are subject to continuing modification as manufacturers redesign products to address MR safety precautions.

Various components of the MR environment can pose a risk to a patient and personnel:
- Static magnetic field (B0, pronounced "B zero"). In clinical neuroradiology practice B0 is usually 1.0, 1.5, or 3.0 Tesla (T).
- Dynamic gradient field (to aid in localization).
- Radiofrequency (RF) field.
- Varying level of sound pressure (noise).
- The magnetic fields can interact with ferromagnetic material resulting in:
  - projectile effects
  - torsion with object twisting
  - burning
  - device malfunction.

Ferromagnetic devices

- Aneurysm clips (not endovascular coils):
  - All documentation of types of implanted clips, dates, etc. *must* be in writing and signed by a licensed physician.
  - *Intracranial aneurysm clips manufactured in or after 1995* – for which the manufacturer's product labeling continues to claim MR Conditional – may be accepted for MR scanning without further testing.
  - *Intracranial aneurysm clips manufactured before 1995* – these require pretesting or careful review of any prior MRI performed by certified personnel.
- Neurostimulators:
  - Deep brain stimulators, vagal nerve stimulators, and other devices with implanted electrodes and battery control systems are typically not compatible with standard MRI.
- Cardiac implantable electronic devices:
  - Include cardiac pacemakers, implantable cardioversion-defibrillator devices, and implantable cardiac monitors.
  - Written documentation of the specific manufacturer, model, and type of each device must be obtained.
  - The MR environment may cause:
    - early battery depletion;
    - programming changes with loss of pacing, abnormal pacing, and induction of ventricular fibrillation;
    - device failure requiring reimplantation, and multiple deaths "under poorly or incompletely characterized circumstances."
- These rules apply regardless of whether the device is presently turned on or off, or has even been removed, leaving implanted electrodes. Simply moving the patient and residual wires across the magnetic gradients within the MR scanner and the play of the time-varying magnetic field gradients across the wires during scanning will induce currents within the in-dwelling wires (Faraday's and Lenz's laws).

- Programmable shunts:
  - MRI may change valve settings and patients need to be checked and the shunt reprogrammed if necessary.

Patients who state they had no difficulties with a prior MRI scan *CANNOT* be considered safe on that basis alone, because their prior study may have been on a scanner of different field strength or one that used less rapidly changing electromagnetic gradients. Further, it is clearly established that wires and implants may show no significant heating at one field strength, but heat to clinically significant levels in seconds at a different field strength *in either direction*: 1.5 T to 3 T or vice versa. When in doubt, delay scanning until safety is assured.

Conclusions

- Performed safely, neuroimaging contributes greatly to the discovery and characterization of the neuropathology responsible for the patient's presenting signs and symptoms.
- Neuroimaging helps to determine the grade of severity, the triage category, and the likelihood that any planned intervention will improve patient outcome.

Images

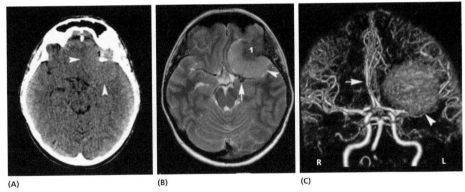

(A)　　　　　　　　　　　(B)　　　　　　　　　　　(C)

Figure 2.1 Terminology. A 26-year-old woman with left sphenoid wing meningioma. (A) Axial non-contrast CT reveals high-density calcifications (1) within a large mass (white arrowheads) that is nearly isodense to gray matter. There is no low-density edema. The mass compresses the adjacent portion of the star-shaped suprasellar cistern. (B) On the axial non-contrast T2-weighted (W) MR image, the mass shows a low signal intensity core (1) of calcification and hyperostosis arising from the left sphenoid wing, a high T2 signal intensity cap of soft tissue with "spoke wheel" texture (arrowhead), and thin film of very high signal CSF at the interface of the tumor with the compressed and displaced brain. Black "flow voids" delineate the vessels of the circle of Willis, documenting displacement and bowing of the left supraclinoid internal carotid artery (white arrow) and the adjacent A1 segment of the left anterior cerebral artery and the proximal M1 segment of the left middle cerebral artery. (C) Contrast-enhanced CT angiography displays the normal vascularity of the brain, the hypervascularity of the tumor (arrowhead), the proximity of the tumor to the M1 segment of the left middle cerebral artery, and the displacement of the A2 segments (arrow) of both anterior cerebral arteries across the midline to the right.

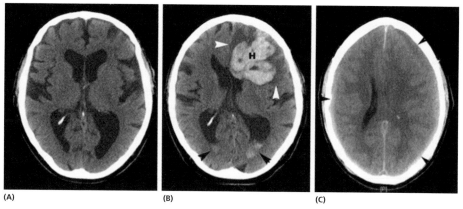

(A)   (B)   (C)

Figure 2.3 Mass. Non-contrast CT scans. (**A, B**) Lobar mass effect in an 86-year-old man. As compared to prior study from the same patient (**A**), the dense hematoma (H) and surrounding low-density edema (white arrowheads) expand the left frontal lobe, compress and displace the left frontal horn, and shift the midline from left to right (**B**). There is only a minor mass effect on the other lobes. High-density blood (black arrowheads) layers are seen within the dependent occipital horns. (**C**) Diffuse mass effect in a 70-year-old man. Bilateral nearly isodense subdural hematomas (black arrowheads) cause a diffuse mass effect effacing all convexity sulci, effacing the interhemispheric fissure, and compressing both lateral ventricles. The slightly larger size of the left subdural hemorrhage shifts the midline from left to right. N.B. Unusually small size of ventricles in an elderly patient mandates search for a cause of diffuse mass effect.

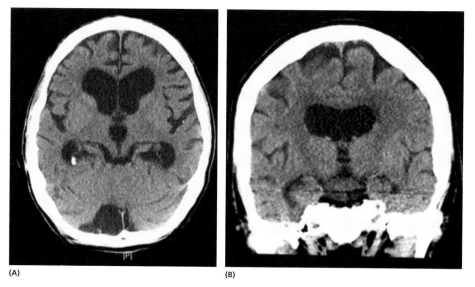

(A)   (B)

Figure 2.4 (**A**) Ventricular enlargement in a 55-year-old man. Axial non-contrast CT. There is disproportionately larger size of the ventricles than the sulci, greater rounding of the ventricular walls, and more acute angulation of the ventricular roof suggesting hydrocephalus. (**B**) A 56-year-old woman. Coronal non-contrast CT. Expansion of the ventricles proportional to the sulci and fissures, less tense curvature of the ventricular walls, lesser expansion of the temporal horns, and a flat callosal angle suggest atrophy.

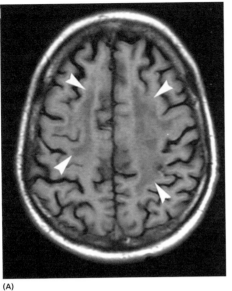
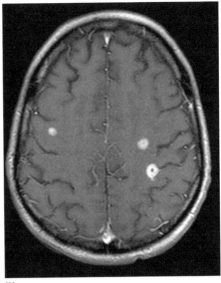

(A)   (B)

Figure 2.5 Contrast enhancement in a 50-year-old man with nocardial abscesses. (A) Axial T1 FLAIR MR shows broad zones (white arrowheads) of low-signal edema within the white matter of both cerebral hemispheres. These surround multiple small foci of even lower signal. (B) After intravenous administration of Gd-chelate contrast agent, passage of contrast agent into the tissue at sites where the damaged blood–brain barrier is "leaky" reveals the multiple nocardial abscesses.

Reading list

Key reading sources for this chapter can be found online at www.mountsinaiexpertguides.com

Suggested websites

American College of Radiology: www.acr.org

Additional material for this chapter can be found online at:
www.mountsinaiexpertguides.com

This includes Figures 2.2, and 2.6–2.11; Tables 2.1–2.17; and a reading list.

CHAPTER 3

Neurophysiologic and Other Neurodiagnostic Tests

Susan Shin[1], Sarah Zubkov[2], Deborah R. Horowitz[1], and David M. Simpson[1]
[1]Icahn School of Medicine at Mount Sinai, New York, NY, USA
[2]Temple University Hospital, Philadelphia, PA, USA

Nerve conduction studies (NCS) and electromyography (EMG)
Role of EMG in clinical practice

EMG studies are an extension of the neurologic examination. Clinicians should consider referring patients in whom they suspect a peripheral nervous system (PNS) disorder. These may include disorders affecting the anterior horn cells, nerve roots, dorsal root ganglion, plexus, peripheral nerve, neuromuscular junction, muscle membrane, and muscle. The test results may help guide management and further work-up, and often can lead to a specific diagnosis. In addition, NCS/EMG yields valuable information regarding the degree of muscle or nerve injury and duration of the illness, and aids in prognosis.

Patient referral

- Patients referred for an EMG study should come prepared with their referral diagnosis and pertinent history and examination findings.
- Prior to the appointment, patients should be given a brief description of what the study will entail, and a caution that the testing may produce some discomfort. Most patients do not find the test excessively painful.
- For patients in whom a neuromuscular junction disorder is suspected, the morning dose of pyridostigmine should be held if safely tolerated.
- Anticoagulants and antiplatelet agents usually do not need to be suspended for needle EMG.

Patient safety

Although nerve conduction studies are rarely associated with serious adverse events, special patient populations may be at higher risk.

- Caution should be taken with patients who have cardiac devices such pacemakers. Furthermore, the risk of electrical injury increases in patients with central lines and wires that come in close contact with the heart. Proximal stimulation sites, like the axilla and Erb's point, should be avoided. The study should not be performed in patients who have external pacemaker wires.
- Electromyography is the invasive portion of the exam that requires a needle electrode to be inserted into a muscle.

The risks with EMG include bleeding, infection, and rarely pneumothorax. A limited EMG can be safely performed on patients on anticoagulation; however, deep muscles where pressure cannot be effectively applied should be avoided.

Mount Sinai Expert Guides: Neurology, First Edition. Edited by Stuart C. Sealfon, Rajeev Motiwala, and Charles B. Stacy.
© 2016 John Wiley & Sons, Ltd. Published 2016 by John Wiley & Sons, Ltd.
Companion website: www.mountsinaiexpertguides.com

Anatomy

The peripheral nervous system consists of motor and sensory neurons and their peripheral nerves, the neuromuscular junction, and muscle. Cranial nerves III to XII are also part of the PNS.

- Primary motor neurons lie within the ventral gray matter of the spinal cord, or anterior horn.
- Cranial nerve motor neurons lie within the brainstem.
- Sensory neurons lie outside the spinal cord in the dorsal root ganglion (DRG):
  - Cells in the DRG are bipolar
    - proximal segment = sensory nerve root
    - distal segment = sensory fibers of the peripheral nerve.
  - Bipolar nature of the sensory neuron is important to neuroanatomic localization
    - lesions proximal to the DRG will produce normal sensory nerve potentials, e.g. radiculopathy;
    - lesions distal to, or including, the DRG will affect the sensory nerve potential, e.g. ganglionopathy, plexopathy, or peripheral neuropathy.
- Mixed spinal nerves are formed by motor and sensory nerve roots that arise from each segment of the spinal cord:
  - Spinal nerves divide into dorsal and ventral rami
    - C5–T1 ventral rami combine to form the brachial plexus, which innervates the upper extremities;
    - L1–S2 ventral rami combine to form the lumbosacral plexus, which innervates the lower extremities.
- The peripheral nerves in the limbs are the distal branches of the brachial and lumbosacral plexuses:
  - Further classified by their diameter, degree of myelination, and by their function
    - Functional classification: motor, sensory, somatic, autonomic.
    - Nerve conduction studies (NCS) measure only the heavily myelinated, fastest conduction fibers.
    - Small fiber neuropathy cannot be diagnosed by NCS/EMG.
    - Consider skin biopsy and epidermal nerve fiber analysis for patients with paresthesias and normal EMG.
- Myotomes = muscles innervated by one nerve root or spinal segment.
- Dermatomes = cutaneous areas innervated by a spinal segment.
- Neuromuscular junction = interface between axon terminals (axolemma) and muscle fibers (sarcolemma); aka motor end plate.
- Nerve terminals form bulbous structures called synaptic end bulbs, which contain vesicles of the neurotransmitter acetylcholine (Ach).

Physiology

The peripheral nerves transmit information from the brain and spinal cord to their end organs (muscles, skin, and viscera). The transmission of information is carried out by a complex set of electrical and chemical events within the nerve and the neuromuscular junction. Nerve depolarization leads to the generation of action potentials. Depolarization at the axon terminals causes calcium channels to open allowing an influx of calcium ions; this causes acetylcholine (Ach) to be released into the neuromuscular junction. Binding of Ach to the Ach-receptor leads to depolarization of the muscle end plate, which then results in a muscle fiber action potential.

Nerve conduction studies (NCS)

Nerve conduction studies consist of electrically stimulating an accessible motor, sensory, or mixed nerve at a given site along its course. A brief electrical current is delivered across the skin, which causes depolarization of axons that lie beneath the stimulation site. This evokes action potentials that travel both proximally and distally from the stimulation site. The evoked motor and sensory action potentials are recorded as a waveform.

Key definitions:

- CMAP = compound muscle action potential
- SNAP = sensory nerve action potential
- NCS = nerve conduction study
- CV = conduction velocity
- Orthodromic – describes potentials that travel in the direction of normal nerve conduction
- Antidromic – describes potentials that travel opposite to the direction of normal nerve conduction.

Motor NCS

Routine motor NCS:

- Upper extremity: median and ulnar.
- Lower extremity: peroneal and tibial.
- Special nerves can be tested in the appropriate clinical setting, e.g. radial nerve for wrist drop.

As regards setting up the test, Figure 3.1 (on the companion website) shows the example of testing the median nerve while recording at the abductor pollicis brevis muscle:

- Surface disk electrodes are placed over the muscle innervated by the nerve that will be tested:
  - Recording electrode over the muscle "belly" (motor end plate).
  - Reference electrode over an electrically silent part such as tendon or bone.
  - An inter-electrode distance of 3 to 4 cm is optimal.
- Ground is placed between the recording and stimulating electrodes.
- Place stimulator over the median nerve at the wrist.

The stimulator delivers a brief electrical pulse of current that causes the nerve to depolarize, which ultimately causes the muscle fibers to depolarize. The summation of all the muscle fiber action potentials underlying the recording electrode is captured as a waveform called the compound motor action potential (CMAP) (Figure 3.2).

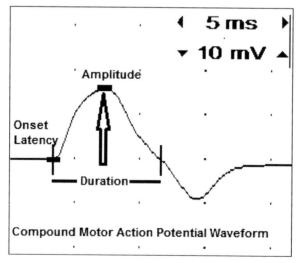

Figure 3.2 Compound motor action potential waveform.

- *Onset latency* = initial upward deflection of the CMAP waveform from baseline:
  - Measured in milliseconds, it reflects the conduction down the nerve, conduction of the muscle, and neuromuscular junction transmission time.
- *Duration* represents the synchrony of the muscle fiber depolarization:
  - May increase in demyelinating conditions that result in slowing of a select number of motor axons.
- Conduction velocity:
  - Calculated by dividing the conducted distance between the distal and proximal stimulation sites by the conduction time between these two points.
  - Requires both a distal and proximal stimulation site in order to exclude the distal motor (or onset) latency, which includes more than just the nerve's conduction velocity.

Conduction block

- Results as a consequence of severe demyelination along the course of a motor nerve causing the nerve impulses to be slowed or partially obstructed.
- Electrophysiologic criterion is a ≥40–50% reduction in the CMAP amplitude:
  - Exception to the rule is stimulation of the tibial nerve in the popliteal fossa.
    - Nerve lies deep making it difficult to stimulate all the nerve fibers (especially in obese patients).
    - May be normal to see up to a 30–40% reduction in the CMAP amplitude.
- Conduction block may be seen in:
  - Focal nerve compression at common entrapment sites;
    - peroneal nerve at the fibular head
    - ulnar nerve at the elbow (Figure 3.3 and Figure 3.4).
  - Acquired, immune-mediated, demyelinating conditions like Guillain–Barré syndrome (GBS) and chronic inflammatory demyelinating polyradiculoneuropathy (CIDP).
    - Figure 3.5 (on the companion website) represents conduction block of the ulnar nerve in the forearm, outside a common area of entrapment.

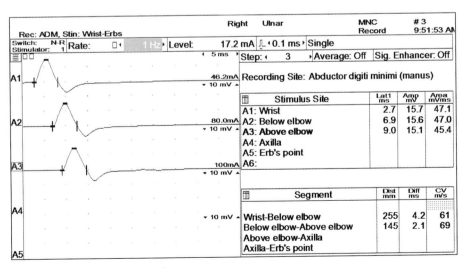

Figure 3.3 Normal ulnar nerve waveforms.

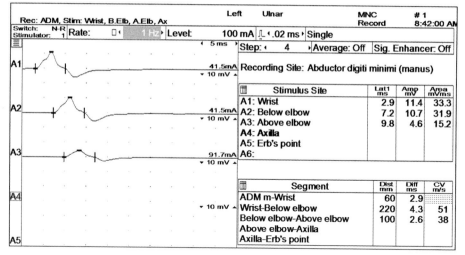

Figure 3.4 Focal ulnar neuropathy with slowed conduction velocity across the elbow and conduction block.

- Conduction block is generally NOT seen in inherited forms of peripheral nerve demyelination like Charcot–Marie–Tooth (CMT) disease type 1.
  - Figure 3.6 (on the companion website) shows uniform slowing of conduction velocities, without conduction block, in a patient with CMT type 1A. Note the markedly prolonged distal latency and slowed conduction velocities, but preserved normal ulnar CMAP amplitudes.
  - This is due to uniform demyelination along the nerve in contrast to acquired demyelinating conditions, which are multifocal and in which a point of severe involvement often leads to conduction block.
- Temporal dispersion results when individual nerve fibers depolarize at different times:
  - Occurs as a normal phenomenon because any given motor or sensory nerve is made up of fibers that vary in their degree of myelination.
  - Is more prominent with proximal stimulation because the small myelinated fibers increasingly lag behind larger myelinated fibers with greater distance.
  - Causes a slight increase in CMAP duration and slight decrease in CMAP amplitude and area in normal motor NCS.
  - Becomes quite prominent in demyelinating lesions that cause slowed conduction velocities, and often accompanies conduction block.

F-waves

- Type of late response demonstrated by applying a supramaximal stimulus over the distal portion of a motor nerve, which causes current to travel both orthodromically and antidromically from the stimulation site.
- F-waves are produced when the antidromic current travels proximally to stimulate a small population of motor neurons in the spinal cord, which then back fire an impulse orthodromically down the nerve to cause a few muscle fibers to depolarize.
- M-wave = initial waveform (CMAP) produced by the orthodromic current.
- F-waves are always smaller in amplitude than the M-wave and vary in morphology and latencies (see Figure 3.7 on the companion website).

- Clinical significance:
  - Sensitive measure in detecting lesions affecting the proximal nerve segment.
    - Structural lesion affecting the nerve root, e.g. herniated disk causing radiculopathy.
    - Immune-mediated demyelinating diseases like acute inflammatory demyelinating polyradiculoneuropathy (AIDP) – prolonged or absent F-responses may be the first abnormalities seen because the proximal segments are usually affected.
- Caveat in interpreting abnormal F-waves:
  - May be affected by a number of factors other than lesions affecting the proximal nerve segment: abnormal nerve conduction velocity, abnormal distal latency, or a very tall patient.

H-reflex

- Another type of late response that provides information about nerve conduction along the proximal segments of a nerve.
- Relies on both sensory afferent and motor efferent fibers, unlike the F-response, which is purely motor.
- Considered the electrophysiologic equivalent to the clinically produced Achilles tendon reflex.
- Elicited by applying a submaximal stimulation to the tibial nerve in the popliteal fossa while recording over the calf muscles:
  - This activates mixed motor and sensory nerves that are insufficient to produce a direct motor response but activates muscle spindle afferents.
  - Sensory fibers carry the impulse to the spinal cord where they synapse with anterior horn cells that transmit the impulse along motor fibers and to the muscle.
  - H-waves attenuate as the direct motor response (M-wave) becomes more prominent with increasing current (see Figure 3.8 on the companion website).
- Clinical significance:
  - S1 radiculopathy
  - Polyneuropathy
  - Absence of H-reflex is an early finding in AIDP.

Sensory NCS

Routine sensory nerve conduction studies:
- Upper extremity: median, ulnar, and radial.
- Lower extremity: sural and superficial peroneal.
- Special nerves can be tested in the appropriate clinical setting:
  - Lateral and medial antebrachial cutaneous sensory nerves are important in investigating brachial plexopathies.
  - Saphenous nerves are important for femoral neuropathy.
  - Medial and lateral plantar nerves for tarsal tunnel syndrome.
  - Dorsal ulnar cutaneous nerve for ulnar neuropathy; wrist versus elbow.

Figure 3.9 (on the companion website) illustrates setting up your test in the case of antidromic median sensory nerve testing with ring electrodes recording over the index finger.
- Ring electrodes are placed over the cutaneous region innervated by the nerve to be tested.
- Ground is placed between the recording and stimulating electrodes.
- Place stimulator over the median nerve at the wrist.
- Test can also be performed orthodromically where the ring electrodes deliver the current and recording occurs over the median nerve.

Important differences between sensory nerve testing compared to motor NCS:

- SNAP amplitude is measured in microvolts compared to CMAP, which is measured in millivolts (see Figure 3.10 on the companion website).
- The small sensory potential is more affected by technical factors:
  - Low limb temperatures (<30°C lower, <32°C upper) produce falsely increased amplitudes and slowed conduction velocities.
  - Electrical noise in the environment.
- Sensory NCS only assess sensory nerve fibers whereas motor NCS reflect the conduction time across the motor nerve, neuromuscular junction (NMJ), and muscle fibers.
- Measurement of the sensory nerve CV only requires one stimulation site:
  - Sensory nerve CV = onset latency/distance between the stimulator and active recording electrode.

Special tests: blink reflex and repetitive nerve stimulation
Blink reflex
- Evaluates the trigeminal and facial nerves and is considered the electrical correlate of the clinically evoked corneal reflex:
  - Afferent limb = sensory fibers of the supraorbital branch of the trigeminal nerve.
  - Efferent limb = motor fibers of the facial nerve.
- Can detect lesions along the reflex arc both peripherally and centrally in the brainstem.
- Test set-up:
  - Recording electrodes are placed over orbicularis oculi muscles bilaterally.
  - Stimulation is given to the supraorbital nerve at the supraorbital notch over the medial eyebrow.
- *R1 response*: The early response represents the conduction time along the afferent pathway of the trigeminal nerve to its sensory nucleus located in the mid-pons, then across disynaptic pathways between the trigeminal sensory nucleus to the facial nerve nucleus located in the lower pontine tegmentum, and finally through the efferent pathway of the ipsilateral facial nerve.
- *R2 response*: The late response represents the synapse in the nucleus of the spinal tract of the trigeminal nerve in the ipsilateral pons and medulla, followed by impulses that travel across multiple synapses in the pons and lateral medulla to both the contralateral and ipsilateral facial nerve nuclei, and then finally across the efferent pathways of both facial nerves.
- Figure 3.11 (on the companion website) depicts a normal blink reflex.
- Figure 3.12 (on the companion website) demonstrates a complete right facial nerve lesion. Note the absent ipsilateral R1 and R2 potentials but normal contralateral R2 potential when the affected side is stimulated. When the unaffected side is stimulated, the ipsilateral R1 and R2 potentials are present but the contralateral R2 potential is absent.

Repetitive nerve stimulation (RNS)
This is an important test in evaluating patients with neuromuscular junction disorders, especially myasthenia gravis.
- Two nerves are usually tested, one distal and one proximal:
  - Ulnar nerve recording over the abductor digiti minimi muscle.
  - Spinal accessory nerve recording over the trapezius muscle.
  - Sensitivity is increased if clinically affected muscles are tested.
- A train of 5 to 10 supramaximal stimuli are given at 2 or 3 Hz and CMAP is recorded as with routine motor NCS (Figure 3.13).

- Positive test if there is a progressive decline in the CMAP amplitude of greater than 10% within the first five stimuli:
  - Smallest CMAP amplitude typically occurs between the second and fourth stimuli.
  - Decremental response may plateau and improve after the fifth stimulus due to mobilization of secondary stores of acetylcholine to the neuromuscular junction.
  - Typically gives a characteristic U-shaped curve to the RNS test, which is highly characteristic of a neuromuscular junction disorder (Figure 3.14).
- Post-exercise (post-tetanic) facilitation:
  - A repair in the decremental response seen after the patient is asked to perform a brief 10-second exercise of the muscle being recorded.
  - The brief maximal contraction of the muscle causes a transient increase in the presynaptic calcium levels, which leads to a temporary increase in acetylcholine release, thus repairing the decremental response.
- Post-exercise (post-tetanic) exhaustion:
  - Worsening of the decremental response due to exhaustion of the acetylcholine reserves over subsequent trains.
  - Usually occurs in trains recorded at around 3 to 4 minutes.

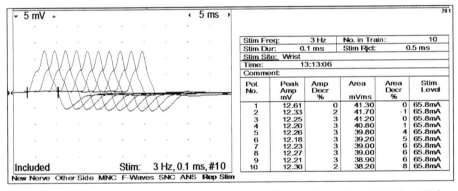

Figure 3.13 Normal baseline recording of left ulnar nerve, repetitive stimulation [Rec: ADM, Stim: Wrist].

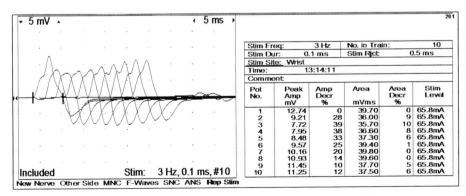

Figure 3.14 Positive decremental response left ulnar rep stim [Rec: ADM, Stim: Wrist].

Rapid repetitive nerve stimulation (RNS) in suspected presynaptic disorders (Eaton–Lambert syndrome, botulism)

- High frequency (10–50 Hz).
- Assesses presynaptic neuromuscular junction disorders like Lambert–Eaton myasthenic syndrome.
- In rapid RNS, more calcium accumulates at the presynaptic terminal because not enough time is allowed for the previously infused calcium to be actively pumped out. This leads to an increased release of acetylcholine quanta due to an increased level of calcium.
- An abnormal increase in CMAP increment (>100%) indicates a presynaptic abnormality.
- Similar findings can be demonstrated with a post-exercise facilitation test.
- Most laboratories prefer using the post-exercise facilitation test over the rapid RNS, which may be uncomfortable for patients.

Electromyography

Electromyography (EMG) follows the NCS testing and is a vital part of the electrophysiologic evaluation. EMG consists of inserting a concentric needle electrode into muscle. The needle detects the electrical potential generated by the myofibers; these are studied to detect abnormalities in the muscle (myopathic) or its innervation (neurogenic). When examining a muscle with EMG, there are several components that will need to be carefully analyzed. These include the presence of spontaneous activity, motor unit recruitment, size, and activation patterns, all of which will be discussed in detail in this section. Although most individuals tolerate the examination, there are varying levels of tolerance. Muscles should be carefully selected prior to starting the examination in order to obtain an accurate diagnosis. See Table 3.1 and Table 3.2.

Spontaneous activity

Analysis of spontaneous activity begins when the needle is inserted into a relaxed muscle. Normal insertional activity is produced as the needle is quickly moved through the muscle generating a brief electrical discharge that lasts less than 300 ms. The presence of insertional activity is important to ensure that the needle is in muscle rather than subcutaneous tissue. Any waveforms that persist after 300 ms are considered abnormal; an exception is when the needle is near the neuromuscular junction where end plate noise or end plate spikes may be detected.

Table 3.1 EMG findings seen in neurogenic conditions.

	Spontaneous activity	MUAP morphology			Firing pattern
		Duration	Phases	Amplitude	Recruitment
Axonal: acute	No	Normal	Normal	Normal	Reduced
Axonal: subacute	Yes	Normal to increased	Increased	Normal to increased	Reduced
Axonal: chronic	No/yes	Increased	Increased	Increased	Reduced
Demyelinating without conduction block	No	Normal	Normal	Normal	Normal
Demyelinating with conduction block	No	Normal	Normal	Normal	Reduced

Table 3.2 EMG findings seen in myopathic conditions.

| | Spontaneous activity | MUAP morphology | | | Firing pattern |
		Duration	Phases	Amplitude	Recruitment
Myopathic: acute	No/yes	Brief	Increased	Small	Normal or early
Myopathic: chronic	No/yes	Brief or long	Increased	Small or increased	Normal or early
Myopathic: end stage	No/yes	Brief or long	Increased	Small or increased	Markedly decreased

Normal spontaneous activity
- End plate noise: characteristic "sea shell" sound on EMG and represents motor end plate potentials.
- End plate spikes: can be seen with end plate noise and result from muscle fiber action potentials:
  - Biphasic morphology with an initial negative deflection and fire irregularly.
  - Should not be mistaken for fibrillation potentials, which are pathologic.

Careful examination of spontaneous activity is one of the most important parts of the needle examination:
- Some discharges, like myotonia, are seen in certain muscle disorders.
- Pattern of spontaneous activity can help localize the anatomic lesion:
  - Muscle membrane irritability restricted to proximal muscles in an inflammatory myopathy.
  - Denervation potentials are seen within a myotome of a radiculopathy.
- Presence of spontaneous activity may provide clues to the time course of a lesion:
  - Fibrillation potentials and positive sharp waves may not be evident for 2–3 weeks after an axonal injury to a nerve.

Abnormal spontaneous activity
- Fibrillation potentials and positive sharp waves:
  - Generated by spontaneous depolarization of muscle fibers and have the same electrophysiologic significance of active denervation.
  - Commonly seen in neuropathic disorders (i.e. neuropathy, motor neuron disease, and radiculopathy) but also in inflammatory myopathies and some muscular dystrophies.
  - Fibrillation potentials look like a brief spike with an initial positive deflection, brief duration and low amplitude:
    - Characteristic sound of a fibrillation potential is described as "rain falling on a tin roof."
    - May become very small in amplitude in end-stage fibrotic muscle.
  - Positive sharp waves have a brief positive deflection followed by a long negative phase:
    - Duration is longer than fibrillation potentials and the amplitude is variable.
    - Sounds like a dull pop on EMG.
  - Firing patterns of both potentials are very regular.
- Fasciculations:
  - Generated by a motor neuron or its axon.
  - Represent spontaneous, involuntary discharges of single motor units.
  - Fire very slowly and with an irregular pattern.
  - Sound like dull pops and have been described as like the sound of "corn popping."

- Frequently associated with motor neuron disease but may be seen in a variety of conditions:
  - Radiculopathies, polyneuropathies, and in benign conditions like benign fasciculation syndrome.
- Complex repetitive discharges (CRDs):
  - Commonly occur in chronic disease states where denervated muscle fibers lie adjacent to one another.
  - Potentials are generated by the depolarization of a single muscle fiber that causes an adjacent denervated muscle fiber to also depolarize; also known as ephaptic spread.
  - The shape (morphology) of the motor potential is due to individual muscle fibers linked together; morphology is identical from one discharge to the next.
  - Sound of a CRD has been described as like a machine gun firing, which may start and end abruptly.
- Myotonia:
  - Generated by muscle fibers and has similar morphology to fibrillation potentials and positive sharp waves.
  - Can be differentiated by characteristic waxing and waning of both frequency and amplitude, which makes it sound like a "revving engine" on EMG.
  - Unique type of spontaneous activity that can be seen with specific disorders:
    - Myotonic dystrophy, paramyotonia congenita, myotonia congenita, and hyperkalemic periodic paralysis.
    - May also be seen in toxic myopathies, acid maltase deficiency, and some inflammatory myopathies.
  - Rarely detected in common neurogenic conditions like radiculopathy or motor neuron disease.
- Myokymia:
  - Generated by either a motor neuron or its axon and appears like grouped fasciculations.
  - Bursts should be of the same individual motor unit but may vary in the number of potentials between bursts.
  - Characteristic sound on EMG is described as "marching soldiers."
  - Presence of myokymic discharges is an important finding in radiation-induced nerve damage and can help distinguish between radiation plexopathy and neoplastic invasion of the plexus.
  - Facial myokymia may be seen in brainstem lesions and in Guillain–Barré syndrome.
- Cramp:
  - High-frequency discharges generated from either a motor neuron or axon.
  - Persistent normal-appearing motor unit potentials bunched together.
  - Clinically, cramps are involuntary contractions of muscles that are quite painful.
  - Seen in benign conditions like cramp fasciculation syndrome, nocturnal cramps, or after exercise as well as metabolic, endocrine, and various neurologic conditions.
- Neuromyotonia:
  - Rare spontaneous activity that has the highest frequency of any discharge generated by a motor neuron or its axon.
  - Consists of repetitive discharges of a single motor unit with decremental amplitude that gives it a characteristic "pinging" sound on EMG.
  - Clinically seen in:
    - Isaac's syndrome.
    - Acquired neuromyotonic syndromes with positive antibodies against voltage-gated potassium channels or contactin-associated protein-like 2 (CASPR2).
    - Neuromyotonia has been reported in myasthenic patients with thymoma and in inflammatory demyelinating polyneuropathies.

Analysis of voluntary motor unit action potentials

The analysis of the motor unit action potential (MUAP) comes after the initial assessment of the insertional and spontaneous activity. A MUAP represents the extracellular compound potential of all muscle fibers within a motor unit. A motor unit is comprised of a motor neuron, its axon, and associated NMJs and muscle fibers. Several elements of MUAPs are diagnostically significant, including the morphology of the waveform, recruitment, and activation patterns.

MUAP duration
- Reflects the number of muscle fibers within a motor unit, and the dispersion of their depolarizations over time.
- Duration can be different in limb muscles compared to proximal and bulbofacial muscles, where they generally have a shorter duration.
- Can also be affected by age and cool limb temperature, which can both increase duration.
- Neurogenic conditions:
  - Chronic neurogenic processes increase MUAP duration as reinnervation occurs and one motor unit innervates many muscle fibers.
  - Long duration leads to a dull and thudding sound on EMG.
- Myopathic conditions:
  - Duration may shorten as there is a loss of muscle fibers.
  - Short duration leads to a crisp sound on EMG.

MUAP polyphasia
- Calculated by counting the number of times a MUAP crosses the baseline (normal MUAP has two to four phases).
- Each muscle has a certain percentage of polyphasic MUAPs that are considered normal; e.g. up to 25% of the units seen in the deltoid muscle may appear polyphasic.
- Once this normal percentage is exceeded, an increase in polyphasic MUAPs is considered pathologic and may be seen in both neuropathic and myopathic conditions.
- The sound of a polyphasic unit produces a high frequency "clicking" sound and represents the asynchronous firing of muscle fibers within a motor unit.

MUAP amplitude
- Not as helpful as MUAP duration in determining motor unit size.
- Can vary greatly among normal individuals.
- Factors that affect motor unit amplitude:
  - Distance of the needle electrode to the motor unit.
  - Increased muscle fiber diameter (e.g. muscle fiber hypertrophy in weight trainers).
  - Increased number of muscle fibers within a motor unit (i.e. seen in reinnervation).
- Increased in neurogenic conditions.
- Decreased in myopathic conditions.

Recruitment, activation, and interference pattern
- Normal muscle force is generated by a combination of:
  1. increasing firing rate of an individual motor unit; and
  2. recruiting additional motor units.
- Reduced recruitment:
  - Occurs in neurogenic conditions.
  - Axonal loss, severe demyelination.
  - Loss in the number of available motor units.

- Early recruitment:
  - Occurs in myopathic conditions.
  - Loss of individual myofibers from a motor unit.
  - Since each individual motor unit can no longer generate the same amount of force, many more motor units must fire early in order to generate the same amount of force.
- Activation refers to the ability to increase the firing rate of MUAPs:
  - It is different than recruitment in that it is a central process.
  - Poor activation can be due to:
    - central causes of weakness (stroke hemiparesis, myelopathy, etc.);
    - pain;
    - lack of patient effort during the examination.
- Complete interference pattern occurs during maximal contraction when multiple MUAPs overlap and no one single MUAP can be distinguished from one another.
- An incomplete interference pattern can occur from reduced motor unit recruitment as well as in poor activation.

BOTTOM LINE
- NCS/EMG is an essential tool when evaluating patients with suspected neuromuscular disorders.
- Understanding the basic electrophysiologic patterns can help the general neurologist localize the neuromuscular problem, guide workup, as well as make a diagnosis.

Electroencephalography

Electroencephalography (EEG) is essential in evaluating patients with suspected seizure disorders and is also useful in encephalopathies. This section will focus on the basics of EEG and touch upon frequently encountered patterns in clinical practice.
- In patients with a history of seizures, longer recordings with activating procedures including photic stimulation, hyperventilation, and sleep can increase study yield. The use of video is helpful in correlating electrographic activity with the patient's behaviors and can help localize seizures.
- Encephalopathies for which EEG is diagnostically useful include toxic metabolic states, rapidly progressive dementias like spongiform encephalopathy, and coma following cardiac arrest.
- Video EEG is crucial in the diagnosis of non-epileptic behavioral events, during which there is no underlying electrographic seizure activity associated with the patient's actions.
- The use of continuous EEG monitoring has greatly impacted the neurologic care of critically ill patients with altered mental status in the ICU by diagnosing non-convulsive status epilepticus that requires treatment with anti-seizure medications, which has often been misattributed to medication effects.
- Continuous EEG is also utilized in monitoring brain function during therapeutic hypothermia following cardiac arrest.
- There are many more applications of EEG, such as in the study of sleep (polysomnography).

Source of EEG potentials
- Surface electrodes applied to the scalp with conductive paste record the postsynaptic potentials (PSPs) generated by the pyramidal cells of the cerebral cortex:
  - PSPs are the summations of countless inhibitory and excitatory postsynaptic potentials.
  - These potentials are likely influenced by thalamic and brainstem reticular formation afferent impulses.

- A minimum of 6 cm² of synchronous cortical activity is needed to generate a detectable scalp potential.
- EEG is a graphic plot of the voltage difference between two different cerebral locations (*y*-axis) plotted over time (*x*-axis).
- Volume conduction:
  - Process by which current flows through the tissues (brain parenchyma, CSF, skull, and scalp) to the recording electrode from the electrical source generator.

Electrode placement and montages

The most commonly used system for electrode placement is the International 10-20 System (see Figure 3.15 on the companion website), so named because electrodes are placed either 10 or 20% of the distance across key landmarks on the head.

The EEG records the potential difference, or voltage, between two electrodes. By convention, a positive potential difference is represented as a downgoing deflection. Thus, if the Fp1-F7 lead produces a downgoing deflection, Fp1 is positively charged compared with F7.

Two leads can be compared using a variety of montages. A common set-up is the longitudinal bipolar (also referred to as "double banana") as shown in Figure 3.16 on the companion website. The tracings in this chapter were obtained using the longitudinal bipolar montage.

Normal EEG patterns

The normal EEG record of an adult in a restful and wakeful state consists of various types of rhythms in an organized fashion, as shown in Figure 3.17.

- Alpha rhythm:
  - Consists of regular, monomorphic waveforms that have a frequency of 8–13 Hz.
  - When it is observed in occipital and posterior parietal regions in a relaxed individual with closed eyes, it is also known as the posterior dominant rhythm.
    - Most prominent in a relaxed, awake state with eyes closed.
    - Attenuates with mental activity or eye opening.
    - Disappears in drowsiness.
  - Slight frequency difference between two hemispheres is common; differences >1 Hz are considered abnormal slowing in the hemisphere with lower frequency.

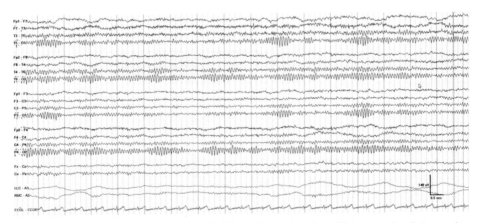

Figure 3.17 Normal awake EEG in 26-year-old adult who is quietly resting with her eyes closed. A posterior dominant rhythm is prominent in the occipital region and there is moderate frontal beta activity.

- Beta rhythms:
  - Frequency is over 13 Hz, usually lower amplitude (10–20 μV).
  - Normally recorded from the frontal regions bilaterally.
  - Commonly accentuated over the fronto-central regions during drowsiness.
  - Increased beta activity may be noted with medications such as benzodiazepines and barbiturates.
- Theta rhythms:
  - Frequency 4–7 Hz.
  - Seen in the temporal regions as individuals become drowsy.
- Mu rhythm (see Figure 3.18 on the companion website):
  - Arc-shaped waves at frequency 7–11 Hz usually seen over centro-parietal regions.
  - Most commonly seen in young adults.
  - Facilitated when individuals scan visual images.
  - Attenuated by passive or active movement of the limb contralateral to the hemisphere generating the rhythm.
- Delta rhythm:
  - Frequency <4 Hz.
  - Occurs normally in sleep.
  - Correlates with periods of decreased pyramidal cell activity.
- Breach rhythm:
  - Focal rhythm (usually central or mid-temporal) corresponding to an area with a skull defect.
  - Waveforms are high voltage and fast frequency (6–11 Hz).
  - Not pathologic, but may be confused with spikes or sharp waves, which must be interpreted with caution in this setting.

Normal sleep patterns

Sleep can be divided into two categories: non-rapid eye movement (NREM) and rapid eye movement (REM) sleep. NREM is further subdivided into stage I, stage II, and slow wave sleep (previously stages III and IV, which are now combined); each has characteristic EEG patterns. Stage II sleep is shown in Figure 3.19.

- Stage I:
  - Drowsiness begins with slow eye rolling movements.
  - Attenuation or disappearance of alpha rhythm.
  - Distinguished from waking if <50% of a 30-second recording contains the waking background alpha activity.
  - Vertex sharp transients (also known as V waves):
    - Bilaterally synchronous, sharply contoured waves of negative polarity at the vertex of the head.
  - Positive occipital sharp transients of sleep (POSTS):
    - Triangular waves in the occipital region that are monophasic or biphasic in morphology.
    - Can occur intermittently, independently, or simultaneously on both sides.
- Stage II:
  - Characterized by presence of sleep spindles and K complexes.
  - Sleep spindles:
    - Short bursts of waxing and waning rhythmic activity 12–14 Hz with a duration >0.5 seconds.
    - Maximal over the central regions.
    - Always appear simultaneously over both hemispheres after 2 years of age.

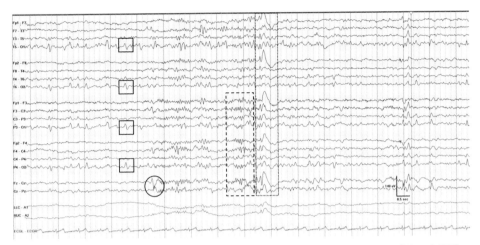

Figure 3.19 Transition between stage I and II sleep EEG. Positive occipital sharp transients of sleep (POSTS; one example in solid box), vertex waves (circled), K complex (in dotted rectangle), and spindles (in dashed rectangle) are seen.

- K complex.
  - High-amplitude, diphasic transients that are often accompanied by sleep spindles.
  - May resemble vertex waves but usually longer in duration and less sharply contoured.
  - Seen in fronto-temporal regions, maximum at the midline.
- POSTS and vertex waves may persist.
- Stage III:
  - Slow-wave, delta sleep.
  - Characterized by 20–50% of a 30-second recording occupied by slow waves of 2 Hz or less.
  - K complexes are often present, sleep spindles may be present or absent.
  - POSTS can usually be seen.
- Stage IV:
  - Characterized by >50% of a 30-second recording occupied by waves of 2 Hz or less.
  - K complexes blend with slow waves.
  - POSTS and spindles are rare.
- Stages III and IV are grouped together as "slow wave sleep."

Artifacts

Recognition of artifacts is crucial in EEG interpretation. Below are some of the most commonly encountered artifacts that originate from the patient.
- Eye blink (vertical eye movement) artifact (see Figure 3.20 on the companion website):
  - The front of the eye carries a positive charge relative to the back.
  - Fp1 and Fp2 are the electrodes positioned above the left and right eyes, respectively. Therefore, the greatest potential difference during vertical eye movements is seen in leads with Fp1 (Fp1-F7, Fp1-F3) and Fp2 (Fp2-F8, Fp2-F4).
  - During eye closure, the fronts of the eyes roll up (Bell's phenomenon) toward Fp1 and Fp2, causing them to see more positive potential difference. This is represented on the EEG as a large downward deflection, maximal in leads involving Fp1 and Fp2.
  - During eye opening, the fronts of the eyes roll down away from Fp1 and Fp2, causing them to see a negative potential difference. This is represented on the EEG as an upward deflection, maximal in leads involving Fp1 and Fp2.

- Eye movement artifact:
  - Leads involving F7 and F8, which are placed laterally to the eyes, will see the greatest potential difference.
  - When the eyes move to the left,
    - leads involving F7 will see a positive potential difference (in a longitudinal bipolar montage, Fp1-F7 sees an upgoing deflection and F7-T3 sees a downgoing deflection);
    - leads involving F8 will see a negative potential difference (Fp1-F8 sees a downgoing deflection and F8-T4 sees an upgoing deflection).
  - Slow rolling eye movements produce smooth deflections (see Figure 3.21 on the companion website).
  - Rapid eye movements produce more irregular deflections. Sometimes, lateral rectus muscle artifact produces a lateral rectus spike (see Figure 3.22 on the companion website).
- Chewing artifact (see Figure 3.23 on the companion website):
  - Chewing produces a combination of signals that includes both muscle artifact (represented as a cluster of fast activity) from contraction of the muscles of mastication as well as slow rhythmical movements of the jaw.
- Glossokinetic artifact (see Figure 3.24 on the companion website):
  - Arises because the tip of the tongue carries a negative charge relative to the back of the tongue.
  - Seen during chewing, talking, swallowing, coughing, sobbing, and sucking.

Activation procedures

Hyperventilation and photic stimulation are activation procedures used to bring out epileptiform discharges in individuals with suspected seizure disorders.

Hyperventilation
- Individuals are asked to breathe deeply for 3 to 5 minutes.
- Theory: presumed to cause hypocapnia-induced alkalosis, which leads to vasoconstriction of cerebral blood vessels and decreases cerebral blood flow.
- Normal response:
  - Generalized, intermittent, slow waves that may begin shortly after the start of hyperventilation.
  - Bilaterally synchronous bursts with sharply contoured waves.
  - Maximum in the anterior or posterior head regions.
  - Response ends within 60 seconds after cessation of hyperventilation.
- May be prominent in children, teenagers, individuals with low serum glucose or cerebral ischemia; rare in older patients.
- Abnormal responses:
  - Prominent asymmetry:
    - May activate focal temporal slowing in temporal lobe lesions.
  - Reappearance of slowing after the background has returned to normal and hyperventilation has stopped.
  - Epileptiform discharges.
    - Activates generalized 3-Hz spike-and-wave discharges seen in absence seizures (Figure 3.25).
    - May activate temporal spikes in temporal lobe epilepsy.

Photic stimulation
- Flashes of light are delivered during the EEG recording at different rates.
- Normal response:
  - Visual evoked potential (VEP).
    - Generated by the occipital lobes; appears ~80–150 ms after a flash of light is delivered.

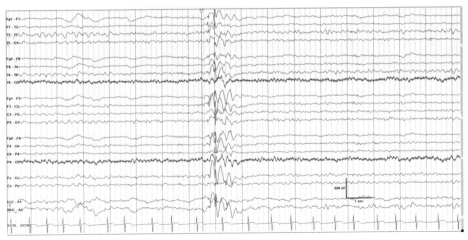

Figure 3.25 A burst of spike-wave discharges is seen in a five-year old boy during hyperventilation.

- Photic driving (see Figure 3.26 on the companion website).
  - Occurs at flash rates greater than 3 Hz, typically 7 Hz or greater.
  - Most reliably evoked at frequencies close to the posterior dominant rhythm.
  - Produces a rhythmic discharge that is time locked to the visual stimulus.
  - Absence of photic driving may not be clinically significant.
- Photomyogenic (formerly photomyoclonic) responses (see Figure 3.27 on the companion website).
  - Brief muscle contractions that are linked to the repetitive flashes of light. Usually involves the orbicularis oculi and frontalis muscles, but may extend to other muscles in the head and neck.
  - Rare phenomenon seen in a few susceptible individuals but clinical significance is uncertain.
- Abnormal response:
  - Marked asymmetry
    - Absence of driving on one side where the other side is well developed may be suggestive of lesions affecting the lateral geniculate nucleus, optic radiations, or the calcarine cortex.
  - Photoparoxysmal response (see Figure 3.28 on the companion website).
    - Also referred to as photoepileptiform or photoconvulsive responses.
    - Epileptiform activity invoked by the flashes of light that does not have a clear relationship to the stimulus frequency and often outlasts the end of stimulation.
    - Maximal over the frontal and central head regions.
    - Most often seen in primary generalized epilepsies, e.g. juvenile myoclonic epilepsy.
    - Photic stimulation should be discontinued after this response is seen, as further stimulation may trigger a generalized convulsion.

Abnormal EEG patterns in epilepsy

A comprehensive review of the classification of seizure types and electroclinical syndromes is beyond the scope of this chapter. The reader is referred to the 2010 Report of the ILAE Commission on Classification and Terminology (see Berg AT, Berkovic SF, Brodie MJ, et al. in Reading list).

- One key concept in classifying epilepsies and their associated electrical discharges is to classify them as either:
  - generalized (occurring in broadly distributed, bilaterally synchronous networks), or
  - focal (originating in one area of the brain).
- Epilepsy syndromes have additionally traditionally been subdivided into:
  - idiopathic (suspected to be of genetic origin);
  - symptomatic (reflecting known cerebral pathology); or
  - cryptogenic (of unknown etiology).

The discussion below highlights the ictal and interictal features of some of the most common generalized and focal epilepsies.

Idiopathic generalized epilepsies

A patient with an EEG consistent with idiopathic generalized epilepsy is shown in Figure 3.29.

- Childhood absence epilepsy (Figure 3.30):
  - Ictal and interictal EEG shows 3-Hz generalized spike-and-wave discharges.
  - Provoked by hyperventilation and hypoglycemia.
  - May be suppressed by treatment.
- Juvenile absence epilepsy:
  - Interictal EEG shows 3–4-Hz generalized spike-and-wave discharges.
- Juvenile myoclonic epilepsy:
  - Icterictal EEG: 4–6-Hz generalized spike-wave and polyspike-and-wave discharges.
  - These patients are sensitive to photic flashes.

Focal epilepsies

- Benign epilepsy of childhood with centrotemporal spikes (BECTS):
  - Interictal EEG: high-voltage centrotemporal spikes.
- Temporal lobe epilepsy:
  - Interictal EEG:
    - In anterior temporal lobe epilepsy, bitemporal sharp/spike-and-wave discharges, either synchronous or independent, can be seen in 25–33% of patients.

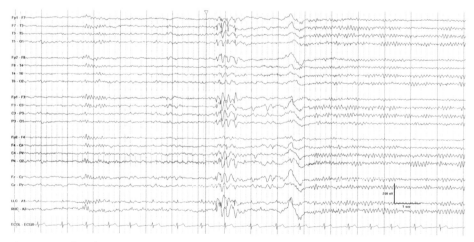

Figure 3.29 Idiopathic generalized epilepsy. There is a single burst of 4-Hz generalized spike and wave interrupting this otherwise normal background.

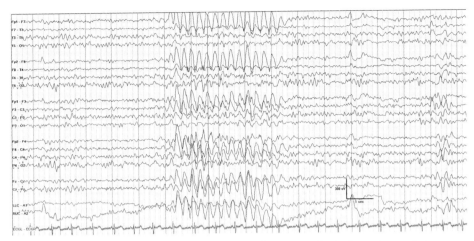

Figure 3.30 Childhood absence epilepsy. There is a burst of 3-Hz generalized spike-and-wave discharges that correlates with a behavioral interruption in this 9-year-old girl.

- In mesial temporal epilepsy, the only clue interictally may be intermittent rhythmic slowing.
- Mid-temporal or posterior temporal interictal discharges are less common.
  - Ictal EEG: varied patterns may be seen.
- Frontal lobe epilepsy:
  - In orbital frontal or mesial frontal epilepsies, interictal and ictal EEG discharges may not be seen using surface electrodes.

Abnormalities not related to seizures
- Continuous focal slowing:
  - Suggestive of a structural defect in the affected area (see Figure 3.31 on the companion website).
- Generalized slowing:
  - Indicative of a diffuse encephalopathy.
  - Sometimes non-specific.
- Frontal intermittent rhythmic delta activity (FIRDA), also known as frontal generalized rhythmic delta activity (frontal GRDA) (see Figure 3.32 on the companion website):
  - Consists of bilaterally synchronous, frontally predominant delta range (0–3 Hz) monomorphic waves.
  - Associated with diffuse encephalopathy, toxic-metabolic conditions, structural brain lesions, or increased intracranial pressure.
  - Not an epileptic pattern and does not predict epilepsy.
  - Non-specific.
- Generalized periodic epileptiform discharges (GPEDs), also known as generalized periodic discharges (GPDs):
  - Consist of diffuse waveforms appearing at a set interval.
  - High association with seizures and status epilepticus.
  - Can be seen in the setting of a toxic-metabolic encephalopathy, in which case they tend to have a triphasic morphology.
    - This can lead to diagnostic confusion as to whether the pattern is related to a seizure or is metabolic.

- Can be seen in the setting of anoxic brain injury, subacute sclerosing panencephalitis (SSPE), and Creutzfeldt–Jakob disease (CJD) (see Figure 3.33 on the companion website).
  - In the context of CJD, these discharges are also referred to as periodic sharp wave complexes.
- Periodic lateralized epileptiform discharges (PLEDs), also known as lateralized periodic discharges (LPDs) (see Figure 3.34 on the companion website):
  - Consist of waveforms appearing at a set interval on one side of the brain.
  - Can be seen in any pathologic lesion and in a wide variety of circumstances.
  - Whether these represent an ictal, interictal, or postictal pattern is not clear.
  - Highly associated with clinical seizures and status epilepticus.

Pitfalls

- Scalp EEG recordings are not 100% sensitive in detecting seizures. As noted previously, a minimum of 6 cm² of cortex with synchronous activity is needed to generate a measurable scalp potential; a seizure focus smaller than this (as is the case with many patients with simple partial seizures) may not be detected on scalp EEG.
- Foci located deep within the brain may not be readily detected by scalp EEG, as is often the case with frontal lobe seizures. Diagnosis may be difficult in these situations but a high level of suspicion must be maintained in stereotyped events.
- The same EEG abnormality may originate from several anatomic areas; imaging studies (MRI) are useful to help identify potential sources for abnormal discharges.

BOTTOM LINE
- Electroencephalography is an important tool in the assessment of patients with known or suspected seizures and altered mental status.
- A basic understanding of normal and abnormal rhythms and their significance is helpful in the approach to treatment.
- EEG is not 100% sensitive, especially in cases of simple partial seizures and frontal lobe seizures, nor is it 100% specific.
- Long-term monitoring in critically ill and unresponsive patients reveals rhythms that often raise more questions than they can answer.
- EEG must be interpreted in the setting of the clinical context.

Evoked potentials

Evoked potentials are electrically generated responses that can be measured in various parts of the nervous system following a particular stimulus. Repetitive stimuli are time-locked and signal-averaged so that the background EEG (i.e. the random activity that may be detected in the environment and would produce an artefactual signal) cancels out and the stimulus-induced signal, which is undetectable in a routine recording, can be resolved. Common evoked potentials include visual evoked potentials, brainstem auditory evoked potentials, and somatosensory evoked potentials.

Visual evoked potentials (VEPs)

- Clinically measure the integrity and function of the optic nerve and retrogeniculate pathways.
- Recorded potential is a large positive waveform that is generated by the occipital cortex in response to a visual stimulus.
- P100 = positive peak that has a latency of approximately 85 to 115 ms (see Figure 3.35 on the companion website).

- VEP recording:
  - EEG electrodes are used to record the cortical potential.
  - The individual is required to maintain visual fixation at the center of a checkerboard pattern.
  - Alternating black and white squares are reversed about 120 times at a frequency of 1 to 2 Hz.
  - Multiple trials are recorded and averaged.
- Delay in P100 suggests conduction defect in the optic pathway anterior to the chiasm in the eye that received the visual stimulus.
- Most commonly seen in optic neuritis.
- Bilateral delay in P100 cannot be accurately localized because it can be due to lesions at or posterior to the chiasm, or widespread cerebral dysfunction.

Brainstem auditory evoked potentials
- Measure the function and integrity of the auditory pathway.
- Repetitive auditory stimulation generates reproducible electrical potentials that are recorded by scalp electrodes (see Figure 3.36 on the companion website).
- The resulting waveforms are generated by specific brain regions and occur at specific latencies and intervals (see Table 3.3 on the companion website and Table 3.4).

Table 3.4 Abnormal brainstem auditory evoked response (BAER) patterns.

Lesion	BAER pattern
Mild–moderate hearing loss	Normal waves III and V, absent wave I
Severe hearing loss	All waves are absent
Brain death	Only wave I (±II) is present
Cranial nerve (CN) VIII	Wave I increased latency
Cerebellopontine angle tumors	Wave I–III increased interpeak latency
Caudal pons to midbrain	Wave III–V increased interpeak latency
Above caudal pons	Waves I and III present, absent wave V

Somatosensory evoked potentials (SSEPs)
- Measure the function and integrity of the somatosensory pathways.
- Electrical potentials are generated by various regions of the ascending sensory pathways in response to peripheral nerve stimulation (see Figure 3.37 on the companion website; timing and causes of SSEP patterns are given in Table 3.5, Table 3.6, Table 3.7, and Table 3.8 on the companion website).

Neuromuscular ultrasound
- Provides good visualization of peripheral nerves and muscles.
- Peripheral nerves best imaged with linear array transducer with a frequency ≥12 MHz.
- Images are captured in real time.
- Echogenicity = ability of a surface to bounce back the sound echo transmitted from the transducer:
  - Hypoechoic surfaces appear dark.
  - Hyperechoic surfaces appear bright.

Clinical applications
- Peripheral nerves:
  - Can appear enlarged and hypoechoic in acquired demyelinating neuropathies as well as focal compressive neuropathies.
  - Figure 3.39 (on the companion website) shows NCS and ultrasound in a patient who presented with a left foot drop, whereas Figure 3.38 (on the companion website) shows a normal right peroneal NCS and ultrasound. The left peroneal NCS reveals slowed conduction velocity across the fibular head and conduction block; ultrasound reveals an enlarged, hypoechoic nerve at the site of compression.
- Muscle:
  - Increased echogenicity can be seen in muscle fibrosis and inflammatory myopathies.
  - Needle guidance.
    - Ultrasound-guided needle placement for electromyography: particularly useful for needle examination of the diaphragm, which carries a high risk of pneumothorax (see Figure 3.40 on the companion website).
    - Targeted delivery of botulinum toxin.

Carotid and transcranial ultrasound
Carotid duplex and transcranial Doppler (TCD) are ultrasound studies that evaluate the vascular supply of the brain. Carotid duplex images the carotid arteries in the neck assessing presence of atherosclerotic plaque and obstructive disease, while TCD evaluates the intracranial vasculature.
- Carotid duplex is a safe and accurate method to diagnose high-grade carotid stenosis and is the most common, least expensive, and least invasive mode for assessing the severity of carotid obstructive lesions.
- Carotid duplex imaging has high sensitivity and specificity, with accuracy approaching 90% for diagnosing greater than 50% stenosis when compared to cerebral angiography. Studies specifically addressing accuracy in diagnosing surgical lesions of greater than 70% as defined by the North American Symptomatic Endarterectomy Trial (NASCET) have also demonstrated high sensitivity and specificity.

Imaging of the carotid vasculature and measurement of blood flow velocity are accomplished using ultrasonography through two basic techniques:
- the pulse-echo technique for two-dimensional (2D) anatomic imaging, and
- the Doppler principle for measurement of blood flow velocity. Duplex ultrasonography or imaging refers to the combination of Doppler ultrasound and real-time 2D, B-mode imaging for simultaneous evaluation of blood vessel anatomy and blood flow characteristics. Initial transmission of the ultrasound signal results in reflected echoes as either stationary tissue boundaries or moving red blood cells are encountered. These echoes are then received by the same transducer that generates the original transmitted signal. The amplitude of the returning echoes that encounter tissue boundaries is used to form the anatomic images, while the Doppler frequency shifts resulting from the encounter with the moving red cells generate velocity information (which correlates with vessel narrowing) through spectral frequency analysis. The internal carotid artery (ICA), external carotid artery (ECA), and the common carotid artery (CCA) are each identified by their distinctive waveform features. The various waveform characteristics used to identify the ICA and ECA are presented in Table 3.9. B-mode and waveform images of a normal carotid bifurcation are shown in Figure 3.41 (on the companion website).

An example of signal transmission during tapping of the ipsilateral temporal artery is demonstrated in Figure 3.42 (on the companion website). This can further assist in correctly distinguishing between the ICA and ECA.

Table 3.9 Characteristics of external and internal carotid arteries.

	External carotid artery	Internal carotid artery
Anatomic location	Anteromedial	Posterolateral
Luminal size	Smaller (3–4 mm)	Larger (6 mm)
Branches in neck	Yes	No
Waveform	High resistance (lower diastolic frequency)	Low resistance (higher diastolic frequency)
Temporal tap transmitted	Yes	No

Table 3.10 Criteria for grading carotid stenosis.

Percent stenosis	Peak systolic velocity (cm/s)	End-diastolic velocity (cm/s)
<50% (mild)	<120 cm/s	<100 cm/s
50–69% (moderate)	120 to 180 cm/s	<100 cm/s
70–99% (severe)	>180 cm/s	<100 cm/s for <80% >100 cm/s for >80%

Peak systolic blood flow velocity increases as the vessel lumen decreases, and these velocity alterations correlate with different degrees of stenosis. Peak velocity will increase within the stenotic segment and continue to increase with the degree of vessel narrowing. This will be followed by an increase in the end-diastolic velocity as the degree of stenosis increases beyond 50%, with significant end-diastolic velocity elevation occurring with narrowing greater than 80%. The degree of stenosis is typically categorized into mild (<50%), moderate (50–69%), and severe (70–99%) – see Table 3.10. Figure 3.43 (on the companion website) demonstrates the various spectral waveforms corresponding to different degrees of carotid artery stenosis.

Complete ICA occlusion can be diagnosed when there is absence of ICA signal but ECA signal remains intact, unless the occlusion also involves the CCA in which case flow may be absent from all three segments (see Figure 3.44 on the companion website). Corresponding hemodynamic changes on TCD are helpful in reliably detecting ICA occlusion or high-grade carotid stenosis (see below).

B-mode imaging is used to directly image the carotid vasculature for information about atherosclerotic carotid disease. The amount of plaque and plaque morphology such as surface irregularities and ulceration can be imaged. This information is important because plaque emboli can be a source of cerebral ischemia even in the absence of significant carotid stenosis. Figure 3.45 (on the companion website) demonstrates various examples of plaque morphology.

Transcranial Doppler is an ultrasound technique that measures blood flow velocity in the intracranial vasculature. As originally demonstrated by Aaslid in 1982, velocity spectra can be obtained from the intracranial vessels using a 2 MHz pulsed ultrasound signal. Range-gating is used to obtain measurements of flow velocity and blood flow direction from a range of selected depths. Vasculature that can be evaluated includes the intracranial carotid siphon, ophthalmic artery, middle cerebral arteries, anterior cerebral arteries, posterior cerebral arteries, vertebral arteries, and basilar artery. TCD can be used to evaluate the intracranial hemodynamic effects of carotid artery stenosis, intracranial artery stenosis, vasospasm following subarachnoid hemorrhage, and traumatic brain injury. It is also used for cerebral emboli detection and determination of brain death.

Vessels are identified with TCD primarily through knowledge of direction of flow, depth of insonation, and flow velocity – for example, the middle cerebral artery (MCA) is located by insonating through the temporal window at 40 to 60 mm depth detecting flow coming towards the probe (see Table 3.11 on the companion website).

Hemodynamic effects of significant carotid obstructive disease can be identified with TCD.

- TCD examination usually remains normal until carotid artery stenosis exceeds 80%, at which point intracranial hemodynamic effects may be realized. These can result in TCD spectral waveform changes as well as specific changes in flow patterns from collateral flow effects. Ipsilateral spectral waveform changes include slowed systolic acceleration, dampened waveform, and lowered flow velocity (see Figure 3.46 on the companion website). If collateral flow occurs via the anterior communicating artery, there will be an increase in flow velocity of the contralateral anterior cerebral artery (ACA) and reversal of flow direction of the ipsilateral ACA. Reversal of flow in the ophthalmic artery occurs if there is collateral flow supplied by the ECA. Collateral flow from the posterior circulation via the posterior communicating artery will result in increased flow velocity in the posterior cerebral arteries (PCAs) and basilar artery. The presence of any of these changes on TCD is highly suggestive of significant proximal extracranial carotid artery occlusive disease (see Table 3.12 on the companion website).
- Intracranial artery stenosis and vasospasm result in increased flow velocity, which can be most reliably diagnosed in the MCAs because of their parallel position to the TCD probe. Significant vessel narrowing can be diagnosed when mean flow velocities are over 120 cm/s, with velocities over 200 cm/s indicating severe vessel stenosis (see Figure 3.47 on the companion website).
- TCD can safely be used to monitor intracranial velocities on a daily basis following subarachnoid hemorrhage (SAH) to assess for development of vasospasm, usually after day 3 of SAH in a significant number of cases.
- TCD can also be used for micro-emboli detection. Emboli cause high-intensity transient signals (HITS), which can be heard as chirps in the velocity spectra (see Figure 3.48 on the companion website).
- Typical patterns of brain death occur on TCD following cessation of intracranial blood flow. These include sharp systolic peaks with absent diastolic flow, and reverberating flow with a "to and fro" pattern (see Figure 3.49 on the companion website).

TCD has been demonstrated to be highly specific and sensitive in diagnosing cerebral circulatory arrest and can be used as a confirmatory test in brain death protocols.

Conclusions

- A variety of neurodiagnostic studies can be used to evaluate patients with neurologic disorders.
- A basic understanding of these tests can help the neurologist come to an accurate diagnosis, and aid in proper workup and treatment for the patient.

Reading list

Key references and reading sources for this chapter can be found online at www.mountsinaiexpertguides.com

---

Additional material for this chapter can be found online at:
www.mountsinaiexpertguides.com

This includes Figures 3.1, 3.5–3.12, 3.15, 3.16, 3.18, 3.20–3.24, 3.26–3.28, and 3.31–3.49; Tables 3.3, 3.5–3.8, 3.11, and 3.12; and a reading list.

PART 2

DIAGNOSIS OF PATIENTS WITH NEUROLOGIC SYMPTOMS

CHAPTER 4

Delirium and Coma

Stephen Krieger
Icahn School of Medicine at Mount Sinai, New York, NY, USA

Background

Delirium, also commonly referred to as encephalopathy or, more broadly, as a form of "altered mental status," is an acute alteration in a patient's level of consciousness, arousal, and alertness, typically manifesting with confusion and disorientation. Coma is a state of profound impairment in the level of arousal characterized by complete unresponsiveness. Delirium and coma are presentations with diverse etiologies and degrees of severity, resulting from dysfunction of both cerebral hemispheres or of the ascending reticular activating system (RAS).

Impact

The prevalence and incidence of delirium and coma are difficult to estimate given their broad range of causes. Delirium is common: a UK study found the prevalence of delirium at hospital admission ranged from 10 to 31%, and incidence of new delirium ranged from 3 to 29%. Delirium was associated with increased mortality at discharge and at 12 months, and increased length of hospital stay (LOS). Another UK-based study found a point prevalence of delirium of about 20% of general hospital inpatients, particularly in those with prior cognitive impairment. Most data on coma incidence stem from traumatic brain injury (TBI) estimates: according to the Centers for Disease Control (CDC), every year at least 1.7 million TBIs occur either as an isolated injury or along with other injuries. The Multi-Society Task Force on persistent vegetative state (PVS) estimates that in the USA there are between 10,000 and 25,000 (i.e. 4–10/100,000 population) in PVS.

Approach to diagnosis
Getting your bearings

Patients presenting with delirium or coma pose a range of diagnostic challenges and require urgent assessment and efficient workup to identify life-threatening causes. The character of the impairment in consciousness should be clearly elucidated, and assessing severity and time course is crucial in planning and expediting the workup and management.

- Both delirium and coma can herald a life-threatening clinical disorder and should be addressed emergently.
- It is important to begin by considering whether delirium or coma is referable either to a medical illness such as a metabolic derangement, systemic infection, drug intoxication, or withdrawal, or is a direct result of an intracranial process.
- If an intracranial localization is suspected, one must consider if this is a supratentorial process affecting both cerebral hemispheres, or a focal process in the brainstem affecting the RAS.

- Delirium and coma may be the manifestations of an acute central nervous system (CNS) infection, and this possibility should be promptly and thoroughly pursued.
- Delirium is acute and should be contrasted with dementia, which is a chronic encephalopathy. The two often coexist.

Key elements of history

Delirium or coma preclude obtaining an accurate history directly from the patient. Patients are rarely the source of key information. Collateral information from family, caregivers, or other medical professionals is crucial to elucidate the time course and predisposing factors.

- The time course is of particular importance: did the confusion or unresponsiveness begin suddenly or insidiously? What is the duration of the symptoms at the point of your clinical encounter? Do the symptoms wax and wane?
- Is there a history of a medical condition that could predispose a patient to a metabolic cause, including liver disease, renal disease, or diabetes?
- Is there a concomitant history of fever or other signs of infection? Is there a history of an immune compromised state (HIV infection or risk factors, chemotherapy) that could predispose a patient to a systemic or CNS infection?
- Is there a history of drug or alcohol use?
- If there is a history of psychiatric illness, one should consider a medication overdose or even a non-physiologic disorder of consciousness.

CLINICAL PEARLS
- A history of pre-existing medical illness and medication/drug/substance exposure or withdrawal is an etiologic clue to the broad category of "toxic/metabolic" causes of delirium or coma. Though not focal intracranial processes, these etiologies are potentially life-threatening and should be pursued by carefully taking into account all organ systems.
- A supra- or infra-tentorial lesion that causes coma is always a life-threatening emergency, and a history suggestive of head trauma, intraparenchymal hemorrhage or infection should prompt an expedited workup to identify and manage an intracranial process.

Key elements of physical examination

- Always begin by assessing and addressing airway, breathing, circulation, and vital signs.
- Look for findings on general examination that may provide a clue to an underlying systemic disease: stigmata of hepatic failure, alcohol or drug use, high blood pressure, HIV.
- A careful mental status examination is crucial. Levels of consciousness range from alert, in which the patient maintains open eyes and responds to verbal stimulation, to coma, where the patient remains completely unresponsive and cannot be aroused even with vigorous stimulation. Evaluate and document descriptively the level of alertness and arousal, attention, orientation, language function, short- and long-term memory, emotional lability, as well as the rationality and content of thought.
- Try to localize the site of the lesion causing impaired consciousness as either a diffuse process or a focal intracranial process. Cranial nerve examination includes assessment of the pupils and their response to light, oculocephalic reflex, response to caloric stimulation, breathing pattern, and corneal, cough, and gag reflexes. Motor examination, reflexes, and sensory examination should be performed as the patient's mental status permits, often by provoking reactions to noxious stimuli.

Table of elements of history and diseases

Disease category	Symptoms	Duration	Other key features
Metabolic causes of delirium and coma			
Includes hypo- and hyperglycemia, hepatic encephalopathy, uremia, and other perturbations in sodium, calcium, thiamine, and other electrolytes	• Impaired arousal, inattention, and confusion, commonly in hospital or critical care settings • Waxing and waning course with periods of lucidity alternating with confusion. May be agitated or combative • Asterixis or myoclonus • Decline into poor responsiveness or coma may indicate cerebral edema, as in severe hepatic encephalopathy	Acute to subacute	History of underlying dementia may predispose patient to metabolically caused delirium (see also Chapters 6 and 7). Seek prior history of metabolic disturbance causing alteration in mental status. History of diabetes and treatment thereof, liver disease (including infectious and non-infectious hepatitis, alcohol abuse), renal disease or dialysis, diuretic use, hepatotoxic or nephrotoxic medications, malnutrition, vitamin deficiency, dehydration
Toxic and withdrawal causes of delirium and coma			
Sedatives including benzodiazepines, opiates, anticonvulsants, antipsychotics, medications with antihistaminergic or anticholinergic properties, alcohol intoxication and withdrawal, and illicit substances including opiate narcotics, marijuana, cocaine, LSD, PCP, ecstasy, ketamine, and many others	Symptoms vary by specific toxic cause but may include: • Inattention, confusion, confabulation, agitation, combativeness, tremor, tremulousness • Itching/formication • Autonomic dysfunction with nausea, sweating, tachycardia, and labile blood pressure	Intoxication typically acute; withdrawal may be subacute and delayed in onset	Medication history is crucial; for the hospitalized patient, review the "medications administered" list. Known history of alcohol use or abuse including type, quantity, frequency of consumption and time since last ingestion; history of drug- or alcohol-related withdrawal or seizure or other complications. History from family members and care providers is essential. If in-hospital intoxication is suspected, review visitor logs and off-floor passes granted

(Continued)

Disease category	Symptoms	Duration	Other key features
Systemic and CNS infections causing delirium and coma			
Includes urinary tract infection (UTI), pneumonia, bacteremia or sepsis; may precede the definitive identification of the source of infection CNS infections including meningitis, encephalitis (such as caused by HSV), brain abscess, or multi-focal or diffuse CNS infections such as neurosyphilis, toxoplasmosis or progressive multifocal leukoencephalopathy (PML).	• Alteration in consciousness, confusion, or lethargy in setting of fever, tachycardia • Meningeal symptoms (including photophobia, phonophobia, nausea/vomiting), or skin rash should prompt immediate concern for CNS infection (i.e. meningococcal meningitis) • Delirium or coma with focal neurologic deficits (aphasia, weakness, loss of sensation, ataxia) may be due to CNS abscess or infectious mass lesion	Acute to subacute. CNS infection may clinically evolve rapidly and decline into coma	History of underlying dementia (see also Chapters 6 and 7) may predispose patient to delirium in setting of a systemic infection, and in such cases disorientation may be the first sign of systemic infection. History of immune-compromised state (HIV, chemotherapy, malignancy, diabetes). Seek out risk factors for bacteremia/sepsis such as intravenous drug use. Geographic location and seasonal variation in infections such as viral encephalitis should be considered. Pursue history of sick contacts, infectious exposures or local outbreaks of meningitis or encephalitis (nursing homes, college dorms, homeless shelters) (see also Chapter 24)
Hypoxic-ischemic encephalopathy			
Cardiac arrest causing failure of brain perfusion; occasionally a patient may be "found down" in coma and the inciting circulatory event is unknown	• A broad range of impairments of consciousness from mild cognitive deficits to persistent vegetative state or coma as a patient evolves from a catastrophic circulatory event • Coma caused by ischemic damage to bilateral cerebral hemispheres and/or the brainstem RAS • Multifocal myoclonus and seizure activity may be present	Acute onset; may decline further after initial insult as cerebral edema and herniation develop. High mortality rate. May have gradual though variable recovery – often a static encephalopathy results	History of catastrophic circulatory event such as cardiac arrest. Cardiac risk factors including arrhythmia, hypertension, congestive heart failure, cardiac output obstruction. Increasing duration of hypoxic or anoxic brain injury may predict poor outcome

Supratentorial lesions causing coma

Intraparenchymal: Cerebral hemorrhage, large territory infarct, tumor, or abscess with related edema Extraparenchymal: Subdural hematoma, epidural hematoma	• Supratentorial lesions causing impairment of consciousness or coma must impair both cerebral hemispheres or indirectly damage the brainstem RAS • A single lesion may cause mass effect on the ventricular system or contralateral hemisphere • Extraparenchymal lesions can cause bi-hemispheric dysfunction by causing uncal or tonsillar herniation • Supratentorial lesions or hemorrhage may obstruct flow of CSF through the aqueduct or fourth ventricle, causing hydrocephalus and raised intracranial pressure yielding coma	Varies by specific etiology – tumor or mass lesion may cause a subacute decline in mental status due to slowly enlarging mass effect; stroke or hemorrhage are acute in onset and may evolve over hours to days. Patients may abruptly slide into coma as intracranial pressure rises if herniation occurs	History of systemic malignancy with potential for brain metastasis (most common primaries are lung, breast, genitourinary, osteosarcoma, melanoma), or history of primary CNS malignancy. History of trauma may be a clue to subdural hematoma; history of alcohol abuse and resultant blackouts may suggest occult head trauma. Hypertension, amyloid angiopathy, or cocaine use are risk factors for cerebral hemorrhage (see also Chapter 20). Fever, focal neurologic deficits, and history or risk factors for bacteremia may indicate brain abscess. Headache, nausea, and vomiting may herald raised intracranial pressure. History of seizures, particularly focal seizures, suggests a supratentorial localization – consider a post-ictal state (see Chapters 5 and 30)

Infratentorial lesions causing coma

Intraparenchymal hemorrhage, ischemic stroke, tumors or infection in the brainstem	• Coma may be caused by lesions directly impairing the brainstem RAS from the medulla through the thalamus • Infratentorial lesions need not be large to cause clinically devastating impairment in consciousness • Cranial nerve involvement (diplopia, dysarthria, dysphagia) and focal neurologic deficits such as a weakness or ataxia	Typically acute in onset, may evolve to deep coma with progressive loss of cranial nerve functions over hours to days	Etiologic features similar to supratentorial lesions, above. History of diplopia, dysarthria, dysphagia, ataxia before clinical decline into coma suggests brainstem localization (see also Chapter 28)

Table of elements of physical examination by disease

Metabolic causes of delirium and coma	Metabolic derangements typically cause delirium or changes in level of consciousness without other focal neurologic signs. Depending on the severity of the metabolic abnormality this can range from mild clouding of consciousness to coma. Note that multiple mild abnormalities can have a cumulative effect and lead to severe encephalopathy
	Patients may have a suppressed level of alertness and arousal, be disoriented, inattentive, and have limited content of thought. Short-term recall is impaired
	• Asterixis and multifocal myoclonus may be present, notably in hepatic encephalopathy
	• Pupillary responses and oculocephalic reflexes should be normal, which is a clue that a focal intracranial process or herniation is not occurring
	• Confusion associated with ophthalmoplegia and ataxia is suggestive of Wernicke's encephalopathy
	• Delayed deep tendon reflex relaxation is the hallmark of hypothyroidism with myxedema coma
	• The general examination may show other evidence supporting specific metabolic causes, e.g. stigmata of hepatic disease (see also Chapters 21 and 36)
Toxic and withdrawal causes of delirium and coma	Symptoms vary by specific toxic cause, but may include inattention, confusion, confabulation, agitation, combativeness, tremor, and tremulousness. Short-term recall is impaired. Pupils may be dilated although the neurological exam is otherwise non-focal
	• Patients in withdrawal from sedating medications or alcohol may have repetitive behaviors, itching/formication, visual (though rarely auditory) hallucinations, and autonomic dysfunction with nausea, sweating, tachycardia, and labile blood pressure
	• In suspected alcohol withdrawal, tremulousness and hallucinations followed by seizures occur within 1–2 days, with delirium tremens manifesting in the subsequent 3–5 days
	• In suspected benzodiazepine overdose, confusion or coma occurs with respiratory suppression, though pupils remain reactive
	• In suspected opioid overdose, coma and respiratory suppression may be accompanied by pinpoint, though weakly reactive, pupils
Systemic and CNS infections causing delirium and coma	Fever, chills, sweats, tachycardia and other manifestations of infection may be present
	Patients with systemic infection causing delirium may exhibit either hyper- or hypoactivity, usually accompanied by inattention, confusion, slow mentation, or cognitive deficits beyond any baseline impairments
	Patients with CNS infections such as meningitis and encephalitis may have alteration in consciousness, confusion, or lethargy in a setting of fever, tachycardia, and meningeal signs (including nuchal rigidity, reflexive thigh flexion upon neck flexion, photophobia, phonophobia, nausea/vomiting). Focal neurologic deficits in this setting (aphasia, weakness, loss of sensation, ataxia) may be due to CNS abscess or infectious mass lesion. Seizures may occur (see also Chapter 24)

Hypoxic-ischemic encephalopathy	Impairments of consciousness ranging from cognitive deficits to deep coma. In cases of bi-hemispheric anoxic injury, there may be no response to vigorous or noxious stimulation, such as nail bed pressure or sternal rub Posturing may occur in response to stimulation: decorticate (flexion of arm, wrist, fingers and extension and plantar flexion in leg) or decerebrate (arms and legs stiffly extended) based on extent of brain injury Cranial nerve dysfunction is referable to the degree of brainstem compromise Prognosis in anoxic coma is poor: no purposeful motor responses at day 1 yields 90% vegetative or severely disabled outcome; this approaches 100% by day 3
Supratentorial lesions causing coma	• Focal neurologic signs such as hemiparesis, hemiplegia, hemineglect, reflex asymmetry with unilateral or bilateral Babinski signs (extensor plantar responses) may be present • Careful observation for signs of raised intracranial pressure (including funduscopic examination for papilledema or hemorrhages), emergent third nerve palsy ("blown pupil", eye deviated down-and-out) are harbingers of herniation • Evidence of head trauma (including raccoon eyes and Battle's sign) may indicate traumatic intracranial hemorrhage including subdural or epidural hematoma
Infratentorial lesions causing coma	Infratentorial (cerebellum, brainstem) lesions are often heralded by other brainstem signs, including cranial nerve deficits (disconjugate gaze and diplopia, facial weakness, tongue deviation, loss of gag reflex), and loss of oculocephalic/cold caloric reflexes • Pupillary responses have localizing value: unilateral dilated (third nerve palsy/herniation); bilateral dilated or poorly responsive (midbrain); pinpoint (pontine) • Note characteristic respiratory patterns of brainstem compromise, including Cheyne–Stokes respiration, central hyperventilation, and ataxic breathing (often a pre-terminal event) (see also Chapter 28) It is important to distinguish coma due to brainstem compromise from the locked-in syndrome, wherein the patient remains fully conscious and sentient, but all motor pathways to the facial musculature and body have been transected. In such a case the patient may be able to blink to command and move the eyes in the vertical direction (due to intact midbrain structures). All patients in coma should be assessed for these retained abilities • No locked-in patient should ever be mistaken for being in coma

CLINICAL PEARLS
• Metabolic causes of delirium and coma are distinguished by a general lack of focal neurologic deficits, intact brainstem and cranial nerve functions, and normal pupillary responses.
• Focal lesions, both supra- and infratentorial, are typically accompanied by focal neurologic signs including hemiparesis, and cranial nerve and pupillary function abnormalities.
• Signs of herniation include an emerging third-nerve palsy ("blown pupil" and down-and-out eye deviation) and should prompt emergent neurosurgical consultation and neuroimaging.
• Test all coma patients for being "locked-in." The difference can be subtle and the implications are enormous.

Diagnostic tests

Metabolic causes of delirium and coma	• Labs: complete blood count (CBC) with differential, basic metabolic profile including glucose, electrolytes, calcium, magnesium, phosphate levels; renal function/blood urea nitrogen (BUN); hepatic function tests including ammonia; arterial blood gases (ABG); thyroid panel, B12, folate, methylmalonic acid, homocysteine • Consider EEG to evaluate for signs of metabolic encephalopathy and non-convulsive seizures • Consider neuroimaging (CT, MRI if source not identified) (see also Chapters 21 and 36)
Toxic and withdrawal causes of delirium and coma	• Labs: blood ethanol level, serum osmolality, urine and serum toxicology, medication overdose panel, therapeutic drug levels (such as anticonvulsants) • Consider diagnostic naloxone or flumazenil administration • Consider CT if concern for concomitant head trauma
Systemic and CNS infections causing delirium and coma	• Labs: CBC with differential, urinalysis and culture/sensitivity, blood cultures, rapid plasma reagin (RPR), HIV • Imaging: CXR, CT head, consider MRI if concern for meningoencephalitis or brain abscess (see also Chapter 24) • Low threshold to perform lumbar puncture (LP) for CSF opening pressure and studies including cell count/differential, protein, glucose, Gram stain, herpes simplex virus polymerase chain reaction (HSV PCR), venereal disease research laboratory (VDRL) test, bacterial antigens, fungal stains/culture, tuberculosis (TB) stains/culture, consider other viral PCRs as indicated
Hypoxic-ischemic encephalopathy	• CT head may help with diagnosis and can reveal extent of cerebral anoxic injury if performed >24 hours after cardiac event • EEG to evaluate brain activity and look for superimposed epileptiform activity
Supratentorial lesions causing coma	• Neuroimaging with CT or MRI to evaluate location/extent/likely etiology of lesion(s). Consider CT or MR angiogram or conventional angiogram to evaluate for source of a hemorrhage • LP for CSF cell count, xanthochromia, and other studies as above • EEG to look for superimposed epileptiform activity and evaluate for non-convulsive status epilepticus
Infratentorial lesions causing coma	• Neuroimaging with CT or MRI to evaluate location/extent/likely etiology of lesion(s)

Recommended diagnostic strategy (Algorithm 4.1)

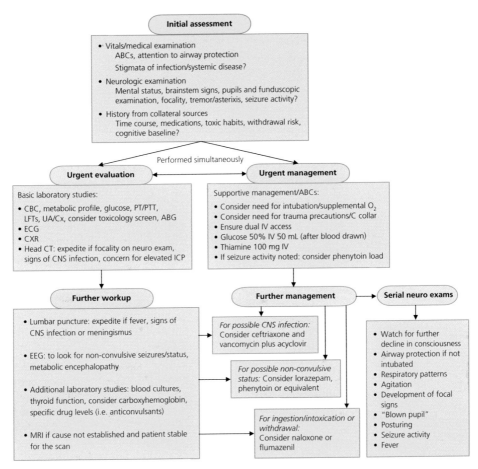

Algorithm 4.1 Differential diagnosis.

BOTTOM LINE
- Delirium and coma both reflect potentially life-threatening situations and should be assessed and managed emergently.
- ABCs are essential, as patients progressing towards coma may need ventilatory support.
- An assessment of likely systemic etiologies (metabolic derangement, toxicity or withdrawal, systemic infection causing delirium) should be made concomitantly with a neurologic examination for focal causes along with obtaining relevant neuroimaging.
- Critical diagnostic possibilities should be considered first, such as: profound hypo- or hyperglycemia or other perilous but correctable metabolic derangements; cerebral hemorrhage or imminent herniation warranting neurosurgical intervention; meningitis or encephalitis warranting urgent antibiotics/antivirals; alcohol withdrawal warranting prompt administration of appropriate benzodiazepines.

Reading list

Key reading sources for this chapter can be found online at www.mountsinaiexpertguides.com

Additional material for this chapter can be found online at:
www.mountsinaiexpertguides.com

This includes a case study, multiple choice questions,
and a reading list.

CHAPTER 5

Episodic Collapse, Loss of Consciousness, Seizures

Lara V. Marcuse and Madeline C. Fields
Icahn School of Medicine at Mount Sinai, New York, NY, USA

Background

In Greek, the literal meaning of syncope is a cutting off. Medically the term syncope refers to loss of consciousness and postural tone resulting from a decrease or cessation of cerebral blood flow. Pre-syncope refers to the symptoms (lightheadedness, visual dimming, giddiness) occurring with decreased cerebral blood which may or may not progress to syncope. As such, syncope and pre-syncope represent an extremely common symptom. Who among us has not experienced a faint, or at least a moment of lightheadedness when standing?

The diagnostic challenge is that cardiac arrhythmias, autonomic insufficiency, as well as neurogenic dysfunction can all result in syncope. Furthermore, while not actually syncope, seizures, vertigo, drop attacks, cataplexy, and transient ischemic attacks can have symptoms that mimic syncope.

This chapter suggests an orderly approach to the workup of possible syncope.

Impact

It is not possible to make an estimate about incidence, economic impact and social impact of this presenting complaint because of the large number of diseases that can have this complaint during their initial presentation.

Approach to diagnosis
Getting your bearings

- The cornerstone of decision-making for the patient with possible syncope is a careful history and physical. This will guide the selection of tests.
- Each individual does not need all tests!
- A history and physical examination may be all that is needed to make the diagnosis.

Key elements of history

Obtain a detailed history from the patient and from an observer (if possible) about the event.

- Does the patient experience a warning or aura prior to the event? If yes, understanding the details of the aura is extremely important. An aura of déjà vu is most consistent with a seizure whereas an aura of lightheadedness is most consistent with neurocardiogenic syncope.
- What triggers the event? Does the event only occur with standing (orthostatic syncope), micturition, or exercise? Can a rapid movement of the head trigger the event (suggestive for benign paroxysmal positional vertigo)? Can heightened emotion trigger the event (syncope, cataplexy)?

Mount Sinai Expert Guides: Neurology, First Edition. Edited by Stuart C. Sealfon, Rajeev Motiwala, and Charles B. Stacy.
© 2016 John Wiley & Sons, Ltd. Published 2016 by John Wiley & Sons, Ltd.
Companion website: www.mountsinaiexpertguides.com

- Is there loss of consciousness (LOC) with the event?
- If there is LOC, is the person confused afterwards? Post-event confusion is more consistent with seizures than with syncope.
- During the event, do witnesses see jerking, foaming at the mouth, or hear a loud cry?
- What other symptoms are associated with the event? Is there confusion, visual loss, headache, panic, vertigo, diplopia, tinnitus, hearing loss?
- Determine prior medical history including seizure risk factors, cardiac history, and stroke risk factors.

Table of elements of history and diseases

	Symptoms	Other key features
Syncope		
Neurocardiogenic (vasovagal)	Often with a prodrome of lightheadedness, sweating, and palpitations. Brief or no confusion after consciousness is regained	Can be triggered by: • Emotion/panic/pain (e.g. the sight of a needle) • Micturition, cough, defecation, exercise • Prolonged standing
Postural orthostatic tachycardia syndrome (POTS)	Lightheadedness, dimming of vision, confusion, and anxiety. Usually no LOC	Symptoms occur upon standing and are relieved upon sitting or lying down
Orthostatic hypotension	LOC occurs with the transition from lying down to sitting or standing	Dehydration- or medication-induced hypovolemia Autonomic dysfunction associated with: • Diabetes • Multiple system atrophy • Parkinson's disease • Neuropathy
Cardiac arrhythmia or disease causing syncope	LOC often without a prodrome	Can have prolonged QT syndrome, congestive heart failure, coronary artery disease, valvular disease, cardiomyopathies. Can have family history of cardiomyopathy or sudden cardiac death
"Convulsive" syncope	Loss of consciousness with a fall followed by a series of body jerks. The initial collapse is with low body tone and not with tonic extension	Syncope of any etiology can result in a few body jerks, particularly if the event is somewhat prolonged. Prolonged hypotension may trigger a true seizure. However, convulsive syncope does not require antiepileptic drugs
Seizures		
Seizure with generalized onset • Generalized tonic clonic • Tonic seizures • Atonic seizures • Myoclonic astatic	LOC triggered by seizure. Can be associated with urinary incontinence and tongue biting. Witnesses may see shaking. There is confusion after the event. Seizures are not positional and may have onset in all positions	There is usually no aura or warning. Interictal EEG may show generalized epileptiform abnormalities

	Symptoms	Other key features
Seizure with partial onset that has secondary generalization	LOC triggered by seizure. Can be associated with urinary incontinence and tongue biting. Witnesses may see shaking. There is confusion after the event	Aura depends on the location of the seizure onset zone. Common auras are deja vu, fear, or visual hallucinations Interictal EEG may show focal epileptiform abnormalities as well as focal slowing
Benign occipital epilepsy	Presents in childhood. Seizures can have autonomic phenomena including asystole causing syncope	EEG will show occipital and generalized spikes interictally
Vertigo		
Benign positional paroxysmal vertigo (peripheral)	Can cause sudden vertigo, causing falls without LOC. Vertigo triggered by head position changes. Vertigo lasts for seconds to minutes	Caused by calcium carbonate crystals in the semicircular canals. Vertigo can be elicited with the Dix–Hallpike maneuver
Ménière's disease (peripheral)	Vertigo can cause falls without LOC. Vertigo lasts for minutes to hours. Nausea and motion sickness are frequently present	Associated with low-frequency progressive hearing loss and tinnitus
Vestibular neuronitis (peripheral)	Vertigo lasts for days with nausea. Patient often feels unwell with difficulty functioning	Often follows a viral illness
Central vertigo	• Sudden onset is suspicious for vascular event • Insidious onset of persistent vertigo is suspicious for a lesion like a cavernoma or a tumor • Migraines can cause an episodic vertigo with or without other symptoms of migraine	Central vertigo due to a lesion is usually milder than peripheral vertigo. Other symptoms or signs may be present with any central vertigo. In the history, assess for double vision, tinnitus, sensory disturbances, motor weakness, or difficulty swallowing. Strokes, TIAs, migraines, vascular malformations, tumors, and multiple sclerosis can all cause central vertigo
Cataplexy/narcolepsy		
	Cataplexy refers to the sudden loss of muscle tone with laughter, terror, or happiness. Usually occurs in individuals with narcolepsy Narcolepsy is uncontrolled sudden onset of REM sleep	Often associated with episodes of sleep paralysis, hypnagogic hallucinations, and excessive daytime sleepiness
Drop attacks		
	Fall without warning and *without* LOC	Etiology is often unclear • Usually elderly • Fall is usually forward • Sometimes associated with brainstem ischemia

(Continued)

	Symptoms	Other key features
Vascular		
Subclavian steal	LOC preceded by exercise of the arm	Rare, unequal pulses, other brainstem symptoms
Vertebrobasilar insufficiency	LOC often with associated diplopia, tinnitus, motor weakness, and/or sensory abnormalities	This tends to occur in older individuals with risk factors for strokes

CLINICAL PEARLS
- Neurocardiogenic syncope, orthostatic hypotension, and POTS: There may be prodrome of diaphoresis and lightheadedness relieved with sitting down.
- Orthostatic hypotension: Symptoms of bradykinesis, resting tremor, and rigidity (Parkinsonism) should be assessed.
- Cardiac syncope: A family and personal history of cardiac disease is important.
- Seizures or epilepsy: Assess for risk factors like traumatic brain injury, brain lesions and prematurity. Post-ictal confusion is expected.
- Cataplexy: Assess for other elements of narcolepsy including sudden onset of sleep, sleep paralysis, and hypnagogic hallucinations.
- Vertigo: Symptom should be true vertigo (spinning, imbalance) as opposed to lightheadedness. Episodic intense vertigo is more consistent with a peripheral lesion. A low-grade sensation of vertigo is worrisome for a central cause.
- Vascular: Determine if there is diplopia, tinnitus, sensory disturbance or motor weakness. Do the symptoms occur when the patient exercises an arm or when the neck is extended?

Key elements of physical examination
- Blood pressure examination
- Cardiac examination
- Vascular examination: palpation and auscultation
- Neurologic examination

Table of elements of physical examination by disease

Syncope	• Check blood pressure and heart rate in the supine, sitting, and standing positions • Careful sensory exam as autonomic insufficiency may occur in the setting of a peripheral neuropathy • Cardiovascular examination. Check for symmetry of peripheral pulses. Is there a cardiac murmur? Examine for rales or lower extremity edema suggestive of congestive heart failure • Neuropathy. Orthostasis may result from pure autonomic neuropathy or a peripheral neuropathy may coexist with this
Seizures	• Focal neurologic deficits • Signs of ongoing seizures such as myoclonus
Cataplexy/ narcolepsy	• Physical examination in patients with cataplexy and/or narcolepsy is generally normal. Those with sleep apnea and severe daytime sleepiness may have obesity or heart failure

Vertigo	• Nystagmus • Hearing acuity • Cerebellar signs • Dix–Hallpike maneuver • Head thrust
Drop attacks	• Examination primarily to exclude other causes of falls without LOC like motor weakness, neuropathy, or ataxia
Vascular	• Pulse and blood pressure in both arms – asymmetric radial pulse and asymmetric blood pressures suggest vascular occlusive disease including subclavian steal syndrome • Carotid bruits • Any focal cerebral deficit

CLINICAL PEARLS
- Orthostatic hypotension: Decrease in 20 mmHg in systolic BP or 10 mmHg in diastolic within 3 minutes of active or passive standing up.
- POTS: Defined as the development of orthostatic symptoms with a heart-rate increment of 30 or more, usually to 120 or more without orthostatic hypotension.
- BPPV: Torsional nystagmus and symptoms of vertigo elicited after a brief latent period with the Dix–Hallpike maneuver.

Diagnostic tests

Tests should be targeted based on the presenting problem, the history, and the physical examination. For example, a young adult who routinely feels faint with phlebotomy may require no further testing if physical examination is normal.

Syncope	EKG, tilt table test, autonomic testing, ECHO, and Holter monitoring. Continuous loop event recording with an implantable device can monitor the heart for several months if an arrhythmia is suspected but not detected on routine tests
Seizures	EEG, long-term monitoring may be necessary
Cataplexy/narcolepsy	Polysomnography. Test may show REM at onset of sleep
Vertigo	ENG, MRI brain with and without contrast to look for cerebellar and brainstem causes (central) and acoustic neuromas, vascular loops, meningiomas, epidermoid tumors, and cholesteatomas (peripheral). Audiology for hearing acuity
Drop attacks	Diagnose by history and physical examination, tests to exclude other causes
Vascular	MRI brain, transcranial/carotid Dopplers, MRA of neck and brain

Table of frequency of each disease

Syncope	Neurocardiogenic syncope: Mean prevalence of 22% in the general population POTS: estimated to be at least 170/100,000
Seizures	10% of population will have a single seizure 1–2% will have epilepsy

(Continued)

Cataplexy/ narcolepsy	Narcolepsy: 1:2000 Cataplexy: uncertain. Majority of individuals with cataplexy have narcolepsy
Vertigo	Vertigo (all types): 40% of individuals by the age of 40 will have vertigo
Drop attacks	Incidence of drop attacks is not clear
Vascular	Posterior circulation strokes: about 20% of all strokes are posterior circulation strokes. Numbers for stroke vary, but about 2–3% of the population will be diagnosed with stroke Subclavian steal syndrome: unknown

Recommended diagnostic strategy

BOTTOM LINE
- Episodic collapse, loss of consciousness, and seizures represent common presenting complaints.
- The cornerstone of diagnosis is a careful history and physical examination. Bedside testing can aid in the diagnoses.
- Appropriate ancillary tests such as EKG, ECHO, Holter monitoring, EEG, polysomnogram, ENG, and MRI are also of significant diagnostic value.

Reading list

Key reading sources for this chapter can be found online at www.mountsinaiexpertguides.com

Additional material for this chapter can be found online at:
www.mountsinaiexpertguides.com

This includes a case study, multiple choice questions, and a reading list.

CHAPTER 6

Dysphasias, Dyspraxias, and Dysexecutive Syndromes: The Non-Memory Cognitive Impairments

Martin Goldstein
Icahn School of Medicine at Mount Sinai, New York, NY, USA

Background
Definition
While memory impairment is the most common complaint for which patients with cognitive symptoms present to physicians, non-memory disorders are also an important category of acquired cognitive dysfunction. Non-memory cognitive disorders can be subdivided into specific syndromes, inventoried in Table 6.1. The most important categories are defined below.

- *Dysphasia* or *aphasia* refers to acquired impairments of expressive or receptive language function. Dysphasia is used for language impairment; aphasia for more complete disruption of language production or understanding.
- *Dyspraxia* or *apraxia* refers to an acquired inability to execute a learned purposeful motor action despite having the motivation and elementary motor ability to perform the task.
- *Agnosia* refers to an acquired impairment of meaningful recognition of intact perception of sensory stimuli.

Impact
- The National Institute of Neurological Disorders and Stroke (NINDS) estimates that at least 1 million people in the USA suffer from aphasia.
- At least 15% of individuals under the age of 65 develop aphasia, with stroke being the most common cause.
- Over 40% of individuals 85 years of age and older develop some form of dysphasia.
- Non-amnestic mild cognitive impairment (MCI) subtypes combined incidence rates average approximately 30 per 1000 person-years.
- Prevalence of non-amnestic MCI ranges from approximately 4% in patients over 50, to over 20% among patients 65 and older.

Approach to diagnosis
- Because neurocognitive disorders are complex and often protean, it is important to describe simply and accurately the deficits observed without imposing diagnostic categories before attempting to formulate a unifying diagnosis.

Mount Sinai Expert Guides: Neurology, First Edition. Edited by Stuart C. Sealfon, Rajeev Motiwala, and Charles B. Stacy.
© 2016 John Wiley & Sons, Ltd. Published 2016 by John Wiley & Sons, Ltd.
Companion website: www.mountsinaiexpertguides.com

Table 6.1 Non-memory cognitive impairments.

Non-memory cognitive domain			Non-memory cognitive syndromes
Attention			Attentional deficit
Linguistic	Auditory		Dysphasias (see Tables 6.4 and 6.5)
	Written	Reading	Dyslexias
		Writing	Dysgraphias
Perceptual processing	Perceptual integration		Dysnavigation, neglect, extinction
	Associative identification		Agnosias
Praxis			Dyspraxias
Executive functions	Agency		Abulia
	Impulse control		Impulse dyscontrol disorders
	Comportmental regulation		Disinhibition
	Task management		Dysexecutive syndromes
	Insight		
	Judgment		
	Decision-making		
	Planning		

- Thorough history acquisition is essential for establishing non-memory cognitive impairment, and detailed multi-system review can narrow differential diagnosis by facilitating etiologic pattern recognition. Non-memory cognitive impairment can be an explicit complaint (i.e. when obvious to the patient, e.g. as in an expressive language disorder), a concern reported by informants but for which the patient is unaware (e.g. comportmental dysregulation in the context of behavioral variant fronto-temporal dementia, or FTD), or occult to patient and even family but incidentally detected on history-acquisition or examination (e.g. a more complex dyspraxia, like driving impairment). An intermediate permutation is when a neurobehavioral issue is identified but mischaracterized (e.g. the abulia or disinhibition of behavioral-variant FTD interpreted as depression or mania, respectively). The potentially nuanced, or even covert, nature of non-memory dysfunction underscores the need to be vigilant for such impairments, and the need to interview a reliable informant when feasible.
- Observe the patient's behavior and interactions in a non-directed manner and formulate hypotheses for more specific testing.
- Be systematic in determining the basis for any cognitive deficits in order to avoid falsely identifying a higher-order abnormality (such as dyspraxia) when the dysfunction is actually due to a lower-order defect (e.g. inattention or paresis). A complex function deficit can only be correctly attributed when the simpler functions on which it depends are intact.
- Be comprehensive: Disorders that produce non-memory cognitive dysfunction are often complexly layered neuropsychiatric spectrum processes – that is, they do not observe historical nosologic boundaries among cognitive, motor, and mood disorders. Consequently, comprehensive multi-neural system assessment is required to adequately capture data crucial for diagnostic precision.
- Adapt the method of cognitive examination and assessment to the setting. A variety of standardized assessment inventories exist to facilitate efficient screening; the most widely used are the Folstein Mini-Mental Status Examination (MMSE; Figure 6.1) and Montreal Cognitive Assessment (MoCA; Figure 6.2). Commercially available computerized neuropsychological screening instruments are available to extend the bedside or office evaluation.

- Consider formal neuropsychological testing: Cognitive metrics using standardized and normed protocols represent the gold standard for characterizing a current neurocognitive profile, thereby informing more precise diagnosis and establishing a quantitative baseline for tracking.

Key elements of history

- What is the age of onset? For example, while Alzheimer's disease is the most common cause of dementia for both younger and older patients, the epidemiology of other causes, like fronto-temporal dementia (FTD), varies significantly with age of onset.
- What has been the temporal course of non-memory cognitive impairment?
- Are there any associated comportmental symptoms? For example, behavioral disinhibition evident to others but not to the patient.
- Are there any reported associated motor or reflex changes? For example, tremors, unsteadiness, gait changes, muscle twitching.
- Is there any family history of cognitive impairment?

The elements of history acquisition important for detecting and characterizing non-memory cognitive impairments, and a neurocognitive review of systems, are outlined in Table 6.2.

Key elements of neurocognitive examination

- Neurobehavioral examination
  - Cognition:
    - language
    - memory (see Chapter 7)
    - perceptual processing
    - praxis
    - executive functions
  - Affective changes:
    - reactivity
    - stability
    - range
    - context-appropriateness
  - Comprehensive neurologic examination.

Aphasias

Table 6.3 provides an inventory of linguistic assessment procedures, and Table 6.4 catalogs dysphasia subtypes. While language is mediated by a complex neural network, the classic modular model of linguistic functional neuroanatomy (Figure 6.3) remains clinically powerful, enabling reasonable correlation of lesion localization with dysphasia subtype, as depicted in Figures 6.4–6.8. Neuropsychological testing should be performed for patients with subtle language deficits to precisely characterize and enable quantitative tracking.

Cognitive disorders can also impact non-verbal communication. These include emotional valence of spoken language and facial expression, comprising important expressive and receptive communicative elements that can become impaired in cognitive disorders.

It is important to distinguish speech disorders, as outlined in Table 6.5, representing dysfunctions of articulation and/or phonation, from linguistic disorders. Historical terms for "speech" abnormalities can be confusing since they sometimes actually involve problems with language rather than speech per se. For example, "telegraphic speech" describes the *linguistic* disturbance sometimes characterizing a Broca's dysphasia. "Scanning speech" refers to the *speech* disturbance associated with cerebellar dysfunction.

Table 6.2 Characterization of current non-memory cognitive dysfunction.

History of present non-memory cognitive dysfunction

Onset and duration	Acute	E.g. dysphasia associated with stroke
	Subacute	E.g. neglect associated with brain tumor
	Insidious	E.g. dyspraxia associated with neurodegenerative process
Course tempo	Static	E.g. executive dysfunction associated with trauma
	Progressive	E.g. executive deterioration associated with amyloid angiopathy
	Step-wise	E.g. agnosia associated with neurodegenerative process
	Continuous	

Neurocognitive review of systems

Neuropsychiatric changes	Affective changes	Reactivity (e.g. blunting)
		Stability (e.g. lability)
		Range (e.g. restriction)
		Context-appropriateness
	Personality changes	
	Impulsive behaviors	
	Compulsive behaviors (punding, gambling, etc.)	
	Food preference changes	
Neurovegetative functions	Sleeping pattern (e.g. sleep-wake cycle disturbances)	
	Daytime wakefulness	
	Appetite (e.g. increased, decreased, food preference changes)	
	Libido	
Elementary neurologic	Vestibular changes	
	Visual changes	
	Auditory changes	
	Olfactory changes (e.g. anosmia)	
	Taste changes (e.g. dysgeusia)	
	Motor changes (e.g. weakness, tremors, rigidity, dyskinesias)	
	Sensory changes (e.g. paresthesias)	
	Gait changes (e.g. tripping, falling)	
Bulbar function	Speech changes (e.g. hypophonia, dysarthria)	
	Swallowing (e.g. dysphagia)	
Neurocognitive risk factors	Headache history (e.g. migraine)	
	Head trauma history?	
	Seizure history?	

Dysautonomias

Current adaptation — Lightheadedness, syncope, etc.

Activities of daily living (ADLs)

Basic
- Feeding
- Bathing
- Toileting
- Dressing
- Hygiene/grooming

Instrumental
- Housekeeping, home safety
- Food preparation
- Health management, medication adherence
- Communication management
- Shopping
- Personal financial management
- Transportation management
- Micrographia, hypergraphia

Handwriting
Driving safety

Neurodevelopmental

Perinatal
Developmental milestones
Handedness

Cardiovascular — Cerebrovascular risk factors?
Endocrine — Endocrinopathies?
Respiratory — Sleep apnea?
Urologic — Urinary dyscontrol?
Gastrointestinal — Bowel irregularity/dyscontrol?
Cutaneous — Pigmentations?
Oncologic history — Cancer history?
Infectious history — Exposures?

Nutrition
Toxin exposure
- Alcohol
- Smoking
- Illicit drugs
- Industrial toxins, heavy metals

Table 6.3 Linguistic assessment.

Linguistic domains	Components		Examples
Fluency	Syntax Rate Phrase length Relational/functor word proficiency Effortfulness		Non-grammatical construction Slowed or pressured Restricted to simple brief constructions Impaired production of "No ifs, ands, or buts about it" Frustrated production (patient knows what he/she wants to say but cannot construct statement); classic for Broca's aphasia
	Generativity	Phonemic/letter	Generates <10 words beginning with the same letter in 60 seconds
		Categorical	Generates <15 words belonging to the same category in 60 seconds
Comprehension	1,2,3-step commands Relational commands		Impaired sequencing Preserved performance of commands using direct active commands but impaired performance of more complex/indirect commands (e.g. "with the pen, touch the light" vs "touch the light with the pen"; latter is more difficult)
Repetition	Simple/complex		"Today is a sunny day" vs "No ifs, ands, or buts about it"
Lexicon	Confrontation naming		Low-frequency item dysnomia (e.g. lapel, clasp)

Table 6.4 Aphasia subtypes.

		Linguistic feature		
		Fluency	Repetition	Comprehension
Dysphasias	Transcortical motor	Abnormal	✓	✓
	Broca	Abnormal	Abnormal	✓
	Conduction	✓	Abnormal	✓
	Wernicke	✓	Abnormal	Abnormal
	Transcortical sensory	✓	✓	Abnormal
	Global	Abnormal	Abnormal	Abnormal

Table 6.5 Speech features and associated impairments.

Component	Abnormality	Example of disease state
Rate	Pressured Tachyphemia Scanning	Mania Parkinson's disease Cerebellar pathology
Articulation	Dysarthria Stuttering	Bulbar pathology Congenital disturbance
Volume	Hypophonia	Parkinson's disease

Table 6.6 Apraxias.

Apraxia subtype	Definition	Examples of praxis assessment tasks
Bucco-oro-facial apraxia	Inability to perform facial movements on command	Whistle, lick lips, wink, cough
Limb-kinetic apraxia	Inability to make fine, precise movements with arm or leg	Manipulate coins, use scissors
Ideomotor apraxia	Inability to perform an action in response to verbal command	Show me how you use a toothbrush, hairbrush, turn a key
Ideational apraxia	Inability to perform sequenced activities	Dressing, eating, bathing
Ocular apraxia	Inability to direct gaze on command	Verbal saccadic command (look left, look right, etc.)
Constructional apraxia	Inability to copy, draw, or construct simple figures	Copy intersecting pentagons

Apraxias

Apraxia refers to an acquired inability to execute a learned purposeful motor action despite having the motivation, comprehension, and motor ability to perform the task. The functional neuroanatomy of praxis is schematically depicted in Figure 6.9. This includes the praxicon, a motor analog of the lexicon. Multiple apraxia subtypes emerge in a variety of cognitive disorders, summarized in Table 6.6.

Disorders of perceptual processing

Perceptual processing involves attentional, integrative, and associational processes applied to the percept generated in each sensory modality's primary cortex. In the case of vision, the functional neuroanatomy of initial post-percept processing is classically organized according to ventral and dorsal streams. The dorsal stream, composed of occipital-parietal association regions, subserves localization, or "where," function. The ventral stream, composed of occipital-temporal association regions, mediates identification, or "what," function. Visual integration of bilateral hemispace is a function of the non-dominant (so, most commonly right) parietal lobe. Figure 6.10 contextualizes levels of integrative visual perceptual deficit, including neglect and extinction.

Visual-spatial screening tests

Key visual-spatial integrative processing screening tasks include:
- left-right orientation
- line bisection
- geometric shape copying
- clock drawing.

Agnosias

Dysfunction of perceptual association processing gives rise to impaired percept recognition, known as agnosia. Tables 6.7 and 6.8 inventory visual and auditory agnosias, respectively. Table 6.9 summarizes disorders of self-awareness such as agnosias regarding body representation.

CLINICAL PEARLS
- Expressive dysphasias are typically accompanied by executive dysfunction.
- Patients are often unaware of dyspraxias and visual agnosias, which are more commonly reported by informants.
- Impaired insight typically accompanies fronto-temporal and parkinsonian degenerative cognitive syndromes.
- Isolated dysnomia suggests semantic dementia.
- Motor signs (e.g. parkinsonian, cerebellar, motor neuron, etc.) are key indicators for the differential diagnosis of cognitive syndromes.
- Mood dysregulation (mania, depression, pseudobulbar affect) commonly accompanies dysexecutive syndromes.
- Dysautonomia can be a key indicator of a parkinsonian neurodegenerative cognitive process.
- Although conventional division of cognitive disorders into cortical and subcortical categories oversimplifies pathogenesis, the relative cortical vs subcortical pattern of cognitive impairment can be extremely informative to differential diagnosis of acquired cognitive disorders (except when in advanced phases):
  - cortical: relatively specific (i.e. focal) cognitive deficits;
  - subcortical: more diffuse cognitive dysfunction, especially with bradyphrenia.

Table 6.7 Visual agnosias.

Type	Stimulus category	Subtype	Clinical distinction	Functional neuroanatomy
Visual object agnosia	Objects	Apperceptive	Cannot match/draw	Bilateral occipito-parietal
		Associative	Can match/draw	Bilateral occipito-temporal
Simultanagnosia	Multiple objects/object features	Dorsal/ apperceptive	Cannot perceive multiple objects simultaneously	Bilateral occipito-parietal
		Ventral/ associative	Cannot recognize multiple objects simultaneously	Dominant fusiform
Prosopagnosia	Faces	Apperceptive	Cannot match faces	Bilateral fusiform
		Associative	Can match faces	Bilateral anterior medial temporal
Color agnosia	Colors	Apperceptive	Cannot perform non-verbal color tasks	Visuo-linguistic disconnection (e.g. posterior corpus callosum)
		Associative	Can perform non-verbal color tasks	Dominant occipito-parietal
Capgras syndrome	Persons to whom patient is emotionally invested	Associative	Misidentification syndrome restricted to emotionally connected persons (e.g. family members)	Disconnection syndrome between limbic and facial recognition (fusiform face area) circuits

Table 6.8 Auditory agnosias.

Type	Stimulus category	Subtype	Clinical distinction	Functional neuroanatomy
Pure word deafness	Speech	Apperceptive/ pre-phonemic Associative/ phonemic	Cannot match phonemes Can match phonemes	Bilateral Heschl– Wernicke disconnection Peri-sylvian
Non-verbal sound agnosia	Non-verbal sounds	Apperceptive Associative	Cannot match sounds Can match sounds	Unclear Unclear
Sensory dysmusia	Musical sounds			Non-dominant > dominant

Table 6.9 Disorders of self-awareness.

Subtype		Definition	Neuroanatomy
Auto-/ somato- topagnosia	Finger agnosia All other	Inability to recognize body parts/locations	Intraparietal sulcus, Brodmann areas 5, 7
Gerstmann syndrome		• Left-right disorientation • Finger agnosia • Dyslexia • Dyscalculia	Dominant angular gyrus
Balint syndrome		• Simultanagnosia • Oculomotor apraxia • Optic ataxia	Bilateral parietal
Anosagnosias	General	Unawareness of deficit (usually neurologic)	Non-dominant parietal
	Hemi-body	Unawareness of hemi-body plegia	Non-dominant parietal
	Anton syndrome	Unawareness of cortical blindness	Non-dominant parietal + bilateral visual occipital cortex

Table of frequency of each disease

While multiple pathogenic processes can yield non-memory cognitive deficits, we focus on those neurologic disorders fundamentally characterized by acquired impairments of non-memory cognitive functions. Table 6.10 inventories heritability, risk factors, and epidemiology of these disorders.

Recommended diagnostic strategy

Diagnostic tests

- Familiarity with the clinical presentations of non-memory cognitive disorders facilitates early identification, which can be crucial to successful management of this diagnostic class, among which are reversible and partially reversible syndromes.
- The diagnostic strategy entails clinical and neuropsychological evaluation, MRI, and routine blood-work for metabolic and endocrinologic disorders that can cause cognitive dysfunction. Additional targeted testing may be performed depending on the specific syndrome and family history.
- The principal clinical features of disorders characteristically showing non-memory cognitive dysfunction are listed in Table 6.11.
- The linguistic characteristics of primary progressive aphasia subtypes are described in Table 6.12.
- Abnormal test results associated with specific cognitive disorders are described in Table 6.13.

Table 6.10 Neurodegenerative cognitive disorders: classification, heritability, risk factors, and epidemiology.

Molecular/ histo-neuropathology	Clinical syndrome		Heritability/ genetics	Other risk factors	Epidemiology	
					Annual incidence	Prevalence
Tauopathies	Fronto-temporal dementia (FTD)	FTD-tau	• Up to half of FTD cases have affected first-degree-relative • Approximately 10% of FTD cases have a single gene mutation, inherited in autosomal dominant manner • Behavioral variant FTD most heritable • FTD-dysphasia and FTD-MND (motor neuron disease) least heritable	Head injury	• ≤5 per 100,000	• ≤30 per 100,000 • FTD-tau likely most common type of FTD
		FTDP-17 (fronto-temporal dementia and parkinsonism linked to chromosome 17)	Autosomal dominant	Unknown	Unknown/rare	Unknown/rare
	Corticobasal ganglionic degeneration (CBGD)		Sporadic	Unknown	≤2 per 100,000	≤10 per 100,000
	Progressive supranuclear palsy (PSP)		Sporadic	Unknown	≤2 per 100,000	≤10 per 100,000

Category	Disorder	Genetics/Etiology	Head trauma		
Mixed amyloidopathies/ tauopathies	Alzheimer's disease (AD) (non-memory predominant presentations)	Sporadic with genetic vulnerability Autosomal dominant	Unknown	See Chapter 27	See Chapter 27
	Chronic traumatic encephalopathy (CTE)	Sporadic with genetic vulnerability	• Single severe trauma → B-amyloid-predominant ApoEe4 • Multiple mild-moderate traumas → tau-predominant	Uncommon Unknown	Uncommon Unknown
Ubiquitin-positive inclusions	FTD-TDP-43 (TAR (trans-active response) DNA-binding protein of 43 kDa)	TARDBP mutations identified in sporadic and familial ALS.	Unknown	Unknown	Second most common FTD type after tau
	FTLD-FUS (fused in sarcoma)	FUS sarcoma gene mutation	Unknown	Unknown/rare	Unknown/rare
	FTD-MND (motor neuron disease)	• Approximately 10% have positive family history • C9ORF72 autosomal dominant subtype of ALS accounts for approximately 40% of familial ALS and these develop FTD	Unknown	Unknown	Unknown

(Continued)

Table 6.10 (Continued)

Molecular/ histo-neuropathology	Clinical syndrome		Heritability/ genetics	Other risk factors	Epidemiology	
					Annual incidence	Prevalence
Synucleinopathies	Parkinson's disease-related dementia (PD-D)		• Majority sporadic • Approximately 15% have positive family history • <10% of early-onset PD with identified genetic mutations (PARK2, PARK7, LRRK2, PINK1, SNCA)	• PD duration • PD severity • Age • Genetic risk factors	• Approximately 2% in general population >65 • Up to 10% of PD cases progress to PD-D per year	• Approximately 10% of all dementia cases • Point prevalence of dementia in PD patient population up to 40% • Cumulative prevalence of dementia in PD >75%
	Dementia with Lewy bodies (DLB)		Majority sporadic	Genetic risk factors (not well defined)	≤4 per 100,000	• ≤400 per 100,000 • Up to approximately 20% of all dementias • Likely second most common neurodegenerative dementia for age >65
	Multiple system atrophy (MSA)	MSA-P (striato-nigral degeneration)	Sporadic	Unknown	≤3 per 100,000	≤5 per 100,000
		MSA-A (Shy–Drager)	Sporadic	Unknown	≤1 per 100 000	≤4 per 100,000
		MSA-C (olivo-ponto-cerebellar degneration)	Sporadic	Unknown	Unknown/rare	Unknown/rare
Trinucleotide repeat disorders	Huntington's disease		• Autosomal dominant • CAG repeat	Unknown	0.38 per 100,000	5–10 per 100,000

		Genetics	Cause		
Spinocerebellar ataxias (SCA)	SCA-3 (Machado–Joseph disease)	• Autosomal dominant • CAG repeat	Unknown	Unknown/rare	Unknown/rare
	SCA-17	• Autosomal dominant • CAG repeat	Unknown	Unknown/rare	<1 per 1 million
Fragile X-associated tremor/ataxia syndrome (FXTAS)		FMR1	Unknown	Unknown/rare	Unknown/rare
Creutzfeldt–Jakob disease (CJD)	Sporadic	Unknown	Unknown	1 per 1 million	85% of CJD cases are sCJD
	Iatrogenic	N/A	Accidental transmission via invasive procedures: • contaminated surgical or laboratory exposure; • tissue transplant (corneal, dural, etc.); • pituitary growth hormones	Rare	<5% of CJD cases
	Variant	Unknown	• Dietary exposure: consumption of food of bovine origin contaminated with agent of bovine spongiform encephalopathy (BSE) has been strongly linked to occurrence of vCJD in humans • Polymorphic codon 129 of PRNP gene is main genetic risk factor for vCJD	Rare	• 175 cases of vCJD reported in UK • 49 cases in other countries
	Familial (Gerstmann–Sträussler–Scheinker)	Autosomal dominant	100% familial	Rare	1–10 per 100,000,000

Spongiform

(Continued)

Table 6.10 (*Continued*)

Molecular/ histo-neuropathology	Clinical syndrome		Heritability/ genetics	Other risk factors	Epidemiology	
					Annual incidence	Prevalence
Leukomalacias	Adult-onset metabolic leuko-encephalopathies	Metachromatic leukodystrophy Adrenoleukodystrophy Polyglucosan body disease Fabry disease	Multiple variants	Unknown	Rare	Rare
Ventricular fluid dynamics	Normal pressure hydrocephalus (NPH)		None known	• Head trauma • Intracranial hemorrhage	<5 per 100,000	Not well known
Mixed	Non-amnestic MCI		Heterogeneous category	Multiple	Approximately 100 per 100,000	≥4% among age >50 ≥5% among age >65 ≥20% among age >85

Table 6.11 Neurodegenerative cognitive disorders: principal clinical features.

Molecular/ histo-neuropathology	Clinical syndrome		Age of onset	Temporal course	Clinical features			
					Cognitive/affective	Motor	Posture/gait	Autonomic/bulbar/ sphincter
Tauopathies	FTD	FTD-tau (Pick's disease)	Mean 58	Gradual progressive	• Dyexecutive • −/+ Primary progressive aphasia (see Table 6.12)	Atypical	Atypical/ late-occurring	Atypical
		FTDP-17	<65	Gradual progressive	Dysexecutive	Parkinsonism	Parkinsonian	−/+
	CBGD		≥60	Gradual progressive	Dyexecutive Dysphasic Asymmetric dyspraxia Alien limb	• Asymmetric parkinsonism • Akinesia • Rigidity • Dystonia • Myoclonus • Frontal release signs • Asymmetric Babinski sign	Postural instability	Atypical
	PSP		Mean 62	Gradual progressive	Dysexecutive	• Supranuclear ophthalmoplegia (especially vertical EOM palsy) • Eyelid dysfunction • Dysarthria • Dysphagia	• Postural instability • Frequent falls	Atypical
Mixed amyloidopathies/ tauopathies	AD		>65	Gradual progressive	Dysmnestic	Atypical	Late-appearing	Atypical
	CTE		Variable	Gradual progressive	Variable	Variable	Variable	Atypical

(Continued)

Table 6.11 (Continued)

Molecular/histo-neuropathology	Clinical syndrome		Age of onset	Temporal course	Clinical features			
					Cognitive/affective	Motor	Posture/gait	Autonomic/bulbar/sphincter
Synucleinopathies	PD/PD-D		Mean 60	Gradual progressive	Dysexecutive	Parkinsonism (asymmetric)	Parkinsonian	Variable, sometimes prominent
	DLB		50–85	Progressive	• Dysexecutive • Visual hallucinations • Consciousness fluctuations • REM behavioral disorder	Parkinsonism	Prominent gait impairment	Variable
	MSA	MSA-P (striato-nigral degeneration)	Mean 54	Progressive	Dysexecutive	Parkinsonism	Parkinsonism	–/+
		MSA-A (Shy–Drager)	Mean 65	Progressive	Dysexecutive	Variable parkinsonism	Variable gait dysfunction	Prominent dysautonomia
		MSA-C (olivo-ponto-cerebellar degeneration)	50s	Progressive	Dysexecutive	Prominent cerebellar dysfunction	Cerebellar gait dysfunction	–/+
Ubiquitin-positive inclusions	FTLDTDP-43		40s–60s	Progressive	Dysexecutive Dysphasic Dysexecutive	Non-characteristic	Non-characteristic	Non-characteristic
	FTD-ALS					UMN signs	Progressive dysfunction	+Bulbar signs
Spino-cerebellar atrophies	SCA-3 (Machado–Joseph disease)		20s–50s	Variably progressive	• Verbal impairment, especially fluency • Visuospatial and constructional dysfunction • Memory deficits	• Slow saccades and saccadic pursuit • Lid retraction-persistent stare • Dysarthria, dysphagia, poor cough • Upper and lower motor neuron signs	Non-specific	Autonomic dysfunction, including cold intolerance, nocturia, and orthostatic symptoms

		Age	Progression				
					• Tongue fasciculations • Tone ranges hypotonia to rigidity • Reflexes absent to exaggerated • Babinski signs • Parkinsonism • Dystonia • Muscle cramps, fasciculations		
Spongiform	SCA-17	3–55	Variable progressive	Non-specific	• Ataxia • Parkinsonism • Dystonia • Spasticity	Motor dysfunction-related	• Dysphagia • Seizures
	CJD	Sporadic/iatrogenic	57–62	Rapidly progressive	Global cognitive dysfunction	Mixed UMN and extrapyramidal signs	Dyspraxic and motor dysfunction-related	Non-specific
		Variant	Much younger	Rapidly progressive	Global cognitive dysfunction	Mixed UMN and extrapyramidal signs	Dyspraxic and motor dysfunction-related	Non-specific
		Familial (Gerstmann–Sträussler–Scheinker)	Slightly younger	Rapidly progressive	• Progressive global dementia • Mood disregulation • Thought content disturbance (psychosis)	Characterized by pyramidal, cerebellar, and parkinsonian features	Dyspraxic and motor dysfunction-related	Non-specific

(Continued)

Table 6.11 (Continued)

Molecular/ histo-neuropathology	Clinical syndrome	Age of onset	Temporal course	Clinical features				
				Cognitive/affective	Motor	Posture/gait	Autonomic/bulbar/ sphincter	
Fragile X-associated tremor/ataxia syndrome (FXTAS)		40s–80s Males >> females	Gradually progressive	• Dysexecutive • Dysmnestic • Mood dysregulation • Personality change • Abulia, reclusiveness	• Late-onset ataxia associated with postural tremor • Moderate parkinsonism • Peripheral neuropathy • Proximal leg weakness	Dyspraxic and motor-related dysfunction	• Autonomic dysfunction • Bladder/bowel incontinence	
Adult-onset metabolic leukoencephalopathies	Multiple subtypes	Variable	Gradually progressive	Mixed cognitive dysfunction	Mixed pyramidal signs	Motor-related dysfunction	Atypical	
Ventricular fluid dynamics	Normal pressure hydrocephalus (NPH)	Typically >50	Gradually progressive	Dysexecutive	Parkinsonism	• Magnetic • Dyspraxic	Urinary incontinence	

Table 6.12 Linguistic characteristics of primary progressive aphasia (PPA) subtypes.

PPA subtypes	Spontaneous speech	Fluency	Motor speech	Single word comprehension	Grammar/sentence comprehension	Sentence repetition	Naming/word retrieval	Reading
Semantic dementia	Grammatically correct Empty and circumlocutory Semantic errors	Preserved	Spared	Impaired	Initially spared, becomes impaired as single word comprehension deteriorates	Spared	Anomia (nouns > verbs)	Surface dyslexia
Progressive non-fluent aphasia	Decreased fluency Articulatory errors Apraxia of speech and/or Agrammatism	Impaired	Impaired	Initially spared, becomes affected in late disease	Impaired for complex sentences	−/+ Impaired	Spared initially but anomic as disease progresses (verbs > nouns)	Phonological dyslexia
Logopenic or phonological variant	Slow output with word-finding pauses Phonemic paraphasias	Impaired	Spared	Relatively spared	Impaired for simple and complex sentences	Impaired	Impaired	Phonological dyslexia

Table 6.13 Neurodegenerative cognitive disorders: principal biomarkers.

Molecular/ histo-neuropathology	Clinical syndrome		Neuroimaging		EEG	Serum markers	CSF markers
			Structural MRI	Functional			
Tauopathies	FTD	FTD-T/Pick's disease FTDP-17	Frontal/ fronto-temporal atrophy ("knife-edge" when advanced)	FDG PET: frontal/ fronto-temporal hypometabolism	–/+ Frontal slowing	GRN DNA test VCP DNA test MAPT DNA test	Tau (phosphorylated)
	CBGD		Cortical atrophy	FDG-PET: variable cortical and subcortical hypometabolism	• Non-specific slowing • Disorganization	None available	None identified
	PSP (PSP-R, PSP-P)		Hummingbird sign	FDG-PET: variable cortical basal ganglia, brainstem hypometabolism	Non-specific	None available	None identified
Mixed amyloidopathies/ tauopathies	AD	Sporadic with genetic vulnerability Autosomal dominant	Cortical atrophy, anteromedial, temporal, and peri-sylvian Predominance	• FDG PET: temporo-parietal hypometabolism • Florbetapir-PET (Amyvid™): +amyloid	• Non-specific slowing • Disorganization • Reduced Amplitude	• ApoE genotype analysis • APP DNA analysis PS-1 DNA test	• $\downarrow$Aβ42 ($\leq$50% nl) • $\uparrow$Phosphorylated tau/total tau
	CTE		• –/+ Trauma-related changes • –/+ Micro-hemorrhages on SWI • –/+ Axonal shear on DTI	• FDG-PET: non-specific • Florbetapir-PET: –/+ amyloidopathy	Variable	None identified, ApoE3, ApoE4 have increased risk	No specific pattern identified

Synucleinopathies	PD/PD-D	Non-specific	Ioflupane-SPECT Dopamine transporter (DaT) scan: reduced putaminal uptake (reflecting dopaminergic neuronal loss); FDG-PET: hypometabolism of dorsolateral putamen	No specific changes	• Typically none • In correct clinical context: alpha synuclein (SNCA) duplication/deletion test, LRRK2 DNA sequencing test, PARK2 (Parkin) DNA sequencing test, PARK7 (DJ1) DNA sequencing test, PARK7 (DJ1) deletion test, PINK1 deletion test, PINK1 DNA sequencing test	No specific marker pattern identified
	DLB	Non-specific atrophy	FDG-PET: +/– posterior cortical hypometabolism	Non-specific changes	None identified	No specific biomarker pattern identified
	MSA MSA-P (striato-nigral degeneration) MSA-A (Shy-Drager) MSA-C (olivo-ponto-cerebellar degeneration)	T2 hyperintensities in pons (hot cross bun sign), middle cerebellar peduncles, cerebellum	FDG-PET: • putamen hypometabolism • cerebellar hypometabolism • thalamic hypermetabolism	Non-specific changes	No specific markers identified	No specific biomarker pattern identified
Ubiquitin-positive inclusions	FTLD-U/TDP	Frontal/ fronto-temporal atrophy	FDG-PET: fronto/ fronto-temporal hypometabolism	Non-specific changes	TDP-43 DNA sequencing test	TDP-43 sequencing test
	FTD-ALS	–/+ Frontal/ fronto-temporal atrophy	MRS: abnormal motor cortex	Non-specific changes	TDP-43 DNA test C9ORF72 DNA test	Non-specific CSF profile

(Continued)

Table 6.13 (Continued)

| Molecular/ histo-neuropathology | Clinical syndrome | Neuroimaging | | EEG | Serum markers | CSF markers |
		Structural MRI	Functional			
Spino-cerebellar atrophies	SCA-3 (Machado–Joseph disease)	Brainstem atrophy	FDG-PET: ↓cerebellum, limbic, basal ganglia metabolism	No specific changes	SCA-3 genetic testing	Non-specific
	SCA-17	Cerebellar atrophy	Cerebellar −/+ other regional hypometabolism	Non-specific changes	TBP (encoding TATA-box-binding protein)	No specific biomarker
Spongiform	CJD	Cortical and BG hyperintensities on DWI	Cortical and BG hypometabolism	Periodic sharp wave complexes	No specific markers identified	Protein 14-3-3
Adult-onset metabolic leukoencephalopathies	Multiple subtypes	White matter T2 hyperintensities	Non-specific changes	Non-specific changes	Multiple subtype-specific	Elevated protein
Ventricular fluid dynamics	Normal pressure hydrocephalus (NPH)	Ventricular dilatation disproportionate to parenchymal atrophy	Non-specific changes	Non-specific changes	N/A	No specific markers

BOTTOM LINE
- Clarify cognitive impairment and neurobehavioral adaptation via detailed history acquisition and informant interviews.
- Perform comprehensive physical examination and neurocognitive assessment.
- Assemble comprehensive problem list regarding cognitive, affective, neurovegetative, motor, and any other relevant systems.
- Formulate differential diagnosis with attention to unifying etiologies.
- Perform targeted neurodiagnostic investigations.
- Identify safety concerns (ADLs, home environment, driving, etc.).

Images

Mini-Mental State Examination (MMSE)

Patient's Name: _____ Date: _____

Instructions: Ask the questions in the order listed. Score one point for each correct response within each question or activity.

Maximum Score	Patient's Score	Questions
5		"What is the year? Season? Date? Day of the week? Month?"
5		"Where are we now: State? County? Town/city? Hospital? Floor?"
3		The examiner names three unrelated objects clearly and slowly, then asks the patient to name all three of them. The patient's response is used for scoring. The examiner repeats them until patient learns all of them, if possible. Number of trials: _____
5		"I would like you to count backward from 100 by sevens." (93, 86, 79, 72, 65, ...) Stop after five answers. Alternative: "Spell WORLD backwards." (D-L-R-O-W)
3		"Earlier I told you the names of three things. Can you tell me what those were?"
2		Show the patient two simple objects, such as a wristwatch and a pencil, and ask the patient to name them.
1		"Repeat the phrase: 'No ifs, ands, or buts.'"
3		"Take the paper in your right hand, fold it in half, and put it on the floor." (The examiner gives the patient a piece of blank paper.)
1		"Please read this and do what it says." (Written instruction is "Close your eyes.")
1		"Make up and write a sentence about anything." (This sentence must contain a noun and a verb.)
1		"Please copy this picture." (The examiner gives the patient a blank piece of paper and asks him/her to draw the symbol below. All 10 angles must be present and two must intersect.)
30		TOTAL

(Adapted from Rovner & Folstein, 1987)

Advantages
- Ease of use
- Extensively validated
- Widely recognized/accepted

Disadvantages
- Insensitivity to mild dementia
- Insensitivity to executive impairment

Method	Score	Interpretation
Single Cutoff	<24	Abnormal
Range	<21	Increased odds of dementia
	>25	Decreased odds of dementia
Education	21	Abnormal for 8th grade education
	<23	Abnormal for high school education
	<24	Abnormal for college education
Severity	24–30	No cognitive impairment
	18–23	Mild cognitive impairment
	0–17	Severe cognitive impairment

Figure 6.1 Mini-Mental Status Examination (MMSE). *Source*: Adapted from Folstein MF, et al. 1975, J Psych Res; 12:189–198. Copyright © 1975 Elsevier.

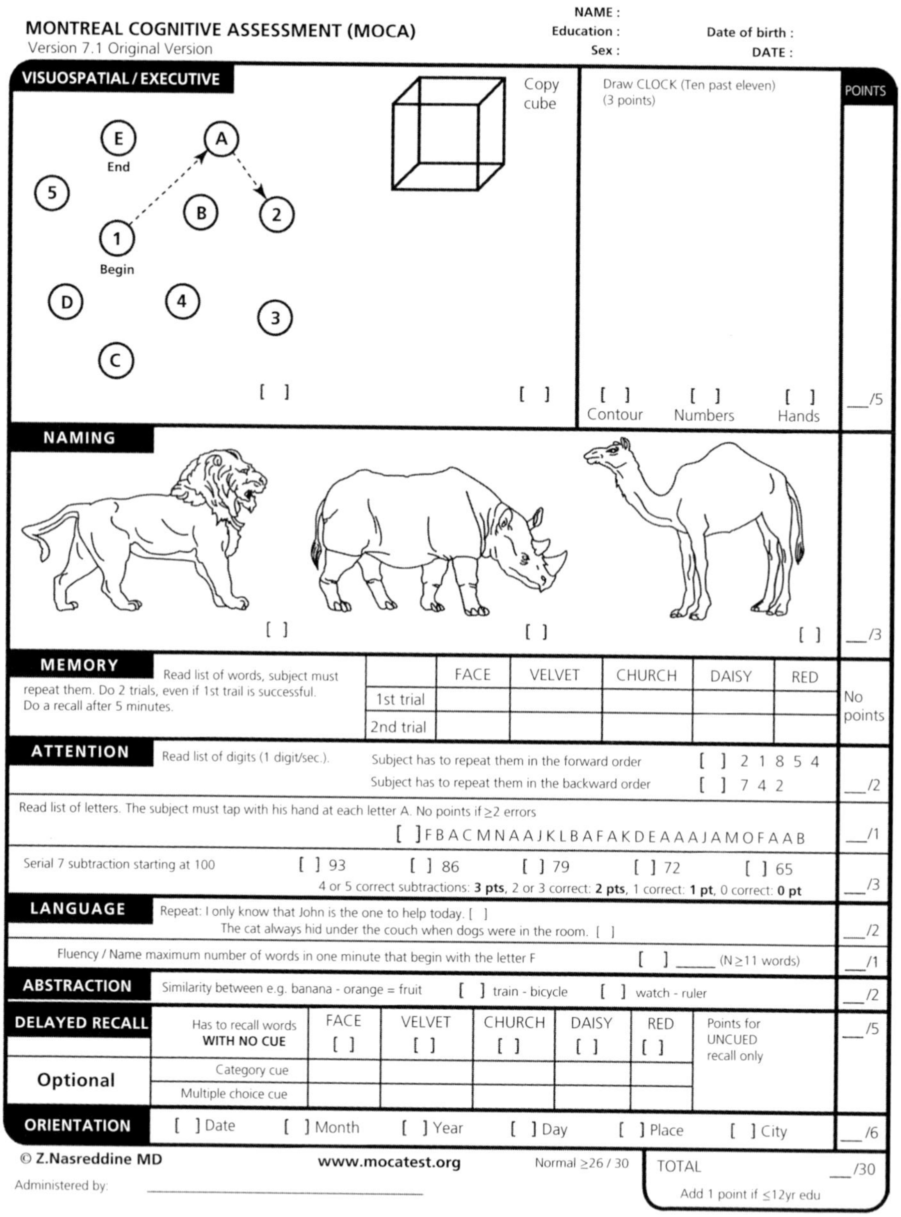

MONTREAL COGNITIVE ASSESSMENT (MOCA)
Version 7.1 Original Version

NAME :
Education : Date of birth :
Sex : DATE :

VISUOSPATIAL / EXECUTIVE — POINTS

[ ]

Copy cube [ ]

Draw CLOCK (Ten past eleven) (3 points)

[ ] Contour [ ] Numbers [ ] Hands ___/5

NAMING

[ ] [ ] [ ] ___/3

MEMORY Read list of words, subject must repeat them. Do 2 trials, even if 1st trail is successful. Do a recall after 5 minutes.

	FACE	VELVET	CHURCH	DAISY	RED
1st trial					
2nd trial					

No points

ATTENTION Read list of digits (1 digit/sec.). Subject has to repeat them in the forward order [ ] 2 1 8 5 4
Subject has to repeat them in the backward order [ ] 7 4 2 ___/2

Read list of letters. The subject must tap with his hand at each letter A. No points if ≥2 errors
[ ] F B A C M N A A J K L B A F A K D E A A A J A M O F A A B ___/1

Serial 7 subtraction starting at 100 [ ] 93 [ ] 86 [ ] 79 [ ] 72 [ ] 65
4 or 5 correct subtractions: **3 pts**, 2 or 3 correct: **2 pts**, 1 correct: **1 pt**, 0 correct: **0 pt** ___/3

LANGUAGE Repeat: I only know that John is the one to help today. [ ]
The cat always hid under the couch when dogs were in the room. [ ] ___/2

Fluency / Name maximum number of words in one minute that begin with the letter F [ ] ____ (N ≥ 11 words) ___/1

ABSTRACTION Similarity between e.g. banana - orange = fruit [ ] train - bicycle [ ] watch - ruler ___/2

DELAYED RECALL

Has to recall words **WITH NO CUE**	FACE [ ]	VELVET [ ]	CHURCH [ ]	DAISY [ ]	RED [ ]	Points for UNCUED recall only
Optional: Category cue						
Optional: Multiple choice cue						

___/5

ORIENTATION [ ] Date [ ] Month [ ] Year [ ] Day [ ] Place [ ] City ___/6

© Z.Nasreddine MD **www.mocatest.org** Normal ≥26 / 30 TOTAL ___/30
Add 1 point if ≤12yr edu

Administered by: ____________

Figure 6.2 Montreal Cognitive Assessment (MoCA). A score of less than 26 is abnormal. *Source*: www.mocatest.org. Copyright Nasreddine Z. MD. Reproduced with permission. Copies are available at www.mocatest.org.

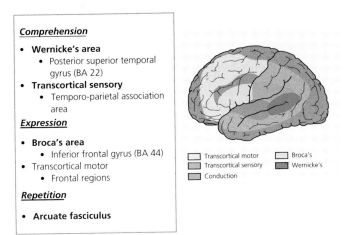

Comprehension

- **Wernicke's area**
  - Posterior superior temporal gyrus (BA 22)
- **Transcortical sensory**
  - Temporo-parietal association area

Expression

- **Broca's area**
  - Inferior frontal gyrus (BA 44)
- Transcortical motor
  - Frontal regions

Repetition

- **Arcuate fasciculus**

☐ Transcortical motor	☐ Broca's
◐ Transcortical sensory	◼ Wernicke's
◼ Conduction	

Figure 6.3 Linguistic neuroanatomic modules. *Source*: Text adapted from Goldstein M, Silverman M. The Neuropsychiatric Examination. Psychiatric Clinics of North America. In: Riggio S, ed. Psychiatric Clin North America 2005;28(3):507–547. Reproduced with permission of Elsevier. Figure from Perkin GD. Mosby's color atlas and text of neurology. St Louis (MO): Mosby; 1998. Copyright © 1998 Elsevier.

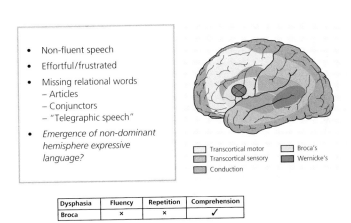

- Non-fluent speech
- Effortful/frustrated
- Missing relational words
  - Articles
  - Conjunctors
  - "Telegraphic speech"
- *Emergence of non-dominant hemisphere expressive language?*

☐ Transcortical motor	☐ Broca's
◐ Transcortical sensory	◼ Wernicke's
◼ Conduction	

Dysphasia	Fluency	Repetition	Comprehension
Broca	✗	✗	✓

Figure 6.4 Broca's aphasia. *Source*: Text adapted from Goldstein M, Silverman M. The Neuropsychiatric Examination. Psychiatric Clinics of North America. In: Riggio S, ed. Psychiatric Clin North America 2005;28(3):507–547. Reproduced with permission of Elsevier. Figure from Perkin GD. Mosby's color atlas and text of neurology. St Louis (MO): Mosby; 1998. Copyright © 1998 Elsevier.

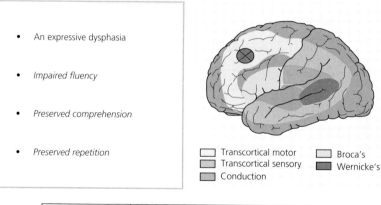

- An expressive dysphasia

- *Impaired fluency*

- *Preserved comprehension*

- *Preserved repetition*

☐ Transcortical motor   ☐ Broca's
▨ Transcortical sensory   ▨ Wernicke's
▨ Conduction

Dysphasia	Fluency	Repetition	Comprehension
Transcortical motor	×	✓	✓

Figure 6.5 Transcortical motor aphasia. *Source*: Text adapted from Goldstein M, Silverman M. The Neuropsychiatric Examination. Psychiatric Clinics of North America. In: Riggio S, ed. Psychiatric Clin North America 2005;28(3):507–547. Reproduced with permission of Elsevier. Figure from Perkin GD. Mosby's color atlas and text of neurology. St Louis (MO): Mosby; 1998. Copyright © 1998 Elsevier.

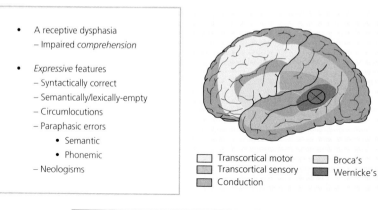

- A receptive dysphasia
  - Impaired *comprehension*

- *Expressive* features
  - Syntactically correct
  - Semantically/lexically-empty
  - Circumlocutions
  - Paraphasic errors
    - Semantic
    - Phonemic
  - Neologisms

☐ Transcortical motor   ☐ Broca's
▨ Transcortical sensory   ▨ Wernicke's
▨ Conduction

Dysphasia	Fluency	Repetition	Comprehension
Wernicke	✓	×	×

Figure 6.6 Wernicke's aphasia. *Source*: Text adapted from Goldstein M, Silverman M. The Neuropsychiatric Examination. Psychiatric Clinics of North America. In: Riggio S, ed. Psychiatric Clin North America 2005;28(3):507–547. Reproduced with permission of Elsevier. Figure from Perkin GD. Mosby's color atlas and text of neurology. St Louis (MO): Mosby; 1998. Copyright © 1998 Elsevier.

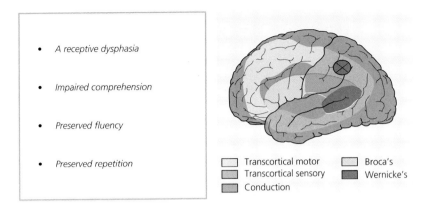

- *A receptive dysphasia*

- *Impaired comprehension*

- *Preserved fluency*

- *Preserved repetition*

Transcortical motor   Broca's
Transcortical sensory   Wernicke's
Conduction

Dysphasia	Fluency	Repetition	Comprehension
Transcortical sensory	✓	✓	×

Figure 6.7 Transcortical sensory aphasia. *Source*: Text adapted from Goldstein M, Silverman M. The Neuropsychiatric Examination. Psychiatric Clinics of North America. In: Riggio S, ed. Psychiatric Clin North America 2005;28(3):507–547. Reproduced with permission of Elsevier. Figure from Perkin GD. Mosby's color atlas and text of neurology. St Louis (MO): Mosby; 1998. Copyright © 1998 Elsevier.

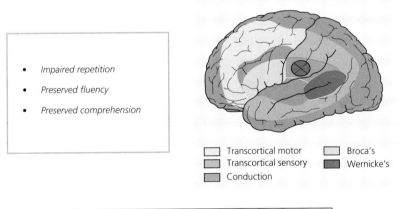

- *Impaired repetition*
- *Preserved fluency*
- *Preserved comprehension*

Transcortical motor   Broca's
Transcortical sensory   Wernicke's
Conduction

Dysphasia	Fluency	Repetition	Comprehension
Conduction	✓	×	✓

Figure 6.8 Conduction aphasia. *Source*: Text adapted from Goldstein M, Silverman M. The Neuropsychiatric Examination. Psychiatric Clinics of North America. In: Riggio S, ed. Psychiatric Clin North America 2005;28(3):507–547. Reproduced with permission of Elsevier. Figure from Perkin GD. Mosby's color atlas and text of neurology. St Louis (MO): Mosby; 1998. Copyright © 1998 Elsevier.

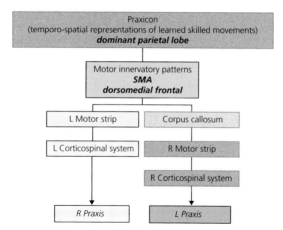

Figure 6.9 Functional neuroanatomy of praxis. SMA, supplementary motor area.

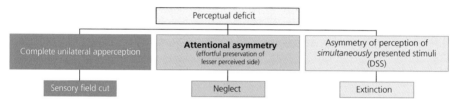

Figure 6.10 Levels of perceptual deficit. DSS, double simultaneous stimulation.

Reading list

Key reading sources for this chapter can be found online at www.mountsinaiexpertguides.com

Suggested websites

National Aphasia Association: www.aphasia.org
NINDS Apraxia Information Page: http://www.ninds.nih.gov/disorders/apraxia/apraxia.htm
The Association for Frontotemporal Degeneration: www.theaftd.org
Cognitive Neuroscience Society: www.cogneurosociety.org
National Institute on Aging: www.nia.nih.gov
Montreal Cognitive Assessment: www.mocatest.org

Additional material for this chapter can be found online at:
www.mountsinaiexpertguides.com

This includes a case study, multiple choice questions,
and a reading list.

CHAPTER 7

Memory Loss and Dementia

Sam Gandy

Icahn School of Medicine at Mount Sinai; and James J. Peters VA Medical Center, New York, NY, USA

Background

- Memory loss, or amnesia, refers to a memory disorder. Memory loss may be an isolated or pure disorder or occur in association with other cognitive dysfunction or dementia. Selected components of memory can be affected, such as retrograde or anterograde amnesia. Amnesia may be confined to a window of time, for example following head injury or transient global amnesia. Amnesia can also refer to an ongoing inability to form and retrieve new short-term memories with or without difficulty in retrieving older long-term memories.
- Dementia is a general term that refers to the persistent loss of any combination of previously intact cognitive functions, such as memory, language, abstraction, and judgment.
- The most common cause of dementia is Alzheimer's disease, a neurodegenerative disorder of the CNS resulting in progressive loss of memory and intellectual functions. It begins in the middle or later years and is characterized by brain neuropathologic changes such as neurofibrillary tangles and neuritic plaques.

Impact

Incidence

The incidence of cognitive impairment is highly aging-related. In the population of age 85 years or older, one-third to one-half have measurable cognitive impairment.

Economic impact

The impact depends primarily on whether the amnestic syndrome is disabling. Numbers vary between studies, but memory disorder costs worldwide have been calculated around $160 billion, while the costs of Alzheimer's disease alone (among memory disorders) in the USA may be $100 billion each year. Amnesia due to head injury can affect younger patients, but function is usually restored following recovery from the initial trauma.

Approach to diagnosis

Getting your bearings

- Exclusion of reversible dementia is the first step in the evaluation.
- Alzheimer's disease may initially present with isolated memory disturbance.
- Fronto-temporal dementia (Pick's disease) typically presents with personality change and language disturbance.
- Sometimes dementia presents as aphasia.
- Acute presentations include transient global amnesia, limbic encephalitis, and infectious encephalitis.

Mount Sinai Expert Guides: Neurology, First Edition. Edited by Stuart C. Sealfon, Rajeev Motiwala, and Charles B. Stacy.
© 2016 John Wiley & Sons, Ltd. Published 2016 by John Wiley & Sons, Ltd.
Companion website: www.mountsinaiexpertguides.com

- Head trauma may be occult, and post-traumatic encephalopathy is increasingly recognized.
- Amnestic mild cognitive impairment (MCI), when restricted to memory, is a frequent harbinger of dementia.
- The transition from MCI to mild dementia is usually considered to be the progression of the amnestic disorder to a point that interferes with daily function.

Key elements of history

- Is this an isolated memory disorder?
- Is it associated with other cognitive deficits?
- Is it a behavioral syndrome with relative sparing of memory?
- What is the onset, time course, and evolution of the syndrome?
- Are there any antecedent precipitants or systemic medical illness?

Elements of history corresponding to particular diseases

The most common reversible cause of dementia is polypharmacy or overmedication with sedatives or antihistamines. Thus, a medication history is critical.

Among those elements of history that may point to other reversible causes of dementia, the following should be sought:

- Nutritional status and history.
- History of cancer.
- Sexual history, history of HIV or syphilis.
- History of thyroid disease.
- History of known intracranial mass lesions.
- History of head trauma including sports and military exposure.
- History of autoimmune disease.

Table of elements of history and diseases

Disease	Symptoms	Duration/tempo	Other key features
Alzheimer's disease	Amnesia for recent events	Subacute-chronic	Often lack of insight, typically noted by a family member. May have a positive family history
Vascular dementia	Varied cognitive deficits, executive function affected more than memory, other focal neurologic symptoms	Evolution over years, classically stepwise onset, associated with strokes, but may be progressive	Vascular risk factors, history of previous stroke(s)
Fronto-temporal dementia	Aphasia, impulse control disorder in addition to memory deficits	Subacute onset, usually in 60s	May have family history of early-onset dementia
Transient global amnesia	Isolated impairment of retrograde and anterograde memory	Acute onset, lasts less than 24 hours	Can be recurrent, may have emotional or physical precipitant (e.g. exertion), possible relation to migraine
Thyroid disorder	Slow recall of recent and past events	Subacute-chronic	Cold or heat intolerance, weight change, tremors, swelling
Depression	Tearfulness, sad affect	Subacute-chronic	Patient may not acknowledge condition

Disease	Symptoms	Duration/tempo	Other key features
Subdural hematoma	History of head injury or anticoagulation	Subacute-chronic, fluctuating symptoms	Trauma history may be absent, particularly with alcohol abuse
Normal pressure hydrocephalus	Falls, slow gait, incontinence, cognitive slowing	Subacute-chronic	Sometimes follows acute neurologic illness (meningitis, trauma, neurosurgery)
Seizures or post-ictal state	Fluctuating consciousness, without or with tonic-clonic component	Intermittent or slowly improving	Post-ictal state can be prolonged (24 h) in elderly and in those with baseline cognitive deficits
Infections (syphilis, Lyme, Whipple's, viral encephalitides)	Without or with fever, systemic symptoms	Acute to chronic	May have associated seizures or meningeal symptoms (neck stiffness, etc.)
Creutzfeldt–Jakob disease	Myoclonus, rapidly progressive dementia	Subacute-acute	Change in personality or behavior
Huntington's disease	Family history, psychosis, depression, chorea	Chronic	Can begin from youth to late life, motor symptoms predominant in young onset
Alcoholism	History of alcohol abuse; prominent memory difficulties, confabulations noted by others	Subacute-chronic	Alcohol abuse may be hidden or unrecognized (e.g. as alcohol-related GI and liver disease episodes)
Heavy metal toxicity	History of occupational exposure (e.g. manganese) or intentional poisoning (e.g. arsenic)	Subacute-chronic	Use of well water
Wilson's disease	Family history, liver failure	Subacute-chronic	
Vitamin deficiency (B12, B6, B2)	Nutritional deficiency, especially in alcoholism	Subacute-chronic	
Medications, polypharmacy	Access to prescription drugs or drugs of abuse	Subacute chronic	Inquire about over-the-counter medications, herbal supplements
Hepatic encephalopathy	Liver disease, jaundice, alcoholism, previous hepatitis	Episodic, subacute-chronic	
Tumors	Postural headache, lobar syndromes (e.g. hemiparesis, hemiagnosia)	Subacute-chronic	Systemic cancer, although may be presenting symptoms
Paraneoplastic syndromes	Acute sensory neuropathy, acute cerebellar syndrome, acute dementia	Subacute-chronic or acute	May precede clinical recognition of cancer
Meningeal carcinomatosis	Cancer history, headache, neck stiffness, symptoms from multiple focal root or cranial nerves	Subacute-chronic or acute	Painful or painless
Sleep apnea	Excessive daytime sleepiness, frequent naps, falls asleep during activities (driving), snoring	Subacute-chronic	Partner critical for history

(Continued)

Disease	Symptoms	Duration/tempo	Other key features
Post-anoxic	History of cardiac or respiratory arrest	Acute	
Parkinson's dementia	Rigidity, tremor, hypomimia	Subacute-chronic	Rare delayed-onset subacute leukoencephalopathy syndrome also occurs
Diffuse Lewy body disease	Falls, gait difficulty, visual hallucinations, personality changes, propensity to adverse reactions to low dose neuroleptics	Chronic	Cognitive features are early and prominent in contrast to Parkinson's dementia
Trauma	History of major or penetrating head trauma	Acute	
Chronic traumatic encephalopathy	Memory loss, executive function loss, personality changes, aggression, depression, apathy	Chronic	History of repeated concussions, may be confused with depression

CLINICAL PEARLS
- Asking the same questions or repeating elements of the history in the same interview is suggestive of dementia.
- Fronto-temporal dementia may cause personality changes or language abnormalities that dominate the presentation.
- Most common differential is Alzheimer's versus vascular dementia. Both may coexist, and vascular dementia also increases risk for Alzheimer's.
- The history is crucial in identifying cognitive disorders that are caused by systemic diseases (secondary dementia) versus primary dementing illness in which the patient is often otherwise healthy.

Key elements of physical examination

The general physical and neurologic examination serves to distinguish:
- Patients with only cognitive deficits (primary dementia, especially Alzheimer's).
- Patients with associated neurologic findings such as aphasia, visual field defects, abnormal reflexes, myoclonus (these may indicate neurologic diseases including cerebral infarcts, diffuse Lewy body disease, Parkinson's disease, ALS-FTD, etc.).
- Patients with evidence of systemic disease who have secondary encephalopathies (thyroid, liver, etc.).

It is important to systematically and quantifiably assess cognitive function. Several simple bed-side assessment tools are available.
- MMSE: The modified mini mental status (MMSE) examination, developed by Folstein, has long been the standard bedside clinical assessment of memory and cognition.
- MOCA: Due to patent issues, many dementia centers and pharmaceutical companies have changed from the MMSE to the Montreal Cognitive Assessment (MoCA). Blank MoCA forms, in various languages, can be downloaded from the MoCA website. MoCAs are used for testing trailmaking, animal naming, construction, copying, short-term memory, and attention.

- Other tools: Three other neuropsychological tests are worth noting for dementia: the Clinical Dementia Rating (CDR), the neuropsychological score (NPS), and the cognitive subscale of the Alzheimer's disease assessment scale (ADAS-COG). While the MoCA is rapidly becoming the bedside assessment of choice, the ADAS-COG remains the gold standard for research on new procognitive drugs.

Table of elements of physical examination by disease

Alzheimer's disease	MMSE abnormal, remainder of examination normal
Vascular dementia	MMSE abnormal, may be focal motor signs
Fronto-temporal dementia	MMSE abnormal, disinhibition or aphasia
Hypo- or hyperthyroidism	May have abnormal body temperature and heart rate. MMSE slow
Depression	Tearfulness, sadness, suicidal ideation, psychomotor retardation, GDS (global depression scale) may be helpful
Subdural hematoma	Altered level of alertness and focal signs. Examination variable and not specific
Normal pressure hydrocephalus	Gait difficulties often more marked than cognitive deficits, timed get-up-and-go test abnormal (although non-specific). Examination improves with high-volume LP or ventricular drainage
Seizures, post-ictal state	Fluctuating consciousness, repetitive movements, shaking or jerks, focal or widespread, may be observed
Infections (syphilis, Lyme, Whipple's, viral encephalitis)	May have fever, systemic signs, general stupor, focal signs
Creutzfeldt–Jakob disease	Myoclonus, classically induced by stimulus such as a loud clap, severe dementia
Huntington's disease	Psychosis, depression, chorea
Alcohol-related dementia	Stigmata of alcohol abuse; ataxia, Wernicke–Korsakoff features (short-term memory loss, confabulations) may be present
Heavy metal toxicity	Parkinsonian features, neuropathy, skin lesions, nail striations
Wilson's disease	Kayser–Fleischer rings (slit-lamp examination), extrapyramidal signs, coarse tremor
Vitamin deficiency (B12, B6, B1)	Neuropathy (B6, B12), myelopathy (B12), eye movement abnormalities, ataxia, confabulatory memory deficits (B1)
Medications	Asterixis, stupor, non-focal examination
Hepatic encephalopathy	Stigmata of liver disease, jaundice, asterixis
Tumors	Signs depend on tumor location, lobar syndromes (e.g. hemiparesis, hemiagnosia), signs of raised intracranial pressure, impaired alertness, papilledema
Paraneoplastic syndromes	Dementia may be associated with sensory neuronopathy, cerebellar syndrome, abnormal movements
Meningeal carcinomatosis	May be associated with evidence of raised intracranial pressure, multiple cranial neuropathies, polyradiculopathy
Sleep apnea	May have short neck, crowded oropharynx, appears fatigued

(Continued)

Post-anoxic	Varies from short-term memory deficit to global cerebral dysfunction; may have myoclonus
Parkinson's dementia	Rigidity, tremor, hypomimia
Diffuse Lewy body disease	Symmetrical parkinsonian features; bizarre behavior may be observed
Trauma	Evidence of penetrating injury or scalp bruising or bleeding
Chronic traumatic encephalopathy	Examination non-specific; may have associated minor motor and reflex findings

---

CLINICAL PEARLS
- With the exception of cognitive deficits, the neurologic examination is typically normal in patients with Alzheimer's disease.
- Consider FTD in patients presenting in their 60s with aphasia and loss of impulse control.
- Acute onset of febrile illness associated with seizures and focal findings should prompt immediate initiation of treatment for herpes simplex encephalitis until the diagnosis is excluded.
- Subacute progression of dementia with associated jerky movements (myoclonus) is suggestive of CJD.

Diagnostic tests

For the reversible causes of dementia, the table below summarizes the tests employed for the confirmation of the various possible diagnoses. Refer to Chapter 27 for the differential diagnosis of dementia.

Alzheimer's disease	Atrophy on MRI; amyloid biomarker in CSF or on amyloid imaging, genetic testing for *APP* (amyloid precursor protein), *PSEN1*, and *PSEN2* (presenilin 1 and 2) may be definitive if mutation detected
Vascular dementia	Evidence of multiple strokes or white matter changes as well as atrophy on MRI; no biomarker evidence for amyloidosis
Fronto-temporal dementia	MRI evidence for frontal or temporal atrophy, PET shows hypometabolism; genetic testing; amyloid studies negative
Hypo- or hyperthyroidism	Thyroid function, normal MRI
Depression	GDS (global depression scale) may be helpful
Subdural hematoma	MRI or CT
Hydrocephalus	Ventricular size on CT or MRI, response to high-volume lumbar puncture or lumbar drain; some centers use CSF flow or radioisotope studies
Post-ictal state, seizures	Video EEG
Infections (syphilis, Lyme, Whipple's, viral encephalitis)	CSF pleocytosis, sometimes elevated CSF protein is the only change. Specific CSF antibodies or polymerase chain reaction (PCR)

Creutzfeldt–Jakob disease	CSF tau, 14-3-3 protein, "hockey stick sign" on MRI
Huntington's disease	Genotyping huntingtin gene (*HTT*)
Alcoholism	Cerebellar degeneration may be present on MRI
Heavy metal toxicity	24-hour urine collection or hair examination for heavy metals
Wilson's disease	MRI will show lenticular degeneration or increased signal; abnormal urine or serum copper studies; serum ceruloplasmin; genetic testing
Vitamin deficiency (B12, B6, B2)	Serum levels of vitamins
Medications, drugs of abuse	Serum drug levels, serum and urine toxicology screen
Hepatic encephalopathy	Serum LFTs, ammonia
Tumors	MRI or CT with contrast
Paraneoplastic syndromes	CSF or serum studies, such as anti-Ro, anti-Hu
Meningeal carcinomatosis	MRI with contrast may show meningeal enhancement, CSF cell count, cytology, flow cytometry
Sleep apnea	Polysomnography
Post-anoxic encephalopathy	Watershed zone infarcts, cortex changes on CT or MRI
Parkinson's dementia	Abnormal DAT (dopamine transporter) scan
Trauma	Abnormal CT or MRI. MRI best for contusions and diffuse white matter axonal injury. CT may be better for acute blood

Table of frequency of each disease

Alzheimer's disease	Nearly 2/3 of all dementia; usually over 75 years old; 1.3% aged 65–69, 2.9% aged 70–74, 5.9% aged 75–79, 12.2% aged 80–84; 50% over age 85 years
Vascular dementia	1/3 of all dementia when including mixed Alzheimer-vascular dementia
Diffuse Lewy body disease	10–25% of dementia
Fronto-temporal dementia	<10% of all dementia; usually under 70 years old
Hypo- or hyperthyroidism	Rare; may be due to autoimmune disease
Depression	5–15% lifetime incidence
Subdural hematoma	7 cases per 100,000 persons (lifetime)
Normal pressure hydrocephalus	1 case per 100,000 persons (lifetime)

(Continued)

Post-ictal state, seizures	Prevalence of epilepsy 4.7/1000 persons
Infections (syphilis, Lyme, Whipple's, viral encephalitis)	Rare, varies by disease
Creutzfeldt–Jakob disease	1 case per 1,000,000 (lifetime)
Huntington's disease	3–7 cases per 100,000 (lifetime)
Alcoholism	5% of the general population are alcoholics; 20% of alcoholics have brain damage
Heavy metal toxicity	0.4% of people have elevated serum lead
Wilson's disease	1 per 30,000 population
Vitamin deficiency (B12, B6, B1)	3% of US population have low B12 levels; clinical significance unknown
Medications	Variable
Hepatic encephalopathy	1.4 per 100,000 population
Tumors	200 per 100,000 population
Paraneoplastic syndromes	Rare; 5% of patients with cancer
Meningeal carcinomatosis	Approximately 3–5% of patients with cancer
Sleep apnea	19 per 100,000 population
Parkinson's dementia	40% of Parkinson's disease
Trauma, traumatic brain injury (TBI)	150 per 100,000 population

Recommended diagnostic strategy

All patients should be tested for any reversible causes of dementia consistent with the presentation as described in the diagnostic test table above. Specialized brain imaging or CSF examination can be helpful for confirming or excluding the diagnoses of Alzheimer's disease, tauopathies, or prion disease. In Alzheimer's disease, [^{18}F]fluorodeoxyglucose positron emission tomography (FDG-PET) brain imaging typically reveals asymmetric biparietal hypometabolism. CSF will reveal reduced levels of Aβ42 and elevated levels of total and phospho-tau.

An important and evolving area is the assessment of MCI and its differentiation from dementia. MCI, particularly when of the amnestic type (memory impairment is present), is often a transition stage between the cognitive decline of normal aging and the more severe deficits associated with Alzheimer's disease. During the last decade, the concept of MCI has become widely accepted. The operational definition involves demonstrable deficits in one domain (memory in some) or multiple cognitive domains, yet without clinically important impact on the patient's function. Multi-domain amnestic or single domain amnestic symptoms of MCI, rather than single or multiple non-amnestic symptoms, are the more probable harbingers of eventual progression to Alzheimer's disease.

The American Academy of Neurology workgroup of specialists identified the following criteria for an MCI diagnosis:

- an individual's report of his or her own memory problems, preferably confirmed by another person;
- measurable, greater-than-normal memory impairment detected with standard memory assessment tests;
- normal general thinking and reasoning skills;

- ability to perform normal daily activities.
  These criteria for MCI are helpful but do not settle some issues facing clinicians, including:
- How much memory impairment is too much to be considered more than normal?
- How much memory impairment is significant enough to be considered a symptom of mild dementia?
- How hard should one look for subtle abnormalities in other areas of thinking?
- How do we know if these other changes are normal aging or worse?

BOTTOM LINE
- Identifying reversible causes of memory loss is paramount.
- The physician's role in supportive care for patients with chronic dementia is crucial.

Reading list

Key reading sources for this chapter can be found online at www.mountsinaiexpertguides.com

Suggested websites

Alzforum: www.alzforum.org
Alzheimer's Association: www.alz.org
Alzheimer's Disease on MedlinePlus: www.nlm.nih.gov/medlineplus/alzheimersdisease.html
Alzheimer's Foundation of America: www.alzfdn.org
Bright Focus Foundation: http://www.brightfocus.org/
Clinical trials: www.clinicaltrials.gov
Fisher Center for Alzheimer's Research Foundation: www.alzinfo.org
HBO The Alzheimer's Project: www.hbo.com/alzheimers
Mayo Clinic: http://www.mayoclinic.org/diseases-conditions/alzheimers-disease/basics/definition/con-20023871
Mount Sinai Alzheimer's Disease Research Center: http://icahn.mssm.edu/research/centers/alzheimers-disease-research-center
Mount Sinai Center for Cognitive Health: http://www.mountsinai.org/patient-care/service-areas/neurology/areas-of-care/center-for-cognitive-health
National Institutes of Health (NIH) website: www.alzheimers.gov
National Institutes of Health (NIH) National Institute on Aging Alzheimer's Disease Education and Referral Center: http://www.nia.nih.gov/alzheimers
WebMD Alzheimer's Disease Health Center: www.webmd.com/alzheimers/default.htm

Acknowledgement

The author thanks Mariel Pullman for her assistance.

Additional material for this chapter can be found online at:
www.mountsinaiexpertguides.com

This includes advice for patients, a case study, multiple choice questions, and a reading list.

CHAPTER 8

Headache

Mark W. Green
Icahn School of Medicine at Mount Sinai, New York, NY, USA

Background

Headaches are common, and 90% of people have had them. The challenge is to distinguish which headaches are primary headache syndromes, and which are symptoms of a secondary medical illness.

Secondary headaches are caused by another medical illness. The headaches can present in many ways depending upon the cause. Headaches that reach full intensity over seconds suggest subarachnoid or other intracranial hemorrhages. Those evolving over hours to days, particularly when associated with fever, suggest meningitis or other infectious causes. Those evolving over weeks to months raise concern over a mass lesion. Periodic, recurring, stereotyped attacks that have been present for some time suggest a primary, rather than a secondary cause.

The "worst headache of my life" should always raise the question of a secondary headache, although in the ED, most are migraines.

Migraine is discussed more fully in Chapter 38.

Approach to diagnosis
Getting your bearings

Primary headaches are likely to be recurrent whereas secondary headaches may have a different presentation. Historically determine an anchor in time for the disorder:
- When did these headaches begin?
- Has there been any recent change in the character and frequency of the attacks?
- How many days per month do you have ANY degree of headache?
- Primary headaches, which are benign, are likely to be recurrent. Secondary headaches are commonly progressive.

Key elements of history
- How many days per month do you have any degree of headache?
- How many days/months are the attacks functionally incapacitating?
- What symptoms accompany an attack?
- How long do the attacks last?
- How disabling are attacks? Do they interfere with routine activities? Do they require bedrest?
- What triggers an attack?
- Is there a family history of similar headaches?

Mount Sinai Expert Guides: Neurology, First Edition. Edited by Stuart C. Sealfon, Rajeev Motiwala, and Charles B. Stacy.
© 2016 John Wiley & Sons, Ltd. Published 2016 by John Wiley & Sons, Ltd.
Companion website: www.mountsinaiexpertguides.com

Table of elements of history and diseases

Headache	Symptoms	Course	Additional features
Brain tumor	Early morning headache; a worsening of a pre-existing headache type Dimness of vision upon arising, diplopia	Gradually progressive over weeks to months Only 5% with brain tumors present with headache	If known or suspected malignancy, metastases are likely; if progressive focal symptoms
Subarachnoid hemorrhage	Sudden onset of a severe head pain, often occipital	Sudden onset, reaching full intensity instantly, may resolve rapidly (low volume bleed) or last days	May occur with exertion or spontaneously
Giant cell arteritis	Scalp pain and tenderness, masseter or tongue claudication	Unremitting, often worse in cold weather	Over age of 60, feels systemically ill, more commonly affects Whites
Meningitis	Throbbing head pain with photophobia, fever	Hours to a few days, depending upon organism	Varies by organism; headache, fever, nuchal rigidity
Pseudotumor cerebri	Progression of pre-existing headaches or new headache that progresses, often sounds in head (pulsatile tinnitus), dimness of vision upon arising or diplopia common Radicular pain as elevated pressure transmitted to root sleeves	May be static or progressive over weeks to months	Commonly obese young women with menstrual irregularities. Noises in the head and pain in the shoulders are common, and upper extremity radiculopathies can occur. Diplopia, often from a VI nerve palsy, is common
Brain abscess	"Brain tumor headache" Impaired sensorium	Progressive over days to weeks	Fever seen with fewer than 50% of cases Cause variable: in young children often complication of otitis media Often a complication of a medical disorder with immunosuppression; seizures common
Low pressure headache	Headaches best or resolved when supine, worse upon arising. May be generalized and dull with nuchal rigidity	Acute onset, may resolve spontaneously May occasionally have a thunderclap onset	May follow a known cause, e.g. lumbar puncture, neurosurgical procedure, or be unknown; can be due to overshunting or use of a carbonic anhydrase inhibitor, or a remote CSF leak
POTS syndrome (postural orthostatic tachycardia syndrome)	Mixture of orthostatic and non-orthostatic headaches	Variable	Commonly thin young females Significant fatigue and palpitations can occur. May appear to have panic attacks

(Continued)

Headache	Symptoms	Course	Additional features
Exertional headaches	Head pain with exertion, including sexual activity, cough, and sneezing	Episodic, often of acute onset with the activity	May be due to tumor or other mass lesion, Chiari or other posterior fossa malformation
Cardiac cephalgia (angina)	Headache upon exertion, pain can be anywhere in head	Subsides with rest. In many cases, the headache subsides with nitroglycerin (most primary headache syndromes will worsen with this agent) Proof is EKG changes suggesting angina correlating with headache	Risk factors for coronary heart disease (CHD)
Carotid/vertebral dissection	New headache; in carotid dissections usually headache in ipsilateral face and neck. In vertebral dissections cervical and occipital pain	May resolve, but can cause cerebral infarction up to a few weeks after onset	Trauma to artery from direct injury or chiropractic manipulation; upper respiratory infection also a risk factor

---

CLINICAL PEARLS
- Brain tumor headaches and headaches of pseudotumor cerebri are both progressive, often increasing with a Valsalva maneuver, cough, or sneeze. They can cause a progression of a pre-existing headache syndrome, rather than a new headache.
- Migraines are typically worse with exertion, so the fact that exertion or leaning forward worsens the pain does not, by itself, suggest a secondary headache.
- Those with giant cell arteritis are almost always over 60 years of age, feel systemically ill with diffuse myalgias, may have jaw or tongue claudication, and pain often in the scalp, which may be tender to touch. Migraine commonly is associated with tenderness of the superficial temporal arteries as well, but has a different clinical pattern including its periodicity.

Key elements of physical examination
- A complete neurologic examination is mandatory in all patients with new or progressive headaches.
- The funduscopic evaluation may be the most important element.

Table of elements of physical examination by disease

Brain tumor	Papilledema; motor, sensory, or visual field defects; may experience transient visual obscurations or photopsias
Subarachnoid hemorrhage	Stiff neck, change in sensorium, neurologic findings vary based on cause and location of the hemorrhage
Giant cell arteritis	Scalp tenderness or allodynia, superficial temporal artery tenderness

Meningitis	Fever, stiff neck, change in sensorium
Pseudotumor cerebri	No localizing neurologic signs. Papilledema, VI nerve palsy, radicular symptoms, occasionally bruits in head on auscultation
Brain abscess	Same as brain tumor, half have fever
Carotid/vertebral dissection	Tenderness along the involved artery, Horner's syndrome in a carotid dissection
Sinusitis	Fever, tenderness overlying affected sinus, location varies based on involved sinus, purulent drainage
Hypertension	Significant elevation in blood pressure, characteristic changes on funduscopic examination

CLINICAL PEARLS
- Subarachnoid hemorrhage often causes meningeal signs of stiff neck; confirmation on CT and then LP if strongly suspected and CT negative. CT is more sensitive than MRI for an acute hemorrhage; if fluid xanthochromic, spectrophotometry is preferred test, if available.
- Meningitis presents over hours to a few days; course very variable depending upon organism: usually fever is seen, photophobia, pain on eye movements, and nuchal rigidity.
- Tenderness over superficial temporal artery is common with giant cell arteritis; scalp is allodynic, carotid artery may be tender.

Diagnostic tests

Brain tumor	Identified on CT or MRI scan, contrast preferred
Subarachnoid hemorrhage	Blood seen in CT scan; LP if negative and strongly suspected
Giant cell arteritis	Elevated CRP, ESR, biopsy of superficial temporal artery; the inflammatory markers are not always predictive of disease activity
Meningitis	CSF changes such as increased WBCs, low glucose, elevated protein; culture might identify organism
Pseudotumor cerebri	Small or normal ventricles on MRI scan, empty sellas, flattening of the posterior globes, protruding optic nerve headaches, and vertical tortuosity of optic nerves can be seen on scan and strongly suggest this diagnosis; normal CSF under elevated pressure is the hallmark (occasionally protein low)
Brain abscess	MRI or CT scan, contrast preferred
Low pressure (orthostatic) headache	Meningeal enhancement, cerebellar tonsils may be displaced downward on CT or MRI, CSF pressure low or unmeasurable. If rhinorrhea present, should be assayed for beta-2 transferrin (proving it is CSF) Cisternography or myelography may reveal source of leak
POTS	Documented with autonomic (tilt table) testing
Exertional headaches	MR to exclude mass and posterior fossa malformations
Sinusitis	Direct visualization, sinus CT (MR less sensitive)
Hypertension	Dramatic elevations in blood pressure, careful funduscopic evaluation

Table of frequency of each disease

Brain tumor	Estimated 70,000 new cases in USA/year (25,000 are malignant, 45,000 benign)
Giant cell arteritis	2 cases/10,000 person years
Meningitis	Varies widely based on causative organism
Pseudotumor cerebri	Incidence ~1.0 per 100,000 in the general population, increasing to 1.6–3.5 per 100,000 in women and to 7.9–20 per 100,000 in women who are overweight
Brain abscess	Incidence of approximately 4 per million population
Subarachnoid hemorrhage	Incidence 6 to 8 per 100,000 person-years
Low pressure (orthostatic) headache	Unknown
POTS syndrome	Unknown but estimated at least 500,000 cases in USA
Cardiac cephalgia	Rare, incidence unknown
Carotid/vertebral dissection	The annual incidence of spontaneous carotid artery dissection is 2.5–3/100,000, while the annual incidence of spontaneous vertebral artery dissection is 1–1.5/100,000

Recommended diagnostic strategy

- If headache severe or of apoplectic onset, consider subarachnoid or intracerebral hemorrhage; occasionally migraines have abrupt onset.
- If progressive over weeks to months, consider mass lesion or pseudotumor cerebri.
- If older than 60 and new headache with systemic symptoms, consider giant cell arteritis.

BOTTOM LINE
- Primary headaches are periodic and recur over long periods of time; migraine often has a positive family history.
- New headaches under age 5 and over age 50 should always be evaluated in more detail, including MRI scan, hematologic evaluation, and possibly a lumbar puncture as these groups have a high incidence of secondary causes.
- Those with a pre-existing primary headache syndrome are at higher risk of developing a headache from a secondary medical disorder; and that headache can be phenotypically similar to the original one with a recent change in its character, frequency, and duration.

Reading list
Key reading sources for this chapter can be found online at www.mountsinaiexpertguides.com

Suggested websites
American Academy of Neurology headache guidelines: https://www.aan.com/Guidelines/Home/ByTopic?topicId=16
American Headache Society: http://www.americanheadachesociety.org/
International Headache Society: http://www.ihs-headache.org/
National Headache Foundation: http://www.headaches.org

Additional material for this chapter can be found online at:
www.mountsinaiexpertguides.com

This includes advice for patients, a case study, multiple choice
questions, and a reading list.

CHAPTER 9

Abnormal Movements and Incoordination

Winona Tse

Icahn School of Medicine at Mount Sinai, New York, NY, USA

Background
Definition

Movement disorders are neurologic diseases in which the principal characteristics consist of abnormal movements. They are traditionally subdivided into two major categories:

1. Hypokinetic disorders, in which there is a paucity of movements, often with associated bradykinesia (slowness of movement), as well as a reduction in the amplitude of movement.
2. Hyperkinetic disorders, in which there is an excess of abnormal involuntary movements.

Notably, abnormal movements may also be seen in diseases of the cerebellum and its pathways, in the form of impaired coordination (ataxia), clumsiness, or tremor. More detailed information can be found in Chapters 25, 26, and 28.

Impact

Movement disorders are common in the clinic population. Essential tremor is one of the most common movement disorders. Its prevalence increases markedly with age (4.6% in people over age 65, 22% in people over age 95). The prevalence of Parkinson's disease (PD) is about 1% from ages 65 to 85, and 4.3% over age 85. PD patients experience progressive disability and a reduced quality of life. The economic burden of PD includes not only the costs related to increased inpatient and nursing home care, but also costs related to caregiver burden and lost work productivity. It has been estimated that the total annual burden of PD in the USA in 2002 was $23 billion, and by 2040 the cost of PD has been forecast to exceed $50 billion. Huntington's disease (HD), the prototypic choreic disorder, is associated with significant psychosocial burden and comorbidity and typically progresses to institutionalization.

Approach to diagnosis
Getting your bearings

- First distinguish whether the movement disorder is:
  - Hypokinetic: includes parkinsonism, spasticity, catatonia, hypothyroidism.
  - Hyperkinetic: includes dystonia, chorea, tremor, tics, athetosis, and ballism.
  - A third category to distinguish is cerebellar-type disorders, which can be either hypokinetic or hyperkinetic.
- Assess whether the movement abnormality occurs at rest, or with volitional activity, is focal or generalized, and whether the movements are repetitive, or random and unpredictable.
- Assess the duration, course, comorbidities, family history, and other neurologic findings.

Mount Sinai Expert Guides: Neurology, First Edition. Edited by Stuart C. Sealfon, Rajeev Motiwala, and Charles B. Stacy.
© 2016 John Wiley & Sons, Ltd. Published 2016 by John Wiley & Sons, Ltd.
Companion website: www.mountsinaiexpertguides.com

Hypokinetic disorders

- *Parkinsonism*: Most cases of hypokinetic disorders are due to parkinsonism. The most common cause of parkinsonism is idiopathic PD, in which there is a combination of signs of slowing and fatiguing of movement (hypokinesia), cogwheel rigidity, tremor, and a gait disturbance, typically consisting of a stooped posture, shuffling gait, and postural instability (see Video 9.1 on the companion website). In contrast to PD, atypical parkinsonism patients will have a more symmetric presentation, a more rapidly progressive course, and a lack of response to dopaminergic treatment. Examples of atypical parkinsonism syndromes include: multiple system atrophy (MSA), in which there is prominent autonomic and/or cerebellar dysfunction; corticobasal ganglion degeneration (CBGD), in which there is a profoundly asymmetric presentation with a rigid, dystonic limb; and progressive supranuclear palsy (PSP), in which there is a supranuclear vertical gaze paresis, axial more than appendicular rigidity, and early postural instability. Patients with Lewy body disease will have parkinsonism in conjunction with early dementia and drug naïve visual hallucinations.
- *Spasticity*: Slowness or paucity of movement may also be due to spasticity, in which there will be a velocity-dependent rigidity described as "clasp knife," which is most easily elicited when moving the spastic limb through a fast range of motion.
- Other causes of slow movements include weakness due to pyramidal disease, which can be elicited by doing a careful motor examination, or catatonia, in which patients may present with fixed abnormal postures (catalepsy), waxy flexibility, and bizarre behavioral abnormalities.
- Slowness of movements may also be due to incoordination (ataxia) or clumsiness of movement (dysdiadochokinesia) such as seen in cerebellar disease. Appendicular ataxia can be elicited by having the patient perform a finger-to-nose maneuver. A patient with cerebellar dysfunction will be unable to precisely pinpoint the target, instead oscillating around the target as it is approached (dysmetria). One can evaluate for dysdiadochokinesis by having the patient do rapid alternating movements. A wide-based, unsteady gait and difficulty with tandem gait are signs of midline cerebellar dysfunction.

Hyperkinetic disorders

- *Tremor* is a rhythmic, oscillatory movement that can affect one or several body parts. Tremors can occur at rest, with posture holding, or with action (see Table 9.1). The rate and amplitude vary depending on the type of tremor. Tremor at rest is classically seen in idiopathic PD. Essential tremor presents with bilateral postural and action hand tremors.
- *Chorea*, *athetosis*, and *ballism*: Chorea consists of irregular, abrupt movements that appear to flow randomly from one body part to another. Movements may affect different muscle groups in an unpredictable pattern. Huntington's disease is a prototypical choreiform disorder. Athetosis refers to slow, writhing, continuous movement, as seen in athetoid cerebral palsy (Video 9.2 on the companion website). Ballism refers to high-amplitude, proximal flinging movements. Athetosis, chorea, and ballism are thought to represent a continuum of hyperkinetic movements, in terms of velocity and amplitude of movements.
- *Dystonia* consists of involuntary, often repetitive muscle contractions that produce abnormal sustained or twisting postures. Dystonia can affect focal body regions or be generalized. Generalized dystonia tends to have onset in childhood or early adulthood, while focal dystonias such as cervical dystonia or blepharospasm have onset in adulthood and tend to remain focal (Videos 9.2, 9.3, and 9.4 on the companion website).
- *Myoclonus* refers to sudden, brief, shock-like movements, which can occur at rest as well as with movements. It can occur focally, in a segmental body region, or may be generalized. It is often stimulus sensitive and exacerbated by volitional movement (Video 9.5 on the companion website).

Table 9.1 Common types of tremors.

Type of tremor	Features
Rest tremor	4–6 Hz, "pill rolling," typically seen in PD
Enhanced physiologic tremor	A fine, high-frequency (8–12 Hz) bilateral tremor seen in outstretched arms, exacerbated by fatigue, anxiety, hyperthyroidism
Essential tremor	4–12 Hz bilateral arm tremors that occur with posture or with action, may have head or voice tremor, alcohol responsive
Cerebellar tremor	1–4 Hz action tremor. Amplitude of tremor increases as movement approaches the target (intention tremor), may have associated ataxia
Dystonic tremor	Seen in limb affected with dystonia, may have variable frequency and amplitude
Rubral tremor (midbrain, Holme's tremor)	Irregular, 2–5 Hz proximal > distal tremor, with resting, postural, and action components

- *Tics* are stereotyped, involuntary, repetitive quick movements that tend to affect one or a few muscle groups in a recurrent pattern. Tics can consist of abnormal movements (motor tics) or abnormal sounds (vocal tics), and are associated with a premonitory sensory urge or discomfort that is alleviated once the tic occurs. They can be suppressed briefly, although a flurry of tics will often emerge afterwards. Examples of tics include eye blinking, sniffing, and shoulder shrugging.
- *Paroxysmal disorders* are hyperkinetic disorders that occur transiently and paroxysmally. These disorders can be brought on by movement (paroxysmal kinesigenic dyskinesia) or induced by fatigue, caffeine, or alcohol intake (paroxysmal non-kinesigenic dyskinesia).
- *Akathisia* is a sense of inner restlessness, in which patients will engage in movements such as body rocking, crossing and uncrossing the legs, and getting out of the chair to pace. Performing the movements alleviates the restless sensations. Akathisia often occurs as an acute drug-induced syndrome, as seen with neuroleptic exposure, or as a tardive phenomenon.
- *Cerebellar ataxia*: Signs of ataxia include dysmetria, dysdiadochokinesis, and a broad-based, unsteady gait. There may be a postural or action tremor that increases in amplitude as the target is progressively approached (intention tremor). There may also be a slow frequency bobbing head movement (titubation).

Key elements of history
- Is there a family history? What is the medication history?
- Was the onset gradual or sudden, and what is the rate of progression?
- What is the predominant movement abnormality? What are the other associated neurologic features?
- Which body parts are affected?
- Do the abnormal movements occur at rest or with movements?
- Is the condition alcohol responsive?
- Are there factors that improve or worsen the movement?

Table of movement disorders and their symptoms

Movement disorder	Symptoms	Course of Illness
Hypokinetic movement disorders		

Parkinsonism:
  1. Idiopathic PD
  2. Atypical parkinsonism:
    • Multiple system atrophy (MSA)
    • Progressive supranuclear palsy (PSP)
    • Corticobasal ganglion degeneration (CBGD)
	1. Combination of tremor at rest, bradykinesia, cogwheel rigidity, and postural instability is seen in idiopathic PD
	2. MSA patients may have dizziness upon standing, bowel/bladder urgency or incontinence, and/or clumsiness of movements and gait. PSP presents with frequent falls early in disease course, and visual problems. Patients with CBGD complain of a "jerky" stiff arm, and may also present with cognitive difficulties
		Parkinson's disease patients have a slowly progressive, chronic course. PD symptom onset is unilateral and spreads to the other side slowly over time. Atypical parkinsonism patients tend to have a more symmetric presentation and a more rapidly progressive disease course than do PD patients

Spasticity	May have slowness of voluntary movement associated with stiffness and muscle spasms	Course of illness usually static and chronic, since spasticity is the result of brain or spinal cord injury
Hypothyroid slowness	May have slowness of voluntary movement associated with stiffness and muscle spasms. Patients may complain of fatigue and weakness, which appears out of proportion to examination. Systemic hypothyroid complaints may also include cold intolerance, weight gain, hair loss, dry skin, cognitive problems, and psychosis	Thyroid replacement treatment should improve symptoms, but neuromuscular and psychiatric complications may take months to resolve
Catatonia	Behavioral syndrome consisting of a combination of immobility, abnormal posturing, mutism, and bizarre behavior. Patients may appear awake but with minimal or no verbal response to questions	Milder cases have generally good prognosis after treatment with benzodiazepines and ECT. Malignant cases require admission to an intensive care unit for autonomic instability and can be associated with permanent morbidity
Hyperkinetic movement disorders		
Tremor	Rhythmic, oscillatory movements of a body part, "shaking"	May occur at rest or with movement of affected body part. Often worsened with stress, anxiety
Chorea	Irregular, quick movements that flow randomly from one body part to another, "dancelike" movements	Course of illness depends on etiology
Athetosis	Writhing, slow continuous movements More sustained and flowing than chorea Non-patterned, unlike dystonia	Course of illness depends on etiology. It is typically static when due to athetotic cerebral palsy

(Continued)

Movement disorder	Symptoms	Course of Illness
Ballism	Severe, large-amplitude, flinging movements	Depending on the underlying cause, hemiballismus generally has a good prognosis. Many patients experience spontaneous improvement over time
Myoclonus	Quick shock-like movements, "lightning quick"	Course of illness depends on etiology
Tics	Abrupt, stereotyped movements that affect one or a few muscle groups in a recurrent pattern, producing abnormal movements (motor tics) or sounds (vocal tic)	Tics due to Tourette's syndrome resolve in adulthood in about half of cases. If persistent in adulthood, their severity often diminishes over time
Dystonia	Sustained contractions of agonist/antagonist muscles producing abnormal twisting postures	Focal dystonia presenting in adulthood tends to remain focal. Childhood-onset dystonia can present focally and quickly generalize. Dystonia can also be categorized as *primary* (dystonia is the main symptom and no secondary cause is found) or *secondary* (dystonia is secondary to another cause), which may include heredodegenerative etiologies (neuronal brain iron accumulation (NBIA), Wilson's disease, etc.)

CLINICAL PEARLS
- Sometimes, a combination of hypo- and hyperkinetic movement disorders can coexist.
- It is important to identify the dominant movement abnormality first, then evaluate the other accompanying movement abnormalities, which will help further hone the diagnosis.
- The age of onset of the illness can be helpful in the evaluation. For example, typical age of onset for Parkinson's disease is 60 years of age, while most forms of generalized dystonia of genetic etiology (e.g. due to DYT1 dystonia) begin in childhood.
- In dystonia, a family history is supportive of a DYT1 or other underlying genetic mutation, especially when the dystonia onset is before age 26.
- Family history is usually present in essential tremor.
- Always evaluate medication history to rule out drug-induced as well as tardive syndromes. Some disorders are very alcohol responsive, such as essential tremor or the myoclonus dystonia syndrome.

Key elements of physical examination

The patient should be observed at rest, with posture-holding with the arms outstretched, as well as in performing actions, such as finger-to-nose maneuvers and rapid alternating movements. Muscle tone and strength should be assessed. Ability to get up from a chair, gait, posture, and postural stability should be assessed. A "pull test" can be done to assess stability of posture. In parkinsonism, gait is short stepped, and shuffling. In more advanced cases, there may be a sudden stoppage while walking, where the patient is unable to initiate a step momentarily (freezing of gait). Gait in cerebellar lesions is wide based and unsteady, with an inability to tandem walk. Evaluation of writing and drawing of a spiral can be helpful. Patients with parkinsonism will typically have small handwriting (micrographia) and small spirals (Figure 9.1) while essential tremor patients exhibit tremor in their handwriting and spiral drawings (Figure 9.2).

Table of movement disorders and physical examination findings

Movement disorder	Velocity/duration of movements	Anatomical distribution and other features
Hypokinetic movement disorders		

Parkinsonism:
1. Idiopathic PD
2. Atypical parkinsonism
  • MSA
  • PSP
  • CBGD
	Movements are both slow in velocity and low amplitude, with progressive fatiguing and decrement in amplitude. There is slowness in initiation of movement (bradykinesia)	PD patients typically present with a unilateral rest tremor, cogwheel rigidity, and slowness of movement. Gait is slow and shuffling, with a stooped posture. In later stages there is postural instability. MSA patients may have orthostatic hypotension on exam, cerebellar abnormalities such as appendicular or gait ataxia, and/or corticospinal tract dysfunction
		PSP patients have a characteristic supranuclear gaze palsy, with an inability to voluntarily initiate vertical saccades. There is also severe increased axial tone with postural instability early in disease course, dementia, and emotional incontinence (pseudobulbar palsy)
		CBGD patients have a severely dystonic arm, sometimes with superimposed myoclonus. There may be signs of focal apraxia ("alien limb") or cortical sensory loss in the affected limb. There may be associated dementia

Spasticity	Is a velocity-dependent increase in muscle tone, a "clasp knife" phenomenon	Due to dysfunction of the corticospinal tract. Tends to affect arm flexors and leg extensors predominantly Associated with other signs of corticospinal tract dysfunction, such as weakness, hyperreflexia, and Babinski's sign
Hypothyroid slowness	Voluntary movements are slowed	Additional signs of hypothyroid state may be present such as low temperature, bradycardia, weight gain, and delayed relaxation of deep tendon reflexes
Catatonia	In addition to prolonged hypokinesis or akinesis, there may also be excessive motor activity, echolalia and mutism	May be seen in setting of psychiatric and medical disorders

(Continued)

Movement disorder	Velocity/duration of movements	Anatomical distribution and other features
Hyperkinetic movement disorders		
Tremor	Velocity and amplitude vary depending of type of tremor	Can affect distal or proximal body parts. Can occur at rest, with posture holding, or with actions Is due to parkinsonism when seen in conjunction with cogwheel rigidity and bradykinesia
Chorea	Quick, non-rhythmic, and non-sustained	Movements are usually distal May occur focally, unilaterally ("hemichorea"), or generalized Can be accentuated by having patient perform a motor activity with an unaffected body part, called "overflow" Typical disorder is Huntington's chorea
Athetosis	Slow, non-patterned Tends to be slower than chorea	Often affects limbs distally but can also affect axial muscles, i.e. face, tongue, head May have "overflow" phenomena (see "Chorea" above) Seen in athetoid cerebral palsy
Ballism	Usually fast, forceful movements	Proximal extremities involved Typically hemibody is involved, i.e. "hemiballismus," but can occur bilaterally or in one limb
Myoclonus	Quick and brief Usually arrhythmic, but can be rhythmic	Can be focal, multifocal, segmental or generalized Can occur at rest or with movements May be stimulus sensitive, i.e. cortical myoclonus can be provoked by tactile or auditory stimuli
Tics	Quick, sudden, intermittent non-rhythmic movements, which are patterned	Typically affects the same set of muscles in a recurrent pattern. Often affects face, eyes, upper arms/shoulders Associated with sensory urge or discomfort prior to the tic, with alleviation after the tic occurs. Can be suppressed momentarily, unlike other hyperkinetic disorders Examples include head shaking, shoulder shrugs, eye blinking, or sniffing sounds
Dystonia	Can be fast or slow, with patterned movements Can occur with action or at rest. Can be task specific	May be focal, segmental, unilateral, multifocal, or generalized May have a "sensory trick" May have task specificity May have "overflow" phenomena (see "Chorea" above)

CLINICAL PEARLS
- While tremor is a hyperkinesia, when it occurs at rest in the setting of bradykinesia, rigidity, and postural stability, it is part of the syndrome of parkinsonism.
- Patients with hypothyroidism have a slowness of muscle contraction and relaxation, resulting in muscle stiffness and slowed movements, as well as a slowed relaxation of their tendon reflexes ("hung up reflex"), seen particularly in the ankle jerks.
- Are the movements jerky or non-jerky? Jerky movements include chorea, myoclonus, tics, and cerebellar ataxia. Non-jerky movements include dystonia and tremor.
- Assess whether the movements are stereotyped, or irregular and random, as well as their velocity and duration.
  - Choreiform movements are irregular and random, while tics and dystonia tend to affect muscle groups in a stereotyped pattern.
  - Dystonia tends to be of longer duration than either myoclonus or chorea, while myoclonus tends to be "lightning-quick."

Diagnostic tests recommended for common movement disorders

Parkinsonism	MRI brain, testing for ceruloplasmin and copper studies (young onset cases), slit-lamp examination, HD gene and HIV testing (young onset cases). Consider DAT scan[a] (to differentiate from essential tremor (ET))
Dystonia	MRI brain, consider levodopa trial and genetic testing for DYT5 dystonia to rule out dopa-responsive dystonia. If familial, consider test for *DYT1* or other DYT mutations. Also consider evaluation of CSF for infection (meningitis, encephalitis), HIV, ceruloplasmin, copper studies, gene testing for SCA, test for NBIA, consider tests for metabolic inherited disorders such as Niemann–Pick disease.
Chorea	If familial, consider HD test, test for SCA 17. If sporadic, consider antistreptolysin titer, MRI brain, antinuclear antibody (ANA), antiphospholipid antibody (Ab), thyroid function tests (TFTs), CBC with platelets (plts), ceruloplasmin, HIV, peripheral blood smear for acanthocytes, anti-CRMP5 Ab in patients with small-cell lung cancer (paraneoplastic)
Myoclonus	MRI brain, CSF, EEG, rule out metabolic abnormalities, i.e. renal function, LFTs, electrolytes, heavy metal screen
Tics	MRI brain, CSF for infection, copper studies
Tremor	Consider test for Wilson's disease (copper studies, ceruloplasmin), thyroid function tests, MRI brain
Ataxia	If familial, consider test for SCAs, Friedreich's ataxia, ataxia telangiectasia, or fragile X tremor ataxia syndrome. If sporadic, consider MRI brain, vitamin E level, CSF for infection, antigliadin Ab, colon biopsy

CRMP = collapsin response mediator protein; DAT = dopamine transporter.
[a] A DAT scan uses injection of [^{123}I]ioflupane, a radioactive imaging agent that serves as a visual marker of dopamine transporter density.

Prevalence of movement disorders (per 100,000 in the population)

Parkinson's disease	102–190
Idiopathic torsion (generalized) dystonia	3.4
Idiopathic adult-onset focal dystonia	30
Essential tremor	300
Tourette's syndrome	30–50
PSP	5.3
MSA	2–5
Huntington's disease	2–12

Recommended diagnostic strategy

See the algorithms 9.1 and 9.2 for the differential diagnosis of the major types of movement disorders.

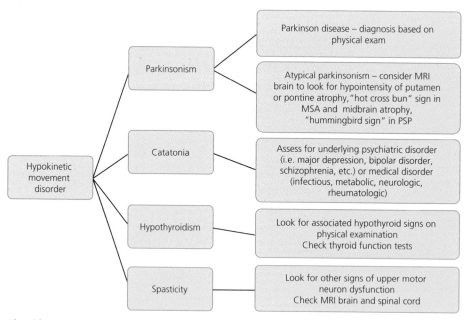

Algorithm 9.1 Hypokinetic movement disorders.

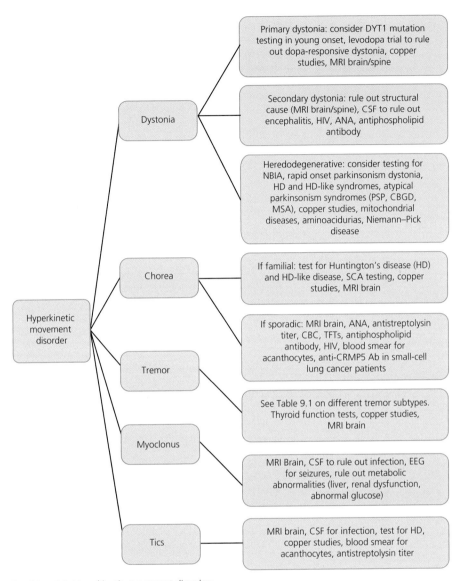

Algorithm 9.2 Hyperkinetic movement disorders.

BOTTOM LINE
- Try to determine the predominant movement abnormality. Is it a hypo- or hyperkinetic movement disorder?
- Evaluate factors such as the regularity and velocity of the movement and provoking factors, as well as which body regions are affected.
- There may be more than one type of abnormal movement present, and hypokinetic and hyperkinetic disorders can coexist in some syndromes.
- Defining the specific movement type will aid in generating the appropriate differential diagnosis, which will lead to the proper diagnostic workup and treatment.

Images

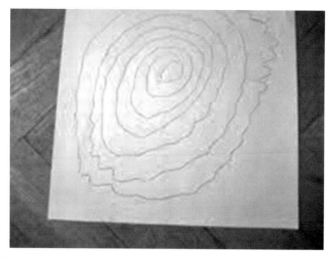

Figure 9.1 Parkinson's disease. This spiral was drawn by a patient with advanced, tremor-predominant Parkinson's disease. The spiral shows re-emergence of tremor near the end of the spiral drawing. There is also a mild asymmetry to the spiral.

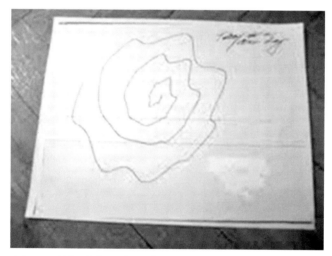

Figure 9.2 Essential tremor. This spiral was drawn by a patient with longstanding essential tremor. His handwritten sentence is illegible due to the tremor.

Reading list

Key reading sources for this chapter can be found online at www.mountsinaiexpertguides.com

Suggested websites

International Parkinson and Movement Disorder Society: www.movementdisorders.org

Additional material for this chapter can be found online at:
www.mountsinaiexpertguides.com

This includes a case study, multiple choice questions, a reading list, and Videos 9.1, 9.2, 9.3, 9.4, and 9.5.

CHAPTER 10

Sleep Disorders, Somnolence, and Fatigue

Charles B. Stacy
Icahn School of Medicine at Mount Sinai, New York, NY, USA

Background
Definition

Sleep disorders refer not only to the direct complaints of difficulty falling asleep and of interrupted, insufficient, or unrefreshing sleep, but also to conditions of which the patient may be unaware since they occur only during sleep.

Somnolence, or sleepiness, can be felt as the increased tendency to fall asleep or as the inability to maintain alertness, both of which may interfere with function. It is common with sleep disorders, but may be the consequence of many other diseases and conditions as well.

Fatigue can refer to a specifically muscular sensation, but more often it encompasses emotional elements or a sense of lack of energy. Mental fatigue may occur separately, but often all aspects are combined into a single experience. To the neurologist, the complaint of fatigue, like that of dizziness, is highly ambiguous, since what it conveys and what mechanisms it implies are so diverse.

Impact

- Sleepiness is reported by 35% of the general population.
- At least 10% of the general population suffers from a sleep disorder that is clinically or socially significant.
- Among sleep disorders, insomnia is the most common, followed by sleep-disordered breathing, then restless legs syndrome or periodic limb movements of sleep.
- In specific populations shift work disorder or jet lag may be prevalent.
- The global economic impact of sleep disorders related to job performance deficits is estimated in direct costs at hundreds of billions of dollars annually, while the indirect toll on exacerbated medical conditions may be equally significant.
- The social impact on quality of life is inestimable, but specific attribution of sleep disorders to situations such as traffic accidents (20%), for instance, has been possible.
- Fatigue has an estimated incidence of 38% in the general population, and 42% among those presenting to a primary care physician. In specific populations such as those with rheumatoid arthritis or multiple sclerosis, the numbers are even higher.
- Lost productivity in the USA attributed to fatigue costs $136 billion annually.
- Fatigue is the major determinant of quality of life for many patients.

Mount Sinai Expert Guides: Neurology, First Edition. Edited by Stuart C. Sealfon, Rajeev Motiwala, and Charles B. Stacy.
© 2016 John Wiley & Sons, Ltd. Published 2016 by John Wiley & Sons, Ltd.
Companion website: www.mountsinaiexpertguides.com

Approach to diagnosis
Getting your bearings
- The complaint of a patient with a sleep disorder may be insomnia, daytime sleepiness, or nocturnal disturbances, and these can occur in any combination.
- The bed partner is an essential source of information.
- Assessment of fatigue should be based on objective parameters of function whenever possible, such as maximum duration of sustained activity or hours of sleep required. When the complaint is muscle fatigue, what is important is not what can be achieved momentarily with maximal effort, but rather any difficulty in sustaining activity during the daily routine.

Key elements of history
- Obtain from the patient or partner objective sleep data such as: bedtime on weekdays and weekends, wake times in both circumstances, delay in sleep onset, number and duration of awakenings, morning feelings of being refreshed or not, morning fogginess or headache, presence and character of snoring, choking, cessation of breathing, behavioral arousals, frequent leg movements or violent bodily activity, and confusion.
- Try to clarify daytime sleepiness as to times of occurrence, specific situations, interference with work, accidents caused by sleepiness, trouble with concentration or recall, and the presence of naps. Enquire about cataplexy, hallucinations, and sleep paralysis.
- List medications taken for medical conditions as well as for sleep.
- Explore bodily symptoms that might affect sleep, such as pain, pruritus, dyspnea, gastric reflux, nasal congestion, or palpitations.
- In the case of fatigue, ask about weakness, endurance, increased need for rest, interference with daily function, the presence of pain, and the present or past use of medications.

Table of elements of history and diseases

Disorder	Symptoms	Course	Circumstances
Insomnia	Delay in sleep onset, frequent awakenings, unrefreshing sleep, daytime somnolence and fatigue	Situational – concurrent stressors Chronic psychophysiologic – more than 6 months	Anxiety, depression, medical illness Poor sleep hygiene, habits
Obstructive sleep apnea	Unrefreshing sleep, snoring, choking, excessive daytime sleepiness	Years of snoring, escalating tiredness	Bed partner notes apnea, choking, snoring; weight gain, cardiovascular disease
Central sleep apnea	Nocturnal arousals, daytime somnolence	Acute altitude sickness or follows course of cardiorespiratory compromise	Cheyne–Stokes respiration, high altitude, respiratory depressant medication
Restless legs syndrome or periodic limb movements of sleep	Arousals, spousal complaints, often restless legs in evening	Chronic, but exacerbated by concurrent factors	Idiopathic, but more with neuropathy, myelopathy, and other conditions causing leg pain
Narcolepsy	Daytime sleep attacks, cataplexy, sleep paralysis, disturbed sleep, hypnogogic hallucinations	Onset at puberty, peak 15–25, then 35–45	Does not always include full tetrad; cataplexy in 60%, REM (rapid eye movement) onset

(Continued)

Disorder	Symptoms	Course	Circumstances
Idiopathic hypersomnia	Daytime sleep attacks	Rare, chronic; several forms; periodic in Kleine–Levin syndrome	No REM-linked phenomena
Sleep in neurodegenerative diseases	Fragmented sleep, daytime somnolence, confusional or hallucinatory episodes	Accompanies course of degeneration	Alzheimer's, fronto-temporal dementia, Parkinson's, multiple systems atrophy, progressive supranuclear palsy, Lewy body dementia, Huntington's, spinocerebellar atrophy type 3
Shift work disorder, jet lag	Somnolence, insomnia, fatigue	Acute and situational	Readjustment time proportionate to dislocation and individual factors
REM behavior disorder	Vivid dreams with life-and-death struggles, spousal or self-injuries	Follows stroke or neurodegenerative disease	May herald neurodegenerative decline
Chronic fatigue syndrome	Debilitating fatigue, unrelieved by sleep or rest, exertional malaise, with many associated systemic symptoms	May follow viral syndrome, onset 25–45, female 2 × male, may improve partly over time	Difficulty concentrating, headache, sore throat, myalgias, arthralgias, sleep disturbance, mood disorder, GI complaints
Fibromyalgia syndrome	Impaired sleep quality in 80%; widespread musculoskeletal pain for >3 months, plus tenderness at 11 or more anatomical soft tissue sites covering all quadrants	Onset may occur with systemic illness, rarely remits, 80% female	Large overlap with chronic fatigue syndrome, but pain and tenderness predominate
Neuromuscular weakness	Fatigue is common presentation	Depends on disorder	See Chapter 15
Systemic disorders (e.g. cardiorespiratory, cancer)	Disease-specific presentations; fatigue and sleep disturbance may strongly affect quality of life	Depends on disorder	Always look for an underlying disorder

CLINICAL PEARLS
- Determine what happens at night, which might be unrecognized or distorted by the patient.
- Define the impact on daily function.
- Understand the context of systemic or neurologic disease.

Key elements of physical examination
- Assess alertness during the interview and in the waiting room.
- Note spontaneous activity or avoidance.
- Observe body morphology – obesity, neck configuration, mandibular position, breathing style.
- Determine neuromuscular condition – strength, tone, bulk, mobility.
- Detect tenderness by manipulation and palpation.

Table of elements of physical examination by disease

Disorder	Examination features
Insomnia	Emotional state, evidence of sleep deficit, effects of hypnotics or stimulants
Obstructive sleep apnea	Obesity, micrognathia, thick or short neck, oral breathing, chronic sleep deficit
Central sleep apnea	No particular habitus; hypersomnolence; evidence of low cardiac output, hypoxia, or neuromuscular disorder
Restless legs syndrome or periodic limb movements of sleep	May show restless legs sitting still; presence of neuropathy, myelopathy, vascular disease, arthritis, or cutaneous disorder in legs
Narcolepsy	Irresistible sleep attacks; attempt to elicit cataplexy
Idiopathic hypersomnia	Sleep attacks; sometimes associated bizarre behavior
Sleep in neurodegenerative disorders	Look for evidence of dementia, parkinsonism, abnormal eye movements, dystonia and dyskinesia, muscle atrophy, weakness, dysarthria or pseudobulbar affect
Shift work disorder, jet lag	No specific features
REM behavior disorder	Signs of CNS dysfunction, including dementia, loss of fine motor control, and personality change
Chronic fatigue syndrome	Dysautonomia (orthostasis, tachycardia); poor muscle tone, dysphoria
Fibromyalgia syndrome	Tender points in all quadrants to palpation at specific sites
Neuromuscular weakness	Paresis, atrophy, myopathic habitus, decline of strength on repetition, loss of voice quality
Systemic disease (e.g. cardiorespiratory, cancer)	Evidence of systemic disease

---

CLINICAL PEARLS
- Observe the behavior and activity of the patient, as well as habitus and breathing.
- Examine for neuromuscular or CNS dysfunction.
- Pay special attention to cardiorespiratory and autonomic features.

Diagnostic tests

Several tests are applicable to sleep disorders in general:

- Polysomnogram – a recording of multiple channels of data to capture the elements of sleep and its disturbances. The elements are: several channels of EEG, eye movement, EKG, respiratory air flow at mouth and nares, chest movement, muscle activity in submental and limb muscles, oxygen saturation, auditory and visual monitors, and (optionally) actigraphy (body motion detection) and esophageal and nasal pressure.
- Multiple sleep latency test (MSLT) – recording of EEG, eye movements, and submental EMG with the subject reclining in a quiet, dark room instructed to allow themselves to fall asleep, in a series of nap opportunities at 2-hour intervals.
- Maintenance of wakefulness test – recording of the above channels while the subject sits in a dim room instructed to resist sleep.

Table of diagnostic tests for specific disorders

Disorder	Tests
Insomnia	Polysomnogram, sleep diary, depression and anxiety rating scales
Obstructive sleep apnea	Polysomnogram, multiple sleep latency test, ENT evaluation, pulmonary function tests, maintenance of wakefulness test for safety concerns, continuous positive airway pressure (CPAP) trial
Central sleep apnea	Polysomnogram, echocardiogram, pulmonary function tests, MRI brain, CPAP trial
Restless legs syndrome or periodic limb movements of sleep	Polysomnogram, may need EMG and NCS, MRI brain or spine
Narcolepsy	EEG (sleep onset REM), polysomnogram, multiple sleep latency test, maintenance of wakefulness test, consider under special circumstances genetic testing, CSF hypocretin assay (low)
Idiopathic hypersomnia	Polysomnogram, multiple sleep latency test, MRI brain, CSF hypocretin (normal)
Sleep in neurodegenerative disorders	MRI brain, polysomnogram, PET scan, CPAP trial
Shift work disorder, jet lag	Polysomnogram, multiple sleep latency test, sleep diary
REM behavior disorder	Polysomnogram, MRI brain
Chronic fatigue syndrome	Polysomnogram, sleep and activities diary, depression and other mood inventories, tilt table test
Fibromyalgia syndrome	Above, plus screening blood tests for rheumatologic disorders, standardized palpatory testing of points in all quadrants
Neuromuscular weakness	See Chapter 15; pulmonary function tests, specifically vital capacity, negative inspiratory force (NIF) and maximum expiratory force (MEF)
Systemic disease (e.g. cardiorespiratory, cancer)	Nocturnal oximetry and EKG monitor, or polysomnogram; hemoglobin, metabolic panel, thyroid functions, echocardiogram

Table of frequency of each disease

Disorder	Frequency
Insomnia	Common (30%), increases with age or illness
Obstructive sleep apnea	4% in men, 1.2% in women, with daytime somnolence and apnea-hypopnea index >10
Central sleep apnea	Rare, depends on concurrent CNS or cardiac disease
Restless legs syndrome or periodic limb movements of sleep	3–5% of population
Narcolepsy	25–50 per 100,000
Idiopathic hypersomnia	Rare
Sleep in neurodegenerative disorders	Incidence increases with severity of each disorder
Shift work disorder, jet lag	One-third of night shift workers; a quarter of those on rotating shifts
REM behavior disorder	0.5%, associated with neurologic disorders
Chronic fatigue syndrome	0.4–1.5%, depending on criteria
Fibromyalgia syndrome	2%, women 4 × more common than in men
Neuromuscular weakness	Depends on specific disorder
Systemic disease (e.g. cardiorespiratory, cancer)	Fatigue extremely common in advanced disease

BOTTOM LINE
- The most complete analysis comes from the polysomnogram, since it details not only the quality and sufficiency of sleep, but also those factors responsible for its disruption.
- Practically, glean as much information as possible from the patient's sleep history and that of the bed partner or other observer.
- Most of these conditions are long-standing, but usually not obvious; index of suspicion is needed to decipher the cause from the complaint.
- The urgency of treatment varies.
- Sleep disorders have a major impact on quality of life and mortality risk.

Reading list
Key reading sources for this chapter can be found online at www.mountsinaiexpertguides.com

Suggested websites
American Academy of Sleep Medicine: aasmet.org
Centers for Disease Control and Prevention information on chronic fatigue syndrome: cdc.gov/cfs

Additional material for this chapter can be found online at:
www.mountsinaiexpertguides.com

This includes a case study, multiple choice questions, and
a reading list.

CHAPTER 11

Visual Loss and Double Vision

Janet C. Rucker

NYU Langone Medical Center, New York, NY, USA

Background
Definition
Visual loss and double vision (diplopia) can be caused by problems in different anatomic locations; thus, the critical first step is to determine the location of the problem prior to considering the possible etiologies. With both chief complaints, determining if the problem is present in one or both eyes is key. The patient with vision loss may describe shadows, blurring, flashes, and areas of missing vision. The patient with a neurologic cause of double vision will generally see two of everything, but occasionally will complain of blurred vision that resolves when either eye is covered.

Impact
It is difficult to quantify the incidence, economic impact, or social impact of vision loss and double vision, given the large number of causes for each symptom. However, given that many conditions causing these symptoms affect young persons and may limit the ability to drive and perform work-related activities, they certainly have a large potential economic and social impact on society.

Approach to diagnosis
Getting your bearings
- The first step in evaluating a patient with vision loss or double vision is to determine if the problem is present in one eye or both eyes.
- Vision loss in one eye is due to either an eye problem or an optic nerve problem.
- Vision loss in both eyes may be due to a simultaneous problem in both eyes, or both optic nerves, or to a problem in the chiasm or retrochiasmal visual pathways.
- For double vision to have a neurologic cause, it should be confirmed that the patient has binocular double vision. In other words, the double vision should resolve completely when either eye is covered.
- It is essential to determine localization for vision loss or double vision before considering the possible underlying causative process.
- Monocular double vision is almost always ocular or psychogenic, not neurologic.

Key elements of history
A thorough history is critical but it is helpful to emphasize the following key questions:
- Is the vision loss or double vision present in one eye or both?
- Is binocular double vision horizontal, vertical, or oblique? Is it worse in a certain gaze direction?
- What is the time course (e.g. acute, subacute, chronic, progressive, stable)?
- Is there pain (e.g. headache, eye pain, pain with eye movement)?

Mount Sinai Expert Guides: Neurology, First Edition. Edited by Stuart C. Sealfon, Rajeev Motiwala, and Charles B. Stacy.
© 2016 John Wiley & Sons, Ltd. Published 2016 by John Wiley & Sons, Ltd.
Companion website: www.mountsinaiexpertguides.com

- Are there any other neurologic symptoms present (e.g. proximal muscle weakness, sensory changes, ptosis, facial weakness, ataxia)?
- Is there a history of medical illness that would predispose a patient to certain problems (e.g. autoimmune disease, malignancy, vascular risk factors, etc.)?

Table of elements of history and diseases

Disease	Symptoms	Duration/tempo	Key features
Vision loss			
Retinal ischemia	Painless partial or complete vision loss in one eye	May be transient (lasting minutes) or acute and persistent (retinal artery infarction). If persistent, vision loss often permanent	History of vascular risk factors (hypertension, diabetes, hyperlipidemia, smoking). If elderly, ask about symptoms of temporal arteritis (headache, scalp tenderness, jaw claudication)
Optic neuritis	Painful central vision loss in one eye. Pain increases with eye movement. May describe loss of color vision	Acute/subacute. Vision loss spontaneously resolves over weeks to months	Young patient. Often, no other neurologic symptoms. May be feature of multiple sclerosis
Non-arteritic anterior ischemic optic neuropathy	Painless vision loss in one eye. Pattern of vision loss may be top or bottom half of vision or all of vision	Acute. Patient often awakens with the vision loss. Vision loss often permanent	Older patient. History of vascular risk factors (hypertension, diabetes, hyperlipidemia, smoking)
Arteritic anterior ischemic optic neuropathy (temporal arteritis)	Severe vision loss in one eye. No eye pain, but headache often present. Severe vision loss may occur in other eye if undiagnosed and untreated	Acute; permanent	Elderly patient. 70% have systemic symptoms, including scalp tenderness, jaw claudication, weight loss, neck pain, myalgias, fatigue
Neoplasm (e.g. optic nerve meningioma or glioma, orbital metastasis)	Vision loss in one eye. Proptosis may be present	Chronic and progressive	Double vision if extraocular muscles or ocular motor cranial nerves involved
Leber's hereditary optic neuropathy	Painless central vision loss in one eye, often followed by the other in weeks to months	Acute/subacute. Permanent, though spontaneous improvement may occur	Classically in young men, though may occur in men > women at any age. Family history with maternal (mitochondrial) transmission
Idiopathic intracranial hypertension	May or may not complain of vision loss. Transient visual obscurations, pulsatile tinnitus, headache. May develop severe vision loss if untreated	Onset often difficult to determine. Often insidious-onset headaches	Obese young women. If other neurologic symptoms present, consider intracranial mass lesion. If atypical patient (thin, male, older), consider cerebral venous thrombosis

(Continued)

Disease	Symptoms	Duration/tempo	Key features
Sarcoidosis	Vision loss in one or both eyes. May affect any segment of visual pathways, from retina to optic nerve to chiasm to intracranial visual pathways. Painless	Subacute	Consider especially in Black patients with recurrent or atypical optic neuritis, though sarcoidosis may occur in other patient populations. If diffuse, may have other neurologic symptoms
Pituitary adenoma and other sellar lesions (meningioma, craniopharyngioma)	Vision loss bitemporally and/or centrally, if optic nerves also involved. Headache frequent	Chronic	May present with abrupt blindness and ptosis with ocular motor deficits in setting of pituitary apoplexy
Stroke	Vision loss in same portion of vision in each eye (homonymous hemianopia). Typically painless	Acute	History of vascular risk factors (hypertension, diabetes, hyperlipidemia, smoking)
Posterior reversible leukoencephalopathy syndrome (RPLS, PRES)	Severe vision loss in both eyes due to bilateral intracranial visual pathway involvement. Often painless	Acute/subacute. Usually reversible	Severe hypertension, eclampsia, certain immunosuppressive agents – e.g. ciclosporin (cyclosporine), tacrolimus. Seizures may be present
Brain tumor	Vision loss in both eyes from papilledema or homonymous hemianopia, headache, seizures, progressive neurologic dysfunction	Subacute	History of systemic malignancy or previously treated brain tumor
Binocular double vision			
Thyroid eye disease	Horizontal or vertical double vision, proptosis, dry eyes, eye swelling, poor eye closure. Occasionally with vision loss from optic nerve compression	Subacute or chronic	May occur with hyperthyroid, hypothyroid, or euthyroid states. Often without known thyroid disorder at time of ocular presentation
Chronic progressive external ophthalmoplegia	Horizontal or vertical double vision. Ptosis. Painless	Slowly progressive	Mitochondrial disease, myopathy, cardiac conduction defects, short stature, hearing loss, diabetes
Myasthenia gravis	Fluctuating double vision – may alternate horizontal and vertical; ptosis, with or without proximal muscle weakness	Acute, subacute, or chronic. Symptoms worsen as day progresses	May occur as isolated ocular myasthenia or in setting of generalized myasthenia. Consider botulism if pupils affected

Disease	Symptoms	Duration/tempo	Key features
Oculomotor nerve palsy (cranial nerve III)[a]	Oblique double vision with or without ptosis. Painful or painless	Acute, subacute, or chronic	Any lesion along course of nerve. Compression by posterior communicating artery aneurysm common – painful, pupil often dilated. Microvascular ischemia common – painful, pupil not involved
Abducens nerve palsy (cranial nerve VI)[a]	Horizontal double vision worse in direction of weak muscle or affected nerve. Painful or painless	Acute, subacute, or chronic	Any lesion along course of nerve. If in isolation and painful in older patient, microvascular ischemia likely. May occur as a false localizing sign in setting of raised intracranial pressure, sometimes bilateral
Trochlear nerve palsy (cranial nerve IV)[a]	Vertical double vision. Painful or painless. Tilting head to one side	Acute, subacute, or chronic	Any lesion along course of nerve. Congenital lesions common – look for long-standing head tilt on old photographs
Skew deviation	Vertical double vision. Typically painless	Acute, subacute, or chronic	Often due to brainstem or cerebellar lesion. Occurs rarely with peripheral vestibular disease
Multiple sclerosis	Horizontal double vision with internuclear ophthalmoplegia may occur. Painless	Acute, subacute, or chronic	Other mechanisms of double vision may occur in multiple sclerosis, including ocular motor nerve palsies and skew deviation

[a] If these cranial nerves are affected in combination, a cavernous sinus lesion is likely. If the optic nerve is also affected, the lesion is likely at the orbital apex.

CLINICAL PEARLS
- Transient painless vision loss lasting minutes in one eye suggests transient retinal ischemia.
- Vision loss in one eye accompanied by pain with eye movements in a young person suggests optic neuritis.
- Abrupt vision loss in an elderly person accompanied by headaches, scalp tenderness, or jaw claudication suggests temporal arteritis.
- Headaches, transient visual obscurations, and pulsatile tinnitus in a young, obese woman suggest idiopathic intracranial hypertension.
- Binocular double vision worse as the day progresses may suggest ocular myasthenia gravis.
- Sudden painful binocular double vision with unilateral ptosis and pupillary involvement should prompt evaluation for an aneurysm.

Key elements of physical examination

A comprehensive neurologic examination is critical but it is essential to remember the following key elements:

- Examination in a patient with vision loss should include the following, tested on each eye separately:
  - Visual acuity – best corrected either with glasses or by having patient look through pinholes.
- Color vision – comparison of color saturation or brightness of a red object between eyes, or formal color vision test plates, if available.
- Pupillary examination to assess for an afferent pupillary defect – the hallmark of an optic nerve problem.
- Visual fields – by confrontation to finger counting or a red object in each quadrant, formal visual fields in an ophthalmology office necessary in many instances.
- Fundus examination for assessment of optic nerve and retina. Look for optic disk swelling or pallor.
- Examination in a patient with double vision should include the following:
  - Range of motion of each eye in the eight gaze positions (up, up and right, right, down and right, down, down and left, left, up and left). Limitations in range may be subtle, but significant.
- Assessment of ocular alignment (e.g. straight, eso = medial deviation, exo = lateral deviation, hyper = one eye higher than the other) in central gaze and in up, down, right, and left gaze. This can be achieved with cover testing, red glass or Maddox rod (see Reading list for references on how to perform these techniques).
- Detailed eyelid examination for ptosis, eyelid retraction, Cogan's lid twitch, lid lag.
- Prolonged upgaze for at least 60 seconds to assess for downdrift of eyes or worsening ptosis.
- Pupil examination, particularly for pupillary dilation in setting of a possible oculomotor nerve palsy.

Table of elements of physical examination by disease

Vision loss	
Retinal ischemia	Examination including fundoscopy may be normal after transient episode. If persistent, decreased visual acuity with retinal swelling and whitening. Macular cherry red spot if central retinal artery infarct. Hollenhorst plaques (carotid emboli, highly refractile, yellow) may be present at peripheral arterial branch points
Optic neuritis	Decreased visual acuity, impaired color vision, central scotoma (Figure 11.1), and afferent pupillary defect in affected eye. Optic disk most often acutely normal, though may be slightly swollen
Non-arteritic anterior ischemic optic neuropathy	Decreased visual acuity – mild or severe, visual field loss that is often in top or bottom half of vision (i.e. altitudinal; Figure 11.2A), afferent pupillary defect, swollen optic nerve in affected eye (Figure 11.2B). Small crowded optic nerve with no central cup in unaffected eye (Figure 11.2C) required for diagnosis
Arteritic anterior ischemic optic neuropathy (temporal arteritis)	Severely reduced visual acuity, afferent pupillary defect, swollen optic nerve (often very pallid white swelling), severe visual field loss in affected eye. Enlarged, tender temporal artery may or may not be present
Neoplasm (e.g. optic nerve meningioma or glioma, orbital metastasis)	Reduced visual acuity, afferent pupillary defect, pale or swollen optic disk (Figure 11.3A,B), and visual field defect in affected eye (Figure 11.3C). Proptosis may be present

Vision loss	
Leber's hereditary optic neuropathy	Decreased visual acuity (often in 20/200–20/400 range) and color vision, afferent pupillary defect, large central scotoma. Optic disk appears swollen (though it is actually pseudoedema) acutely and becomes pale after weeks to months
Idiopathic intracranial hypertension	Visual acuity often normal. Visual fields with enlarged blind spots or peripheral constriction. Swollen optic nerves (papilledema)
Sarcoidosis	If involves optic nerve, decreased visual acuity and color vision, afferent pupillary defect, visual field defect. Optic nerve may be acutely normal or swollen. Uveitis often present on ophthalmologic examination. If involves chiasm, bitemporal hemianopia. If involves intracranial visual pathways, homonymous hemianopia
Pituitary adenoma and other sellar or parasellar lesions (meningioma, craniopharyngioma)	Bitemporal hemianopia most common (Figure 11.4A,B). May involve optic nerves and cause decreased acuity and color vision, central visual field defects, and pale optic disks
Stroke	Homonymous hemianopia (Figure 11.5A,B)
Posterior reversible leukoencephalopathy	Severe visual acuity and color vision loss equal in both eyes. Bilateral homonymous hemianopias. Normal pupils and fundus examination
Brain tumor	Papilledema or homonymous hemianopia.
Binocular double vision	
Thyroid eye disease	Limited range of motility – impaired elevation and abduction early. Eyelid retraction, swollen eyes, proptosis
Chronic progressive external ophthalmoplegia	Diffusely limited range of motility, bilateral ptosis. No proptosis or eye swelling
Myasthenia gravis	Any pattern of eye movement range limitation or ocular misalignment. Ptosis – unilateral or bilateral or even in isolation. Normal pupils. Fatigability of the eyelids or eyes with prolonged upgaze. Cogan's lid twitch. Orbicularis oculi weakness
Oculomotor nerve palsy (cranial nerve III)	Any combination, complete or partial, of limited elevation, depression, or adduction of the affected eye; ptosis; pupillary enlargement with decreased reactivity. With a complete palsy, the eye position is down and out
Abducens nerve palsy (cranial nerve VI)	Impaired abduction of affected eye with resultant eso-deviation of eyes
Trochlear nerve palsy (cranial nerve IV)	Impaired depression of the affected eye, especially in an adducted position – though may appear normal. Hyper-deviation of affected eye that is worse in lateral gaze in direction away from affected eye (adduction), in downgaze and with head tilt toward affected eye. Better with head tilt away from affected eye. Resting head tilt may or may not be present
Skew deviation	Full range of motion of eye movements. Vertical deviation of the eyes, often unchanging in different gaze positions
Multiple sclerosis	Internuclear ophthalmoplegia common. Impaired adduction of one eye with abducting nystagmus in the opposite eye. Convergence may or may not be intact

CLINICAL PEARLS
- Embolic material from the carotid artery may be visible in the retinal vasculature in patients with transient vision loss from transient retinal ischemia.
- Vision loss with pain upon eye movement in a young person with an afferent pupillary defect and normal optic disk appearance strongly suggests optic neuritis.
- In older patients, the presence of severe vision loss in ischemic optic neuropathy with optic disk swelling should prompt evaluation for temporal arteritis.
- Bilateral swollen optic disks with normal visual acuity are most often papilledema, due to raised intracranial pressure.
- Bitemporal hemianopia signifies a lesion at the chiasm.
- Homonymous hemianopia signifies a lesion in the retrochiasmal visual pathways.
- Diplopia accompanied by proptosis, swollen eyes, and retracted eyelids signifies an orbital process, such as thyroid eye disease.
- Examination hallmarks of ocular myasthenia include variable ocular misalignment, ptosis, and fatigability.
- Skew deviation should be considered when a vertical misalignment is present that does not conform to the proper pattern for a trochlear nerve palsy.

Diagnostic tests

Vision loss	
Retinal ischemia	Vascular risk factor and carotid assessment: Doppler ultrasound, MR or CT angiogram. If negative, echocardiogram. Consider ESR and C-reactive protein to screen for temporal arteritis in older patients
Optic neuritis	MRI brain with contrast to assess for intracranial demyelinating lesions and prognosticate multiple sclerosis risk. MRI orbits with contrast to look for confirmatory optic nerve enhancement
Non-arteritic anterior ischemic optic neuropathy	Vascular risk factor assessment. Sleep study for sleep apnea. Tests for embolic sources are not indicated
Arteritic anterior ischemic optic neuropathy (temporal arteritis)	ESR, C-reactive protein, complete blood count. Temporal artery biopsy
Neoplasm (e.g. optic nerve meningioma or glioma, orbital metastasis)	MRI orbits with contrast (Figure 11.3D). May need lumbar puncture if suspect infiltrative malignancy
Leber's hereditary optic neuropathy	Genetic testing for common mitochondrial DNA mutations. EKG
Idiopathic intracranial hypertension	MRI brain. MR venogram of head essential if atypical patient (thin, male, older) to rule out venous sinus thrombosis. Lumbar puncture to assess opening pressure, rule out spinal fluid infectious or neoplastic process, and assess headache response to transient lowering of intracranial pressure
Sarcoidosis	Chest imaging – chest CT with contrast preferred. Lumbar puncture. Whole body gallium or PET scan. Biopsy proof ideal – lacrimal, parotid, or mediastinal lymphadenopathy most common biopsy sites
Pituitary adenoma and other sellar lesions (meningioma, craniopharyngioma)	MRI brain with contrast (special protocol). Endocrine evaluation
Stroke	MRI brain with diffusion-weighted imaging
Posterior reversible leukoencephalopathy	MRI brain. Blood pressure monitoring
Brain tumor	MRI brain with contrast

Binocular double vision	
Thyroid eye disease	Orbital imaging – CT or MRI orbits. Thyroid function studies and thyroid antibody tests. Endocrine evaluation
Chronic progressive external ophthalmoplegia	Mitochondrial nuclear DNA mutation assessment on serum. Muscle biopsy with mitochondrial testing. EKG
Myasthenia gravis	Edrophonium (Tensilon) test, ice pack or rest test. Acetylcholine receptor antibodies. EMG with repetitive stimulation and single fiber
Oculomotor nerve palsy (cranial nerve III)	MRI brain with contrast. MR or CT angiogram of head – conventional angiogram if high suspicion for aneurysm and non-invasive testing negative. If palsy persists and imaging is negative, lumbar puncture. Vascular risk factor assessment if microvascular
Abducens nerve palsy (cranial nerve VI)	MRI brain with contrast. If palsy persists and imaging is negative, lumbar puncture. Vascular risk factor assessment if microvascular
Trochlear nerve palsy (cranial nerve IV)	MRI brain with contrast. If palsy persists and is not congenital, lumbar puncture. Review of old photographs for long-standing head tilt to suggest congenital etiology
Skew deviation	MRI brain with diffusion-weighted imaging
Multiple sclerosis	MRI brain with contrast

Table of frequency of each disease

Vision loss	
Retinal ischemia	Central retinal artery occlusion incidence: 1/100,000 Transient monocular vision loss (TMVL) incidence: 1.5/100,000 in 3rd decade 32/100,000 in 7th decade Annual incidence of stroke after TMVL: 2–2.8%
Optic neuritis	Incidence: 1–5/100,000 Prevalence: 115/100,000 Most common acute optic neuropathy in patients under the age of 50 years
Non-arteritic anterior ischemic optic neuropathy	Incidence: 2.3–10/100,000 Most common acute optic neuropathy in patients over the age of 50 years
Arteritic anterior ischemic optic neuropathy (temporal arteritis)	Incidence: 0.57/100,000 Most common cause of vision loss in temporal arteritis
Neoplasm (e.g. optic nerve meningioma or glioma, orbital metastasis)	Optic nerve sheath meningioma (ONSM): 2% of orbital tumors, 1–2% of meningiomas 90% are secondary, arising intracranially primary ONSM – middle-aged women Optic nerve glioma: 1.5–3.5% of orbital tumors 1% of intracranial tumors 65% of intrinsic optic nerve tumors
Leber's hereditary optic neuropathy (LHON)	Prevalence of vision loss from LHON: 3.2/100,000 80–90% male predominance Prevalence of harboring primary LHON mutation: 11.82/100,000
Idiopathic intracranial hypertension	Incidence of idiopathic intracranial hypertension: 0.9/100,000 3.5/100,000 in women aged 20–44 years 13/100,000 if 10% over ideal body weight 19/100,000 if 20% over ideal body weight

(Continued)

Vision loss	
Sarcoidosis	Prevalence in USA: 10–40/100,000 Central nervous system affected in 5–10%
Pituitary adenoma and other sellar lesions (meningioma, craniopharyngioma)	Pituitary adenoma: incidence of incidental microtumor approaches 30% in older persons 6–12% of symptomatic intracranial tumors
Stroke	Homonymous hemianopia in stroke: 40% occipital lobe 30% parietal lobe 25% temporal lobe 5% optic tract or lateral geniculate nucleus
Posterior reversible leukoencephalopathy	Infrequent
Brain tumor	Papilledema present in 40% of patients, on average. It is present in up to 80% of patients with midline tumors
Binocular double vision	
Thyroid eye disease	Clinical signs present at some point in disease course in 25–50% of patients with thyroid disease, disabling form in 3–5%
Chronic progressive external ophthalmoplegia	Present in 95% of patients with mitochondrial myopathy, presenting feature in 2/3
Myasthenia gravis	Incidence: 3–30/100,000
Oculomotor nerve palsy (cranial nerve III)	30% of ocular motor cranial nerve palsies 17–35% microvascular 18% aneurysmal 19% neoplastic
Abducens nerve palsy (cranial nerve VI)	40–50% of ocular motor cranial nerve palsies 30% microvascular 30% neoplastic
Trochlear nerve palsy (cranial nerve IV)	20–30% of ocular motor cranial nerve palsies 29–67% congenital Trauma – common cause of acquired palsy
Skew deviation	Common cause of vertical diplopia, but less common than trochlear nerve palsy
Multiple sclerosis	Internuclear ophthalmoplegia is a common hallmark of multiple sclerosis

BOTTOM LINE
- Determine if vision loss and double vision involve one eye or both and localize the lesion prior to considering differential diagnosis.
- Identify patients with retinal ischemia, as they are at high risk for permanent vision loss and stroke.
- Identify patients with vision loss in one eye from temporal arteritis, as they have high risk of complete irreversible blindness from loss of vision in the contralateral eye.
- Obtain formal visual field testing in all patients with papilledema.
- Remember that any pupil-involving third nerve palsy requires definitive exclusion of a posterior communicating artery aneurysm.

Images

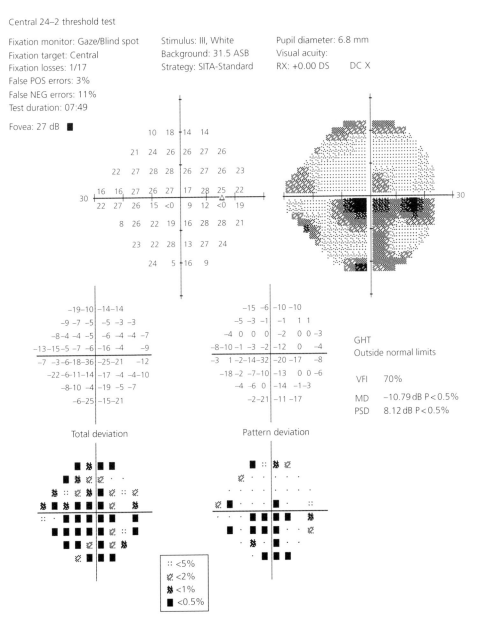

Central 24–2 threshold test

Fixation monitor: Gaze/Blind spot
Fixation target: Central
Fixation losses: 1/17
False POS errors: 3%
False NEG errors: 11%
Test duration: 07:49

Stimulus: III, White
Background: 31.5 ASB
Strategy: SITA-Standard

Pupil diameter: 6.8 mm
Visual acuity:
RX: +0.00 DS   DC X

Fovea: 27 dB ■

```
                10  18  14  14
            21  24  26  26  27  26
        22  27  28  28  26  27  26  23
    16  16  27  26  27  17  28  25  22
30  22  27  26  15  <0   9  12  <0  19                                    30
         8  26  22  19  16  28  28  21
            23  22  28  13  27  24
                24   5  16   9
```

Total deviation
```
   -19-10 -14-14
  -9 -7 -5  -5 -3 -3
 -8-4 -4 -5  -6 -4 -4 -7
-13-15-5 -7 -6 -16 -4      -9
 -7 -3-6-18-36 -25-21    -12
 -22-6-11-14 -17 -4 -4-10
  -8-10 -4 -19 -5 -7
   -6-25 -15-21
```

Pattern deviation
```
   -15 -6 -10 -10
  -5 -3 -1  -1  1  1
 -4  0  0  0 -2   0 0 -3
-8-10 -1 -3 -2 -12  0   -4
 -3  1 -2-14-32 -20 -17  -8
 -18 -2 -7-10 -13  0 0 -6
  -4 -6  0 -14 -1 -3
   -2-21 -11 -17
```

GHT
Outside normal limits

VFI   70%

MD   −10.79 dB P<0.5%
PSD   8.12 dB P<0.5%

Total deviation

Pattern deviation

:: <5%
▨ <2%
▨ <1%
■ <0.5%

Figure 11.1 Central scotoma in the right eye of a patient with acute demyelinating optic neuritis. The patient was a young woman with painful vision loss in one eye. In addition to the central scotoma, examination revealed decreased visual acuity and color vision with an afferent pupillary defect and a normal optic nerve appearance in the right eye.

(A)

Central 24–2 threshold test

Fixation monitor: Gaze/Blind spot Stimulus: III, White   Pupil siameter: 4.0 mm
Fixation target: Central   Background: 31.5 ASB   Visual acuity:
Fixation losses: 0/16   Strategy: SITA-Standard RX: +0.00 DS –1.75 DC X 4
False POS errors: 0%
False NEG errors: 0%
Test duration: 05:45

Fovea: 37 dB

```
                  26  28  23  27
              28  28  29  29  28  33
          29  28  29  30  29  29  29  31
      25  29  30  31  32  32  30  27  27
  30
      <0   8  14  <0  <0  30  26  <0  23
          <0  <0   0  <0  <0  <0  <0  26
              <0  <0  <0  <0  <0  <0
                  <0  <0  <0  <0
```

```
Total deviation                        Pattern deviation

        -1   0   -4   0                        -1   1   -3   1
    0  -2  -1  -1  -1   4                    0  -2   0   0  -1   5
  0  -2  -2  -2  -2  -2  -1   2           1  -1  -2  -2  -1  -1  -1   2
-2   0  -1  -1   0   0  -2      -3       -1   0  -1  -1   0   1  -1      -2
-29 -22 -18 -35 -35  -3  -6     -7       -29 -22 -17 -34 -34  -2  -6     -6
-31 -33 -32 -34 -34 -34 -33 -4          -31 -33 -32 -34 -34 -33 -32 -3
  -32 -33 -33 -33 -33 -32                 -31 -32 -33 -33 -32 -32
      -31 -32 -32 -32                         -31 -31 -31 -31
```

GHT
Outside normal limits

VFI 62%

MD –15.45 dB P<0.5%
PSD 16.44 dB P<0.5%

Total deviation   Pattern deviation

:: <5%
⚥ <2%
✳ <1%
■ <0.5%

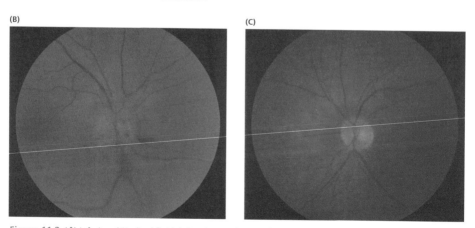

Figure 11.2 (**A**) Inferior altitudinal field defect in a patient with non-arteritic anterior ischemic optic neuropathy (NAION). (**B**) Disk edema with peripapillary hemorrhage in the right eye of a patient with NAION. (**C**) Normal, but crowded, optic disk in the left eye of the patient in B, with NAION in the right eye. Color versions of (**B**) and (**C**) are available on the companion website.

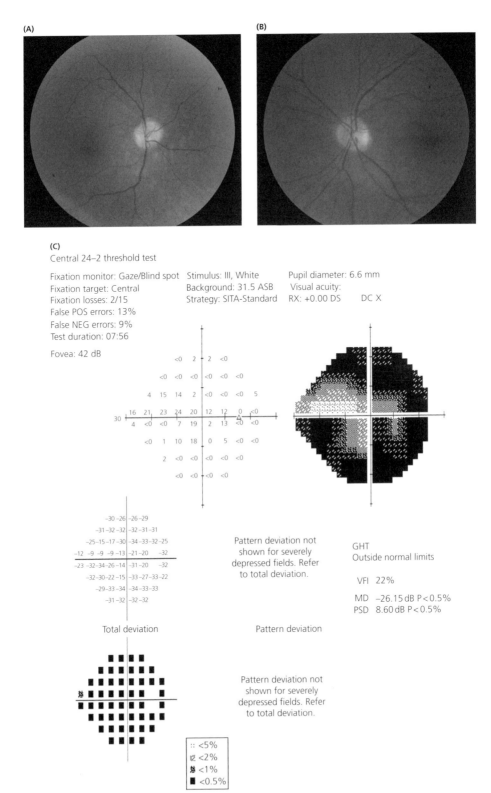

(A)

(B)

(C)
Central 24–2 threshold test

Fixation monitor: Gaze/Blind spot   Stimulus: III, White   Pupil diameter: 6.6 mm
Fixation target: Central   Background: 31.5 ASB   Visual acuity:
Fixation losses: 2/15   Strategy: SITA-Standard   RX: +0.00 DS   DC X
False POS errors: 13%
False NEG errors: 9%
Test duration: 07:56

Fovea: 42 dB

Pattern deviation not shown for severely depressed fields. Refer to total deviation.

Total deviation

Pattern deviation

Pattern deviation not shown for severely depressed fields. Refer to total deviation.

GHT
Outside normal limits

VFI   22%

MD   −26.15 dB P<0.5%
PSD   8.60 dB P<0.5%

:: <5%
<2%
<1%
<0.5%

Figure 11.3 (**A**) Pale right optic disk in a patient with an optic nerve sheath meningioma. (**B**) Normal left optic disk color for comparison. (**C**) Humphrey visual field with severe field loss from optic nerve compression by retrobulbar meningioma. Color versions of (**A**) and (**B**) are available on the companion website.

(D)

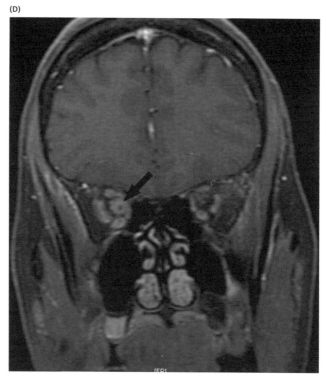

Figure 11.3 (*Continued*) (**D**) Coronal fat-saturated T1-weighted orbital MRI with contrast demonstrating a right optic nerve sheath meningioma (arrow). Note the circumferential thickening and enhancement of the optic nerve sheath surrounding the optic nerve (the small dark spot in the center).

(A)

Central 24–2 threshold test

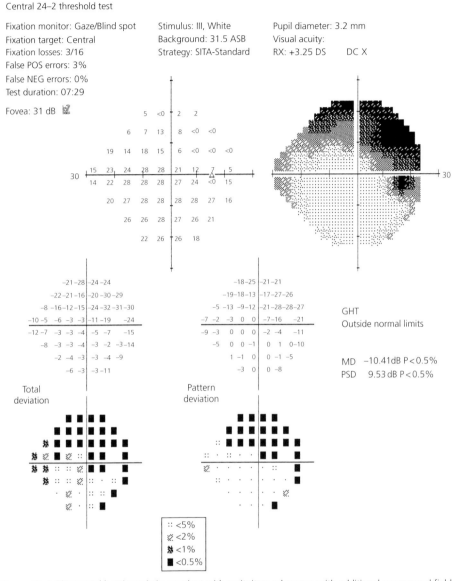

Fixation monitor: Gaze/Blind spot
Fixation target: Central
Fixation losses: 3/16
False POS errors: 3%
False NEG errors: 0%
Test duration: 07:29

Fovea: 31 dB

Stimulus: III, White
Background: 31.5 ASB
Strategy: SITA-Standard

Pupil diameter: 3.2 mm
Visual acuity:
RX: +3.25 DS   DC X

GHT
Outside normal limits

MD   −10.41dB P<0.5%
PSD   9.53dB P<0.5%

Total deviation

Pattern deviation

:: <5%
⊠ <2%
⊠ <1%
■ <0.5%

Figure 11.4 Bitemporal hemianopia in a patient with a pituitary adenoma, with additional superonasal field loss in the right eye from optic nerve compression. Right eye (**A**), left eye (**B**).

(B)

Central 24–2 threshold test

Fixation monitor: Gaze/Blind spot
Fixation target: Central
Fixation losses: 1/16
False POS errors: 1%
False NEG errors: 0%
Test duration: 08:26
Fovea: <0 dB ■

Stimulus: III, White
Background: 31.5 ASB
Strategy: SITA-Standard

Pupil diameter: 3.5 mm
Visual acuity:
RX: +3.25 DS　　DC X

```
              <0   <0   <0   17
          <0   <0   <0  | 12   16   16
       <0    2    4    0  |  8   24   22   22
     <0,   6   <0   <0  | 29   27   27   27   25
30 +  <0   <0    5   <0  | 18   28   26   25   20 + 30
     <0   13   13   18  | 18   28   27   21
           8   19   13  | 21   26   23
               12    9  + 20   16
```

```
      -27 -28 -28  -9                    -24 -25 -25  -6
   -29 -30 -30 -16 -12 -12            -26 -26 -27 -13  -9  -9
 -30 -27 -25 -30 -22  -6  -7  -6      -26 -23 -22 -27 -19  -2  -4  -2
 -31       -33 -33  -3  -4  -3  -1   0    -27       -29 -30   0 -1   0   2   3
 -31       -26 -34 -14  -4  -5  -3  -6    -28       -23 -30 -11 -1  -1   0  -3
 -31 -17 -18 -14 -14  -3  -3  -7      -28 -13 -14 -10 -10   1   0  -3
   -21 -11 -17  -9  -4  -6            -18  -8 -14  -6 -1  -2
     -17 -21   -9 -13                    -14 -17   -6  -9
```

Total   Pattern
deviation   deviation

GHT
Outside normal limits

MD　−15.39 dB P<0.5%
PSD　11.55 dB P<0.5%

:: <5%
✗ <2%
✤ <1%
■ <0.5%

Figure 11.4 (*Continued*)

(A)

Central 24–2 threshold test

Fixation monitor: Gaze/Blind spot	Stimulus: III, White	Pupil diameter: 3.6 mm
Fixation target: Central	Background: 31.5 ASB	Visual acuity:
Fixation losses: 4/16 xx	Strategy: SITA-Standard	RX: –2.50 DS DC X
False POS errors: 10%		
False NEG errors: 6%		
Test duration: 07:54		

Fovea: 20 dB ■

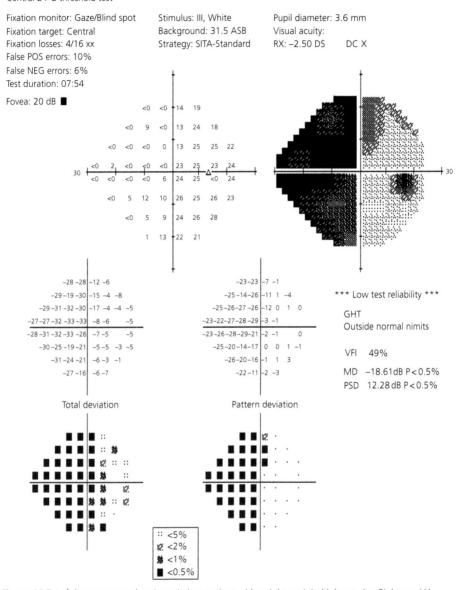

Total deviation

Pattern deviation

*** Low test reliability ***

GHT
Outside normal nimits

VFI   49%

MD   –18.61dB P<0.5%
PSD   12.28dB P<0.5%

:: <5%
▨ <2%
▩ <1%
■ <0.5%

Figure 11.5 Left homonymous hemianopia in a patient with a right occipital lobe stroke. Right eye (A), left eye (B).

(B)

Central 24–2 threshold test

Fixation monitor: Gaze/Blind spot
Fixation target: Central
Fixation losses: 1/15
False POS errors: 6%
False NEG errors: 13%
Test duration: 07:02

Fovea: 29 dB ■

Stimulus: III, White
Background: 31.5 ASB
Strategy: SITA-Standard

Pupil diameter: 3.2 mm
Visual acuity:
RX: −3.50 DS −1.75 DC X 101

		0	0	22	20		
	<0	3	6	24	27	26	
<0	0	<0	8	26	28	25	19
<0	0	<0	<0	27	27	24	23	18
<0	<0	<0	<0	27	26	25	26	19
	<0	0	0	0	26	27	26	26
		<0	0	<0	16	21	23
			<0	<0	16	12

Total deviation

```
      -25 -25 | -3 -5
   -29 -24 -22 | -5 -2 -1
-29 -28 -31 -22 | -4 -2 -4 -8
-30    -32 -33 | -4 -4 -6 -6 -7
-31    -33 -33 | -5 -5 -6 -3 -7
-31 -30 -31 -31 | -6 -4 -4 -2
   -31 -30 -32 | -14 -8 -6
      -31 -31 | -13 -16
```

Pattern deviation

```
      -21 -21 | 1 -1
   -25 -21 -18 | -1 2 3
-25 -24 -27 -18 | 0 2 0 -4
-27    -28 -29 | -1 0 -2 -2 -3
-27    -29 -29 | -1 -1 -2 1 -3
-27 -26 -27 -27 | -2 0 0 2
   -27 -26 -28 | -10 -5 -2
      -27 -27 | -9 -12
```

GHT
Outside mormal limits

VFI   51%

MD   −15.97 dB P<0.5%
PSD   13.42 dB P<0.5%

Total deviation

Pattern deviation

```
:: <5%
𝕩 <2%
𝖇 <1%
■ <0.5%
```

Figure 11.5 (*Continued*)

Reading list
Key reading sources for this chapter can be found online at www.mountsinaiexpertguides.com

Suggested websites
The Neuro-Ophthalmology Virtual Education Library: novel.utah.edu

---

Additional material for this chapter can be found online at:
www.mountsinaiexpertguides.com

This includes advice for patients, a case study, multiple choice questions, and a reading list.

CHAPTER 12

Vertigo, Dizziness, and Hearing Loss

Bernard Cohen and Eric Smouha
Icahn School of Medicine at Mount Sinai, New York, NY, USA

Background

Vertigo involves a sense of rotation of self or surround, and it indicates that the subject has difficulty either in the peripheral or central vestibular system. The neural activity that is responsible for the vertigo arises in the semicircular canals, in particular in the lateral semicircular canals. Thus, in this chapter, we will emphasize the function and dysfunction of the semicircular canals when dealing with the causes of vertigo. We also note a condition that arises from dysfunction of the vestibulo-ocular reflex (VOR), the mal de debarquement syndrome (MdDS).

Dizziness is a less precise term because it includes lightheadedness, imbalance, and disequilibrium. Lightheadedness may signify orthostatic hypotension. Imbalance implies a disturbance of gait, and may be the after effect of a vestibular disorder reflected in vestibulospinal pathways, or a primary neurologic disorder in the motor, sensory, or cerebellar systems. Dysequilibrium is less specific, but indicates difficulty in the control of movement and balance.

Although vertigo and imbalance can be caused by central and peripheral lesions, the emphasis in this chapter will be on the effects of lesions of the peripheral apparatus. They are more common and can be classified more readily, although similar symptoms can occur from lesions that affect the vestibular nuclei, other portions of the brainstem, the cerebellum, the spinal cord, peripheral nerves, and central pathways. Consideration of these conditions, however, is beyond the scope of this chapter.

Hearing loss arises from diseases of the ear or auditory nerve. Tinnitus is usually accompanied by hearing loss, and implies an inner ear disorder.

Definitions

- *Vertigo*: Sense of movement of the subject or the visual surround.
- *Dizziness*: Giddiness, a general term that may encompass all the descriptors that follow.
- *Lightheadedness*: Faintness, fear of loss of consciousness.
- *Dysequilibrium*: Either momentary or prolonged loss of orientation.
- *Imbalance*: Gait disturbance, unsteadiness, veering, falling or fear of falling.
- *Orthostatic hypotension*: Blood pressure normally increases or is stabilized when standing to maintain blood flow to the brain. If blood pressure falls, subjects may feel faint, i.e. they become dizzy; such symptoms frequently occur in older patients on arising from bed. Orthostatic hypotension is defined as a decrease of 20 mmHg in systolic BP or 10 mmHg in diastolic BP within 3 minutes of assuming an upright position. Neural activity that produces the increase in BP when arising originates in the otolith organs and is transmitted to the cardiovascular system by the vestibulo-sympathetic reflex. The cause of orthostatic hypotension is still unclear, but it

Mount Sinai Expert Guides: Neurology, First Edition. Edited by Stuart C. Sealfon, Rajeev Motiwala, and Charles B. Stacy.
© 2016 John Wiley & Sons, Ltd. Published 2016 by John Wiley & Sons, Ltd.
Companion website: www.mountsinaiexpertguides.com

is known that it involves failure of the vestibulo-sympathetic reflex to appropriately activate blood pressure.

- *Hearing loss* is a self-explanatory term:
  - *Conductive hearing loss* is a mechanical impairment of hearing, arising from the ear canal or middle ear (tympanic membrane, malleus, incus, or stapes).
  - *Sensorineural hearing loss* (SNHL) is perceptive deafness, and arises from the inner ear cochlea, or the auditory nerve or central auditory pathways.
  - *Mixed hearing loss* is a combination of conductive and sensorineural loss.
  - *Tinnitus* is ringing or buzzing in the ear, static, or head noise.

Presenting complaints

- Dizziness or vertigo and/or nausea (see definitions above).
- Loss of hearing, or trouble with conversation or ringing in ears.
- Note that hearing loss in children may present with speech delay or learning disability, and that older adults may deny any problem with their hearing and be referred for evaluation by a spouse or relative.

Impact

- Incidence: Dizziness accounts for 3% of primary care visits for patients 25 years and older and 3% of all emergency department visits.
- The 1-year prevalence of vertigo in a recent study in a large Western European nation was about 5%.
- MdDS is uncommon, not rare, and occurs predominantly in women.
- Social impact: Severe persistent vertigo can force patients to be confined to bed for prolonged periods. Severe vertigo has a strong impact on socialization, and may be a cause of disability.
- MdDs is disabling and can cause loss of ability to work.
- According to the National Institutes of Health, hearing loss affects 36 million US citizens, with 25 million experiencing tinnitus. Most people will have some degree of hearing loss by the age of 65. Many will not seek medical help even when it is available. In elderly persons, hearing loss causes loss of social connectivity and can worsen dementia. Cochlear implantation has effectively restored hearing to millions of people with profound hearing loss who could not otherwise be helped.

Approach to diagnosis

- History:
  - Determine if the patient is dizzy or vertiginous.
  - If vertigo – determine the time of onset and duration of the vertigo. Determine whether it is intermittent or whether it is long-lasting, whether the vertigo occurs when moving the head into specific positions, whether balance is impaired, and if there was nausea and vomiting, tinnitus, or transient loss of hearing.
  - If one suspects MdDS, determine if it began after a trip such as a cruise or occurred spontaneously, and if the oscillating motion is persistent, or disappears during car rides but reappears promptly after the ride is over.
- Examination:
  - If dizzy, one should consider orthostatic hypotension, and take blood pressure, lying and standing.

- If vertigo, check for spontaneous nystagmus, imbalance, past-pointing, stepping test (marching up and down in place for one minute with eyes closed and arms extended), and head thrust test. If available, use Frenzel glasses (high-positive diopter lenses that eliminate visual fixation) to check for spontaneous or positional nystagmus. If Frenzel glasses are not available, use the ophthalmoscope to view the retina of one eye while the other eye is covered. If there is spontaneous nystagmus, the slow phases will be detected by drift of the retina. When you view the back of the eye, the direction of the slow phases will be opposite to those seen from the front of the eye. Determine whether there is a positional component to the generation of vertigo using side-down and Dix–Hallpike head-hanging positional maneuvers. Confirm with eye movement test (video-oculography).
- For suspected MdDS: check frequency of rocking, swaying, or bobbing (should be in the range of 0.1–0.3 Hz). Check for lateral movement on the Fukuda stepping test. If possible, look for vertical nystagmus with head rolled to side.
- Hearing loss: assess conversational ability, examine the ears, use tuning forks to determine conductive versus sensorineural loss, and obtain an audiogram. The audiogram will determine the hearing threshold in decibels by frequencies and measure the speech discrimination score.

Getting your bearings

- Dizziness is a relatively vague term and is a frequent medical complaint. It is important to separate dizziness from vertigo, which is a specific sense of rotation of the subject or of the visual surround.
- An accurate history of the characteristics of episodes of dizziness or vertigo is essential for diagnosis.
- The history and physical examination can usually establish the cause of dizziness or vertigo. Additional supplementation by audiometry, video-oculography (VOG), and/or occasionally MRI or 3D temporal bone CT scans can help establish the diagnosis.
- Vertigo can be transient and related to specific head positions (benign paroxysmal positional vertigo, BPPV), of longer duration (episodic vertigo, Ménière's disease), or of extended duration (labyrinthitis). It can be treated with medications, injection of gentamicin, surgery, or physical therapy maneuvers, depending on the cause.
- Hearing loss can be conductive (arising from the external or middle ear), sensorineural (arising from the cochlea or auditory nervous system), or mixed.
- Audiometry will determine the type of hearing loss and guide the diagnostic workup.
- A physical examination will identify the causes of conductive hearing loss. The pattern of the audiogram is helpful for determining the cause of sensorineural hearing loss.
- Unilateral sensorineural hearing loss, with or without associated ipsilateral loss of vestibular function, raises the possibility of an acoustic neuroma. Auditory brainstem responses (ABR, synonymous with brainstem auditory evoked potentials, BAEP) are useful for evaluating the central auditory pathways, and an MRI of the internal auditory canals should be obtained.

Key elements of history

- History is critical to classifying dizziness. When taking the history, determine whether the symptoms are dizziness or vertigo (spinning or movement). There also might be associated "imbalance" (gait disturbance), "dysequilibrium," or "lightheadedness" (faintness or feeling of impending faint).

- Determine the first onset of vertigo.
- Determine whether it is constant or episodic; if episodic, describe the duration and frequency.
- For patients with *hearing loss*: Time of onset, progression, one ear or both, concomitant tinnitus or dizziness, family history of deafness, history of noise exposure or exposure to ototoxic medications (aminoglycosides, loop diuretics, cisplatin, or other chemotherapy agents).

Table of elements of history and diseases

Disease	Symptoms	Duration	Other characteristics
Diseases causing dizziness or vertigo			
Orthostatic hypotension	Sense of dizziness or faintness when arising from bed, lasting for several minutes; no sense of rotation of self or the visual surround	3–5 min	Dizziness abates if subject lies down; more common in elderly patients
Benign paroxysmal positional vertigo (BPPV)	Rotatory vertigo, brief duration, occurring in specific head positions, especially when turning over in bed or looking up at the ceiling or down at the floor	45 s to 2 min; can be intense, but may be mild, decrescendo of symptoms over time	Patient normal between attacks. Most common in postmenopausal women. Can also occur after head injury in men or women. Balance is normal between episodes
Episodic vertigo	Rotation of self or surround, nausea, vomiting, poor balance, headache, intolerance to light and sound, without hearing loss	Occurs suddenly, lasts for 30 min to 1–2 h	Patients feel weak after conclusion of episode; no unique physical findings; has been called migrainous vertigo, but occurs only infrequently in conjunction with migraine headaches. There is no indication that there is vascular dilatation, as in the original description of migraine headaches
Ménière's disease	Rotation of self or surround, nausea, vomiting, commonly have tinnitus and reduction in hearing in affected ear, balance can be normal between attacks	3–12 h	Most often unilateral; affects both hearing and balance (hearing loss is predominantly at low frequencies) Patients are nauseated and enervated after attacks and truly miserable because they have severe motion sickness
Labyrinthitis, vestibular neuritis	Sudden onset of vertigo, accompanied by nausea, vomiting, loss of balance, usually forces the patient to bed	Lasts for days or weeks with decreasing severity of symptoms, but may be permanent	May be viral in origin or involve occlusion of vasculature to the peripheral vestibular apparatus

(Continued)

Disease	Symptoms	Duration	Other characteristics
Bilateral loss of vestibular function	Insidious onset and no true vertigo; imbalance, dizzy when turning head to the side and unable to maintain visual fixation during head turns; absence of prolonged vertigo or nystagmus; may have brief lightning (5–10 s) attacks of vertigo without motion sickness Gait impairment may require cane or walker Vision unclear during head movement Symptoms are frequently disabling	Progressive onset over years – tempo slow but inexorable	May have history of aminoglycoside use or cisplatin chemotherapy
Superior semicircular canal dehiscence	Dizziness induced by loud sound (Tullio's phenomenon) or pressure on the tragus	Months or years	Ear fullness, autophony; occasionally conductive hearing loss
Acoustic neuroma	See below	See below	See below
CNS lesions	Associated symptoms, such as diplopia, slurred speech, paresis, sensory loss, and incoordination depend on location of lesion	Variable	Vascular disease, multiple sclerosis, neoplasms
Peripheral nervous system lesions	Dysequilibrium, falls, may be associated with sensory loss, weakness	Usually insidious and chronic	Peripheral neuropathy, multiple sensory deficits of the elderly
Diseases causing hearing loss			
Chronic otitis media	Otorrhea, history of ear infections	Months to years	Eardrum perforation or retraction pocket
Otosclerosis	Progressive conductive hearing loss in younger adult	Months to years	Absent stapedial reflexes, positive family history
Genetic hearing impairment	Speech delay in young child, progressive hearing loss in childhood	Months to years	Positive family history
Presbyacusis	Social isolation, difficulty with conversation	Years	Bilateral symmetrical involvement
Acoustic neuroma	Unilateral hearing impairment, inability to understand phone in one ear	Months to years, although occasionally hearing loss is sudden	Tinnitus, disequilibrium or imbalance, and headache. May also have reduction in vestibular function and vertigo
Sudden sensorineural hearing loss	Unilateral sensorineural hearing loss of sudden onset	Onset less than one day	Unilateral tinnitus, vertigo resembling acute labyrinthitis

CLINICAL PEARLS

- If patients state that they have vertigo when turning over in bed, that the vertigo is rotatory, lasts for one to several minutes, and is related to a particular head position, then it is BPPV. Perform an Epley maneuver to cure.
- If patients have vertigo and imbalance for days or weeks, it is generally labyrinthitis.
  - Check for spontaneous nystagmus in darkness and lateral movement on stepping test; get VOG and start vestibular rehabilitation.
- If episodes last from 30 minutes to 2 hours and there is no change in hearing, it is episodic vertigo. Consider acetazolamide or methazolamide.
- If the vertigo lasts for 3–12 hours and involves hearing, it is Ménière's disease.
- If vertigo lasts longer than a day, it is labyrinthitis or vestibular neuritis.
- If patients get dizzy when talking on the telephone or with loud sounds (Tullio's phenomenon), think of superior canal dehiscence.
- If patients have prolonged dizziness when lying on one side and the nystagmus is horizontal, think of BPPV from the lateral canals.
- If the direction of the quick phases of nystagmus during BPPV is reversed – i.e. instead of being upward and rotatory toward the affected ear is downward and rotatory instead – think of anterior canal BPPV.
- There is a high rate of spontaneous remission of BPPV, probably due to many head movements that the patients make. If elderly patients have arthritis of the neck, the BPPV may be very severe and last for many years. Expect severe motion sickness when an Epley maneuver is done on these patients. Benzodiazepines (i.e. GABA agonists) are helpful in ameliorating the motion sickness.
- Patients with bilateral vestibular loss cannot walk in the sand.
- Patients with bilateral vestibular loss never become motion sick.
- If patients report faintness or loss of consciousness, they have orthostatic hypotension, not vertigo.

Key elements of physical examination

- Look for nystagmus on direct forward gaze. Use Frenzel glasses if available. If not, use your ophthalmoscope to view one eye while the other eye is occluded. Spontaneous nystagmus can be detected by movement of the retina. Remember, the back of the retina moves in a direction opposite to the front of the eye.
- Direction of slow phases of horizontal nystagmus point to side of peripheral lesion.
- Failure to suppress vestibular nystagmus coupled with a failure to produce optokinetic nystagmus at higher stimulus velocities (>20 degrees per second) indicates central disease in the visual system and may point to a lesion of the flocculus.
- If you suspect labyrinthitis, get the patient to do a short, fast horizontal head turn toward the side of the lesion, i.e. a head thrust, to look for loss of visual fixation. This will be manifest by the patient making a saccade back to the fixation point at the end of the head turn. Loss of fixation on head thrust occurs after severe peripheral labyrinthine lesions, and establishes the cause of vertigo to be peripheral, not central (brainstem). Very helpful at the bedside.
- Check stepping test, tandem walking, and static and tandem Romberg tests. Spontaneous nystagmus is always accompanied by lateral movement on the stepping test in the direction of the slow phases of nystagmus due to co-activation of vestibulo-ocular and vestibulo-spinal

pathways. Tandem walking and tandem Romberg are tests that evaluate gait and imbalance.
- Get the patient to adopt head-hanging positions to check for BPPV. The quick phases of nystagmus point to the affected ear and the involved semicircular canal – usually the posterior semicircular canal of the dependent ear.
- Check hearing, because a concomitant loss of hearing may suggest Ménière's disease or the presence of an acoustic neuroma.

Table of elements of physical examination by disease

Disease	Physical findings
Diseases causing dizziness or vertigo	
Orthostatic hypotension	Failure of the vestibulo-sympathetic reflex to elevate blood pressure when standing. If patient is hypertensive, there may not be any overt increase in blood pressure and the patient may not have serious orthostatic hypotension. Normotensive patients should have a blood pressure rise of 10–20 mmHg upon standing. If instead blood pressure falls, it is likely that the patient will be dizzy and could faint. The faintness can be immediately reversed if the patient lies flat again
Benign paroxysmal positional vertigo (BPPV)	Due to otolith degeneration. Otoliths are composed of $CaCO_3$ and a protein matrix. The protein dissolves, leaving $CaCO_3$ "stones," which then fall, most commonly, into the adjacent posterior canal. Then every time the head is turned to an appropriate position, the "stones" shift in the canal, causing deflection of the hair cells, signaling to the brain that here is sudden movement in the plane of the posterior canal, i.e. in the pitch plane, with severe, sudden, short-lived vertigo. The Dix–Hallpike maneuver (repositioning patient from a sitting position to reclining with head-hanging and chin to left or right) elicits upward rotatory nystagmus with quick phases toward the affected side in patients with BPPV involving the posterior semicircular canal on one side. Lasts 30–45 s. Patient generally frightened, but not nauseated during the vertigo attack. Balance generally OK when not having vertigo. Negative stepping test, maintains gaze fixation during head thrust (normal head thrust)
Episodic vertigo	May have weak spontaneous nystagmus and/or a slight decrease in function on caloric exam on one side. Otherwise, no specific physical findings. Diagnosis is essentially made on history. Although unknown, it is more likely that the pathologic process involves transient electrolyte imbalances of the endolymph of the semicircular canals, similar to the pathologic process in Ménière's disease
Ménière's disease	Patient may have decreased hearing in affected ear that becomes worse during attacks. Generally has spontaneous nystagmus during episodes, with slow phases directed toward or away from the affected ear. Marches to side of lesion on Fukuda stepping test. May be asymptomatic between attacks. Both ears may be affected in some cases. Dangerous because patient could become totally deaf if disease progresses. The pathologic process appears to be an electrolyte imbalance, and there is large expansion of the canals with degeneration of the nerves as the disease progresses. Unfortunately treatment is directed toward reducing the effects of the disease, rather than at the root of the problem. The presence of vertigo and tinnitus with decreased hearing during the attacks makes the diagnosis

Disease	Physical findings
Labyrinthitis, vestibular neuritis	Patient has spontaneous nystagmus with slow phases toward side of lesion. Canal paresis on caloric exam; marches to side of lesion on stepping test; also has past-pointing toward the side of the lesion. If there is significant loss of semicircular canal function, patient will be unable to maintain gaze in space during rapid head thrust toward the side of the lesion. In the acute phase, patients have been treated with steroids with some indication that it may partially ameliorate the effects of the labyrinthitis Check for involvement of the ipsilateral facial nerve and vesicles (as in herpes zoster, Ramsay Hunt syndrome). If facial nerve involvement consider immediate treatment with steroids to reduce swelling of the seventh and eighth nerves in the facial canal
Bilateral loss of vestibular function	The function of the vestibulo-ocular reflex, which originates in the semicircular canals, is to stabilize gaze in space during head movement. Thus, no matter how fast the head is rotated, gaze can be maintained stably on visual targets. In the absence of the vestibulo-ocular reflex, however, it is impossible to maintain stable gaze during head movement. May have positive head thrust test and absent caloric responses. The diagnosis is confirmed by loss of 4–5 lines of visual acuity when the head is in motion while viewing a Rosenbaum chart. Gait is ataxic on attempting tandem walking with veering to both sides. Cannot do tandem Romberg with eyes open or closed. Hearing is generally normal. Severe, bilateral vestibular loss occurs after gentamicin intoxication, but patients can recover with intensive rehabilitation over 1–2 years
Superior semicircular canal dehiscence	Vertigo and eye deviation induced by pressure on the tragus (fistula test) or loud sound (Tullio's phenomenon). The pathologic process is thinning or loss of the superior portion of the anterior canals, which project into the middle cranial fossa. Get 3D CT scan of temporal bone. Can be treated surgically by closing the superior canal dehiscence with muscle
Acoustic neuroma	See below
Diseases causing hearing loss	
Chronic otitis media	Eardrum perforation or scarring, middle ear effusion; keratin mass implies cholesteatoma
Otosclerosis	Tuning forks: Weber lateralizes toward side of loss, Rinne test negative in affected ear, implying conductive hearing loss
Genetic hearing impairment	Examine for facial dysmorphism, preauricular or anterior neck pits, eye abnormalities, skin, bone, or joint abnormalities
Presbyacusis	Bilateral symmetric sensorineural hearing loss on audiometry, without other physical findings
Acoustic neuroma	Unilateral hearing loss, impairment of gait and balance, facial hypesthesia, loss of corneal reflex, facial nerve twitching, nystagmus rare. The pathologic process is neurofibroma (i.e. benign tumor of the nerve sheaths) of the eighth cranial nerve. If unchecked, can grow to affect the flocculus, which lies just over the eighth nerve, causing a loss of ocular pursuit and an inability to suppress the vestibulo-ocular reflex during head turns. A large acoustic neuroma can also impact pontine structures including the trigeminal and facial nerves, causing severe imbalance along with other signs of pontine involvement. Treatment is surgical excision, stereotactic radiotherapy, or serial follow-up with MRI, in selected cases. Surgery strives to preserve facial nerve function, and hearing when possible
Sudden sensorineural hearing loss	Weber lateralizes away from affected ear. May have vestibular signs similar to labyrinthitis. Hearing loss is sudden and permanent

---

CLINICAL PEARLS

- The head thrust test is very useful at the bedside in cases of acute vertigo because it helps separate lesions of the labyrinth from those of the root entry zone in the vestibular nuclei in the brainstem. This portion of the vestibular nuclei receives input from the semicircular canals.
- Patient sensation of zooming (sensation of moving rapidly forward) or looming (sensation that sound source is moving closer to the patient) can be caused by pressure of the vertebral arteries against the root entry zone in the pons. It is likely that these symptoms arise from activation of the otolith system.
- In general, nystagmus is a sign of semicircular canal involvement and not of involvement of the otolith organs. The otolith organs sense orientation in space, and can generate sensations of looming and/or tilt. They can also produce compensatory eye movements for rapid changes in head position. The otolith organs provide the major input to the vestibulo-sympathetic reflex, which causes the increase in blood pressure upon standing from a recumbent position. Thus, deficient otolith input to the vestibulo-sympathetic reflex may contribute to orthostatic hypotension.
- MdDS can be relieved in about 75% of cases by rolling the head at the frequency of rocking while viewing a full-field visual stimulus moving slowly against the direction of movement in the Fukuda stepping test.

Diagnostic tests

Disease	Diagnostic test
Diseases causing dizziness or vertigo	
Orthostatic hypotension	Blood pressure measurements when supine and standing, tilt table test
BPPV	Head-hanging positions with chin to left or right (Dix–Hallpike maneuver)
Episodic vertigo	There is no specific diagnostic test; lateral movement during stepping test may be seen if damage to semicircular canals
Ménière's disease	Caloric test and audiogram. Electrocochleography (ECoG) may be abnormal. Although canal dysfunction can occur first, it is important to note that the diagnosis cannot be made without a change in hearing
Labyrinthitis, vestibular neuritis	Head thrust test, caloric testing, stepping test (i.e. marching up and down in place with eyes closed and arms extended) – turning to one side during the stepping test denotes lesion involving semicircular canal on that side. Spontaneous nystagmus on VOG, with visual fixation suppression. Unilateral loss of caloric function
Bilateral loss of vestibular function	Loss of visual fixation during head movement while viewing visual acuity chart (critical for diagnosis), caloric test shows bilateral loss of caloric (lateral semicircular canal) function, rotational chair test shows bilateral loss of vestibulo-ocular reflex, and patient is severely imbalanced on Romberg and tandem Romberg tests

Disease	Diagnostic test
Superior semicircular canal dehiscence	CT scan of temporal bone in oblique sagittal plane will demonstrate loss of bone over superior semicircular canal. Vestibular evoked myogenic potential (VEMP) will show reduced threshold on affected side
Acoustic neuroma	See below
Suspected central vestibular damage (persistent vertigo with a reduction of semicircular canal function on one side may be central)	Rule out with MRI with special attention to posterior circulation
Possible lesion of the posterior inferior cerebellar artery (dizziness, nystagmus, loss of swallowing, and imbalance)	Rule out with CT or preferably MRI
Dissection of the vertebral artery (sudden onset of vertigo after minor neck manipulation or trauma, e.g. after leaving the hairdresser)	Rule out with CT angiogram, MRI/MRA with dissection protocol or ultrasound

Diseases causing hearing loss

Chronic otitis media or cholesteatoma	Audiometry will show conductive hearing loss. Tympanometry will be flat if fluid or perforation is present. CT may demonstrate middle ear pathology
Otosclerosis	Audiometry will show conductive hearing loss, with decreased bone conduction at 2 kHz ("Carhart notch"). Tympanometry normal, acoustic reflexes absent
Genetic hearing impairment	Audiogram: bilateral or unilateral sensorineural loss. CT scan of temporal bones may show enlarged vestibular aqueduct or other cochlear dysplasia. Screening tests should include eye exam, EKG, and renal function testing. Genetic testing for connexin-26 mutation should be obtained in young children with bilateral severe SNHL and positive family history of deafness
Presbyacusis	Audiometry will show bilaterally symmetric sensorineural hearing loss
Acoustic neuroma	Audiometry will show unilateral sensorineural loss with poor speech discrimination. Auditory brainstem responses will be absent or delayed. MRI of internal auditory canals will demonstrate the tumor
Sudden sensorineural hearing loss	Audiometry will show unilateral sensorineural loss; severity is correlated with prognosis (mild = good, severe = poor). MRI of internal auditory canals should be obtained to rule out acoustic neuroma

Recommended treatment strategy

Disease	Treatment
Diseases causing dizziness or vertigo	
Orthostatic hypotension	Liberalize salt intake, alpha agonists, mineralocorticoids, or lifestyle changes
BPPV	Do Epley maneuver (particle repositioning maneuver) to cure. Posterior semicircular canal occlusion can be performed in rare refractory cases
Episodic vertigo	Treat with acetazolamide or methazolamide. Check electrolytes frequently for possible development of acidosis. Small doses of benzodiazepines are a useful adjuvant. Low-salt diet
Ménière's disease	Low-salt diet is essential, less than 2000 mg/day. Acetazolamide or methazolamide. Check electrolytes frequently for possible development of acidosis. Benzodiazepines are also a useful adjuvant. Steroids during crescendo, by oral or intra-tympanic route. Consider intra-tympanic gentamicin injection in the affected ear. Consider endolymphatic shunt surgery or vestibular nerve section in refractory cases, or labyrinthectomy when hearing is not serviceable
Labyrinthitis, vestibular neuritis	Start vestibular rehabilitation as soon as possible and get patient out of bed. If facial nerve is also involved (Ramsay Hunt syndrome), start steroids immediately. Steroids may or may not be of use in acute labyrinthitis. Benzodiazepines are useful to reduce vertigo. Meclizine (diphenhydramine) can also be used in acute stages
Bilateral loss of vestibular function	Start vestibular rehabilitation as soon as possible. Prognosis is guarded
Superior semicircular canal dehiscence	Surgical occlusion of superior semicircular canals
Mal de debarquement syndrome (MdDS)	Direct patient to medical center that can treat with full-field visual motion while slowly rocking head at frequency of rocking, swaying, or bobbing
Diseases causing hearing loss	
Chronic otitis media	Tympanoplasty surgery for eardrum perforation; myringotomy tube for middle ear effusion; tympanomastoidectomy for cholesteatoma
Otosclerosis	Stapedectomy surgery, or hearing aid
Genetic hearing impairment	Hearing aid at earliest age of detection, cochlear implant for severe/profound loss
Presbyacusis	Hearing aids
Acoustic neuroma	Surgical excision or stereotactic radiotherapy
Sudden sensorineural hearing loss	Prednisone, 1 mg/kg/day, for 10 days. Consider intra-tympanic steroid administration

BOTTOM LINE
- For patients with dizziness or vertigo, accurate diagnosis determines treatment. Effective treatment can be administered in most cases.
- Episodic vertigo is effectively treated with acetazolamide; monitor for acidosis.
- Acetazolamide or methazolamide are sometimes effective in suppressing Ménière's attacks and patients can sometimes obtain relief for months or years. If both ears are affected, treat conservatively to maintain hearing.
- Bilateral vestibular loss can be chronic and disabling, but physical therapy can lessen the disability.
- A workup for acoustic neuroma should be initiated in any case of unilateral sensorineural hearing loss.
- A hearing test should be obtained in any child with speech delay. If hearing loss is detected, it should be treated and the child should be followed closely to prevent learning impairment.
- Most conductive hearing losses can be treated surgically. A hearing aid is an effective alternative. Most sensorineural losses can be treated with hearing aids, or cochlear implant when severe.
- Sensorineural hearing loss in an elderly patient can contribute to dementia, and should be treated with hearing aids or even cochlear implant when appropriate.
- Sudden sensorineural hearing loss is an otologic emergency, and should be treated as early as possible with high-dose steroids. Intra-tympanic steroids are occasionally given. The prognosis is mixed: patients with severe sensorineural impairment do not often recover.

Reading list
Key reading sources for this chapter can be found online at www.mountsinaiexpertguides.com

Additional material for this chapter can be found online at:
www.mountsinaiexpertguides.com

This includes advice for patients, a case study, multiple choice questions and a reading list.

CHAPTER 13

Facial Weakness, Slurred Speech, and Difficulty Swallowing

Hailun Wang[1] and Kenneth W. Altman[2]
[1] Icahn School of Medicine at Mount Sinai, New York, NY, USA
[2] Baylor College of Medicine, Houston, TX, USA

Background
Definition

Slurred speech (*dysarthria*) indicates a defect of speech articulation and intelligibility, in contrast to a disorder of language production (*aphasia*). *Facial weakness* refers to reduction in the contraction of any of the muscles supplied by the facial nerve, whether reflexive or volitional. Difficulty swallowing is termed *dysphagia*.

Impact

Eating, speaking, and expressing ourselves through facial expression all play an enormous role in our daily lives. Quality of life is significantly decreased in patients who are unable to communicate effectively due to dysarthria. And difficulty with swallowing is associated with high levels of morbidity and mortality related to malnutrition, dehydration, and the effects of aspiration, especially in the elderly population.

Approach to diagnosis
Getting your bearings

While the symptoms of facial weakness, dysphagia, and dysarthria can be related to one another, they often present independently of each other and are caused by largely disparate pathologies. Facial weakness, slurred speech, and difficulty swallowing are closely related in the neurology patient as these are common symptoms in stroke patients, for example. There is a broad differential for these three disorders including both neurologic and mechanical causes.

- In approaching facial nerve paralysis, the severity of weakness and etiology will dictate the prognosis and likelihood of improvement.
- Dysphagia can be caused by disruption of any of the three phases of swallowing (oral, pharyngeal, and esophageal), although cognition and the role of the larynx should also be recognized.
- Causes of dysarthria can be categorized as central or peripheral.

Key elements of history

A detailed history should always be obtained with special emphasis on the following.

Mount Sinai Expert Guides: Neurology, First Edition. Edited by Stuart C. Sealfon, Rajeev Motiwala, and Charles B. Stacy.
© 2016 John Wiley & Sons, Ltd. Published 2016 by John Wiley & Sons, Ltd.
Companion website: www.mountsinaiexpertguides.com

Facial paralysis

- Duration of symptoms: acute, subacute, or chronic?
- Pre-existing neurologic disease: e.g. stroke, myasthenia gravis, multiple sclerosis?
- Pre-existing systemic and endocrine disease: diabetes mellitus, hyperthyroidism, hyperostoses, sarcoidosis, pregnancy, sexually transmitted diseases?
- Other associated symptoms: otalgia, hearing loss, tinnitus, vertigo, fever, rash, eye pain, blurred vision?

Dysarthria

- History of stroke, neuromuscular disorders (autoimmune disorders, myasthenia gravis, multiple sclerosis, amyotrophic lateral sclerosis)?
- Distinguish from dyskinesia (secondary to medication effects).
- Differentiate among dysarthria (a voice disorder with loss of neuromuscular control), aphasia (a language disorder), and apraxia (disorder in planning the sequence of and coordination of tongue movements).

Dysphagia

- Acute vs chronic?
- Solids vs liquids, progression from solids to liquids (suggestive of obstructive lesion)?
- Associated symptoms: odynophagia (inflammatory/infectious), coughing/choking (aspiration), regurgitation of digested vs undigested food (gastrointestinal obstruction, Zenker's diverticulum), voice changes/globus sensation (laryngeal involvement, laryngopharyngeal reflux), neurologic symptoms (central etiology), presbypharynges?
- Smoking, alcohol (risk factors for head and neck malignancy), recent weight loss, fevers?
- Pre-existing systemic disorders: hypothyroidism, autoimmune disorders (scleroderma/CREST (calcinosis, Raynaud's phenomenon, esophageal dysmotility, sclerodactyly, and telangiectasia), Sjögren's, sarcoidosis)?
- History of chemotherapy or radiation to head and neck (esophageal stricture, radiation-induced mucositis)?

Table of elements of history and diseases

Facial paralysis	Symptoms	Other key features
Idiopathic (Bell's palsy)	Acute in onset, unilateral (upper and lower divisions), posterior auricular pain, otalgia, hyperacusis, dysgeusia	Although very rare, bilateral paralysis can occur. Bell's palsy more often affects pregnant women, diabetics, and otherwise immunocompromised people
Infectious etiologies	Viral prodrome, otalgia, otorrhea	90% of cases of malignant otitis externa are found in diabetics and those immunocompromised, with pain out of proportion to physical examination

(Continued)

Facial paralysis	Symptoms	Other key features
Trauma, iatrogenic	Immediate onset (transection) vs delayed (edema)	Hearing loss (otic capsule involvement), vertigo
Neoplastic	Pain, other cranial palsies	Facial paralysis is typically a late presentation
Neurologic	Unilateral (stroke) vs bilateral (myasthenia, Guillain–Barré), extremity weakness	

Key elements of physical examination

A complete neurologic examination as well as a head and neck examination should be performed with special emphasis on the following:

Facial paralysis
- Otologic examination: vesicular rash, evidence of otitis externa or media, tuning fork examination.
- Cranial nerve examination: CN VII (facial expression), CN X (palatal elevation, voice), CN XII (tongue movement).
- Associated weakness or reflex changes in extremities.

Dysphagia
- Full cranial nerve examination (see also "Facial paralysis" above).
- The otolaryngologist can perform functional endoscopic evaluation of swallow (FEES): flexible fiberoptic laryngoscopy allowing for evaluation of lesions and masses, oral and pharyngeal phases of swallowing, vocal fold mobility and closure, and aspiration risk (penetration of food or liquid bolus past the laryngeal inlet, pooled secretions in the larynx), sensation in the larynx.

Dysarthria
- Quality of speech: rate, pitch, nasality, intelligibility, volume, vocal quality.
- Focus on CN V, VII, IX, X, and XII.
- Oral cavity: tongue (e.g. hypotonia vs hypertonia, fasciculations, limited ROM), palatal elevation, oral competency.

Table of elements of physical examination by disease (see also Tables 13.1, 13.2, 13.3, 13.4, 13.5, and 13.6)

Facial paralysis	Otoscopy, tuning forks, cranial nerve examination; sensory, motor, cerebellar testing; examine external auditory canal for purulent otorrhea, granulation tissue along osseous-cartilaginous junction (malignant otitis externa), vesicles
Dysarthria	Oral cavity, oropharyngeal examination (muscle atrophy, fasciculation), cranial nerve exam (especially IX, X, XII), bedside speech pathology evaluation, consider ENT referral for flexible laryngoscopy
Dysphagia	Cranial nerve examination (VII, IX, X, XII)

Table 13.1 Facial nerve paralysis grading system: House–Brackmann scale.

Grade	Description
Grade I – Normal	Normal facial function
Grade II – Slight dysfunction	Gross: slight perceptible weakness on close examination At rest: normal symmetry and tone In motion: slight asymmetry, complete eye closure with minimal effort
Grade III – Moderate dysfunction	Gross: obvious but not disfiguring asymmetry At rest: normal symmetry and tone In motion: weak mouth and forehead function, complete eye closure
Grade IV – Moderate/severe dysfunction	Gross: disfiguring weakness At rest: asymmetry In motion: forehead (none), incomplete eye closure, asymmetric with maximal effort
Grade V – Severe dysfunction	Gross: disfiguring weakness At rest: asymmetry In motion: barely imperceptible motion, forehead (none), eye closure (incomplete), mouth (slight movement)
Grade VI – Total paralysis	No movement

Table 13.2 Facial weakness: diseases, treatment, and prognosis.

Disease	Treatment	Prognosis
Idiopathic (Bell's palsy)	Acute phase: oral antivirals and steroids are controversial, eye protection (e.g. eye bubble, Lacri-Lube®, artificial tears) Rare surgical decompression	Incomplete paralysis more likely to recover fully than complete paralysis. 85% improvement, 70% full recovery
Infectious		
Herpes zoster oticus (Ramsay Hunt syndrome)	Antivirals, high-dose prednisone, eye protection, analgesics, vestibular suppressants (if symptoms severe)	Good prognosis for nerve recovery although may be incomplete if severe palsy. Children more likely to fully recover than the elderly
Otitis media	Amoxicillin × 7–10 days, supportive care (analgesics, decongestants)* CT temporal bone to rule out coalescent mastoiditis	Good prognosis with full recovery if aggressive treatment of infectious disease
Necrotizing otitis externa (malignant otitis externa)	Anti-*Pseudomonas* coverage, otic drops, hyperbaric O_2, surgical debridement if failed medical therapy CT temporal bone to rule out coalescent mastoiditis	
Trauma		
Penetrating (transection of branches), blunt force trauma (temporal bone fracture)	Total paralysis: facial nerve exploration with decompression (temporal bone fracture) or surgical reanastomosis (penetrating) within 48–72 h CT temporal bone, and consider carotid angiography depending on vector of trauma Incomplete/delayed paralysis: serial ENoG (electronystagmography), steroids	Primary anastomosis, grafting: >90% of patients have some return of function, 70–75% with good results

(Continued)

Table 13.2 (Continued)

Disease	Treatment	Prognosis
Iatrogenic		
Otologic surgery, neck dissections, salivary gland excisions, local anesthetic	Injury noted intraoperative: primary anastomosis, cable grafting Noted postoperative: observe, steroids, electrodiagnostic testing	Delayed onset and incomplete paralysis usually results in complete recovery
Neoplastic		
Vestibular schwannoma, cholesteatoma, parotid tumors, meningioma, glioma, paraganglioma	Surgical excision	Extrinsic compression and shorter duration are better prognostic factors Poor functional recovery if nerve transected
Neurologic		
Stroke	Supportive care, myofeedback	Spontaneous remission
Myasthenia gravis (MG), Guillain–Barré (GB)	IVIG (intravenous immunoglobulin), immune modulators, thymectomy (MG), supportive care (ventilation – GB)	Prognosis typically good for systemic diseases

*Choice of antibiotic depends on resistance in the local community and culture direct therapy if draining.

Table 13.3 Facial repair and reanimation.

Nerve repair (paralysis <12–18 months)	End-to-end anastomosis, interpositioning, crossover grafting, upper eyelid gold weight implantation
Static procedures (paralysis >12–18 months)	Fascial or allograft slings, browlifts, rhytidoplasty, canthoplasty, gold weights
Dynamic procedures (paralysis >12–18 months)	Local muscle transposition (temporalis, masseter), free nerve muscle grafts

Table 13.4 Neurologic components of swallowing.

Phase of swallowing	Component of swallowing	Localization
Cortical	Cognitive awareness, central motor control	Cerebral hemispheres, brainstem
Oral (voluntary phase)	Seal around mouth Mastication Saliva mixing with food bolus Propulsion of food bolus	CN VII CN V CN IX, VII (parasympathetics) CN XII
Pharyngeal (reflexive phase)	Posterior pharyngeal receptors Nasopharyngeal closure Base of tongue propulsion Closure and elevation of larynx	CN IX, X CN X CN XII CN X
Laryngeal	Vocal fold closure Cricopharyngeal relaxation	CN X CN X
Esophageal	Relaxation of cricopharyngeus Peristalsis of striated/unstriated muscles	CN X CN X

Table 13.5 Common etiologies of dysphagia and their treatment.

Etiology	Treatment
Neurologic	
Neurovascular (stroke – cortical, subcortical, brainstem), neurodegenerative (Parkinson's, multiple sclerosis), systemic (GB, MG), motor neuron disease (ALS)	Swallowing exercises, head and body positioning (head of bed elevation), dietary restrictions (e.g. honey thickened liquids), feeding tube (G-tube or PEG)
Systemic disorders	
Muscular, myopathies (muscular dystrophy, polymyositis), connective tissue disorders (CREST), hypothyroidism	Same as neurologic etiologies above
Miscellaneous	
Gastrointestinal (GERD, achalasia, Zenker's, Plummer–Vinson), neoplastic (obstruction, extrinsic compression, status post resection), infectious (laryngitis, esophagitis, Chagas tonsillitis), iatrogenic, trauma (surgery, chemoradiation), caustic ingestion, foreign body	Medications (PPI, antibiotics), endoscopy (removal of foreign body), esophageal dilatation (strictures, stenosis), surgical resection (neoplasm), feeding tube (G-tube or PEG)

Table 13.6 Etiologies of dysarthria.

Etiology	Voice quality
Spastic (upper motor neuron: e.g. stroke)	Hypernasal, harsh, slow rate, monopitch
Flaccid (lower motor neuron: e.g. bulbar palsy)	Hypernasal, breathy quality to voice
Ataxic (cerebellar lesion)	Slow rate, scanning (separation of syllables), excessive variation in rhythm and volume
Hyperkinetic (e.g. Huntington's, organic voice tremor, Tourette's syndrome)	(Dependent on etiology): variations in pitch, unsteady or rhythmic alterations in rate and loudness
Hypokinetic (e.g. Parkinson's)	Decreased loudness, slow rate, monopitch
Mixed (most common, e.g. ALS, multiple sclerosis)	Slow rate, hoarseness (harsh), hypernasal, monopitch

CLINICAL PEARLS

Facial paralysis
- Difference between House–Brackmann grade III and IV is the presence or absence of full eye closure.
- Facial nerve paralysis associated with numbness, viral prodrome, otalgia, altered taste, hyperacusis commonly seen in Bell's palsy and Ramsay Hunt syndrome.
- Idiopathic Bell's palsy is a diagnosis of exclusion.

Dysphagia
- Disruption of any of the three phases of swallowing (oral, pharyngolaryngeal, esophageal) can cause dysphagia, in addition to cortical and laryngeal dysfunction.
- Stroke is the leading neurologic cause of dysphagia (>50% of patients with stroke will have dysphagia upon initial presentation).
- Neurologic causes of dysphagia, including neurovascular or neuromuscular etiologies, can affect multiple phases of swallowing (e.g. tongue base weakness, loss of pharyngeal

sensation, vocal cord paralysis, weakness, generalized weakness and lack of coordination, poor laryngeal elevation). This also occurs with advancing age in the absence of a specific neurologic disorder.
- Non-neurologic-related dysphagia is usually related to a mechanical obstruction to the swallowing mechanism, including benign tonsil hypertrophy, true neoplasm, cricopharyngeal muscle hypertonicity, and gastroesophageal reflux.
- Pneumonia accounts for one-third of all stroke-related deaths, of which aspiration is a presumed risk factor.
- Dysphagia patients should be referred to ENT or speech pathology for a functional endoscopic evaluation of swallow (FEES).

Dysarthria
- Dysarthria is strictly a motor speech disorder, not to be confused with a problem with language and word finding (aphasia), or with planning and coordination of speech (apraxia), and does not include speech disorders from anatomic abnormalities (e.g. cleft palate).
- Etiologies resulting in dysarthria often affect swallowing as well (dysphagia).

Diagnostic tests
Facial paralysis
- History and physical examination are the cornerstones of diagnosis.
- Imaging:
  - CT temporal bone – best for assessing bony integrity of fallopian canal, indicated when there is clinical evidence of temporal bone disease.
    - MRI with and without gadolinium – better for soft tissue evaluation; indicated if suspicion of cerebellopontine angle lesions/masses (e.g. vestibular schwannoma) or in cases of paralysis without improvement after 4–6 months from onset.
- Ancillary studies:
  - Electrophysiologic testing
    - EMG.
    - Electroneuronography (ENoG) – electrical stimulation of the facial nerve at or near the stylomastoid foramen and recording the motor response at or near the nasal-labial fold is a reliable prognostic indicator during the first 2 weeks of onset.
  - Audiogram – cases of trauma, preoperative assessment.
- Blood tests:
  - CBC – inflammatory process
  - VRDL – syphilis
  - ACE level – sarcoidosis

Dysphagia
- Imaging:
  - Flexible endoscopic evaluation of swallowing (FEES).
  - Modified barium swallow (MBS): videofluoroscopy visualizing oral, pharyngeal, and laryngeal phases of swallow with different food consistencies, allows for evaluation of penetration or frank aspiration of contrast into airway.
  - Esophagram, barium swallow: evaluate esophageal phase (degree of motility), evaluate esophageal lumen (obstructing masses, reflux, diverticuli).

- Ancillary studies:
  - Chest X-ray (pneumonia)
  - Manometry
  - Direct laryngoscopy and esophagoscopy (high suspicion for neoplasm).

Dysarthria

- Imaging:
  - Patients typically present after suffering a neurologic event.
  - Dependent on suspected central or peripheral etiology.

BOTTOM LINE

- Facial paralysis, dysphagia, and dysarthria may all be present in the same patient from a single neurologic cause, but these symptoms can also arise independently and be due to a number of disparate etiologies.
- Dysphagia in stroke patients and the elderly poses a high risk of morbidity and mortality. Evaluation and treatment in conjunction with speech language pathologists (determination of safe diet vs NPO status) is recommended to prevent complications (e.g. aspiration pneumonia, pneumonitis).

Reading list

Key reading sources for this chapter can be found online at www.mountsinaiexpertguides.com

---

Additional material for this chapter can be found online at:
www.mountsinaiexpertguides.com

This includes advice for patients, a case study, multiple choice questions, a reading list.

CHAPTER 14

Difficulty Walking

Ruth H. Walker
James J. Peters Veterans Affairs Medical Center, Bronx, NY, USA

Background

Difficulty in walking can be due to disruption of motor function at a multitude of sites along the neuraxis, impairment of sensory proprioceptive input, or non-neurologic causes, such as bone or joint pain or dysfunction. Here we focus upon potential neurologic causes of problems with gait.

Social impact

- Gait disorders are a common neurologic problem, particularly in the aging population, and can have a significant functional impact, both physical and psychosocial.
- Falls can lead to physical injury, such as hip fracture or subdural hematomas, especially in the older population.
- Impaired gait leads to limited mobility and increased dependence, and can result in isolation, depression, and loss of independence. Fear of falling further compounds the problem. If the person lives with family or other caregivers, there are social stresses for all involved.

Approach to diagnosis

Getting your bearings

- How quickly did the problem develop and is it progressive?
- A thorough neurologic examination will often provide an indication of the cause of the problem, e.g. parkinsonism, peripheral neuropathy, or cerebellar disease.
- Close observation of the patient walking is essential and typically very informative.

Key elements of history

- What is the time course of disease progression? A sudden onset, for example, is consistent with the diagnosis of a stroke. Most neurodegenerative disorders are slowly progressive. Subacute progression may indicate an expanding intracerebral mass lesion or spinal stenosis.
- Are there concomitant medical conditions, e.g. cardiovascular disease, diabetes mellitus, dementia?
- Are there problems with bowel or bladder function?
- Is the patient aware of focal weakness?
- Are there associated neurologic symptoms affecting other functions?
- Is the patient falling?
- Is there any family history of a similar problem with walking?

Mount Sinai Expert Guides: Neurology, First Edition. Edited by Stuart C. Sealfon, Rajeev Motiwala, and Charles B. Stacy.
© 2016 John Wiley & Sons, Ltd. Published 2016 by John Wiley & Sons, Ltd.
Companion website: www.mountsinaiexpertguides.com

Table of elements of history and diseases

Disease	Symptoms	Duration/tempo	Circumstances/other key features
Stroke (see Chapter 20)	Unilateral limb weakness or ataxia, facial weakness, altered speech	Sudden onset, gradual improvement	Unilateral localizing symptoms
Parkinsonian disorders (see Chapter 25) Parkinson's disease (PD)	Slowed, shuffling gait; difficulty getting up from chair, turning in bed; loss of sense of smell; foot cramps; voice softer and monotonous; smaller handwriting; difficulty with fine motor tasks	Gradual onset, progression over years	Specific other features may indicate atypical parkinsonism Asymmetric limb onset, e.g. resting tremor, bradykinesia, foot dystonia
Progressive supranuclear palsy Multiple system atrophy		Gradual onset, progression over years (but more rapid than PD)	Falls within 5 years of disease onset; emotional lability
Corticobasal syndrome		Gradual onset, progression over years (but more rapid than PD)	Falls within 5 years of disease onset (see Chapter 25)
Dementia with Lewy bodies		Gradual onset, progression over years	Dementia, visual hallucinations within first 5 years; marked sensitivity to antipsychotics; fluctuations in mental status and alertness
Vascular parkinsonism		Stepwise progression, over years	Vascular risk factors
Drug-induced parkinsonism		Onset related to administration of the causative medication	Dopamine D2-receptor blocker, e.g. antipsychotics both typical and atypical, anti-nausea medications
Intracerebral lesion (e.g. tumor, multiple sclerosis (MS))	Unilateral weakness or ataxia	Varies with disease	Unilateral localizing features; may be multifocal in MS
Cerebellar disease (see Chapter 28)	Wide-based gait	Gradual onset, progression over years; subacute	May have family history of similar disease or history of toxic exposure (e.g. alcohol, phenytoin, lithium)
Gait apraxia	Difficulty initiating stride, gait freezing	Gradual onset, progression over years	May have frontal signs or be otherwise normal
Peripheral motor neuropathy (see Chapter 32)	Foot drop, often bilateral	Gradual onset, progression over years; subacute; acute	Diabetes; other diseases associated with peripheral neuropathy. If also upper motor neuron signs, consider ALS
Peripheral sensory neuropathy (see Chapter 32)	Wide-based but variable gait, worsened with eyes shut	Gradual onset, progression over years; subacute	Diabetes; other diseases associated with peripheral neuropathy

(Continued)

Disease	Symptoms	Duration/tempo	Circumstances/other key features
Myopathy (see Chapter 33)	Lurching gait due to hip adductor and flexor weakness	Gradual onset, progression over years; subacute	Family history, drug exposure (e.g. statins, corticosteroids)
Psychogenic	Variable features, inconsistent exam	Variable. May have sudden unexplainable onset or remission	Evidence of psychosocial stress, although patient may deny; anxiety on walking, may be as much as 20% of neurology clinic gait disorder patients
Normal pressure hydrocephalus	"Magnetic" gait	Gradual onset, progression over years	Should not have significant features of parkinsonism; urinary incontinence is a classical feature; dementia with disease progression; 1:200 of patients older than age 65
Spinal cord lesions (compressive or intrinsic [see Chapter 18])	Depends upon level of lesion	Variable with etiology	Sensory symptoms, weakness, incontinence
Cervical stenosis	Spastic gait, often wide-based but variable	Gradual, subacute, or acute	May involve arms (sensory, motor)
Lumbar stenosis, radiculopathy	Pain in lower back, often radiating into buttocks, hip, or leg; focal leg or foot weakness	Gradual, subacute, or acute	Claudication. May have bowel or bladder incontinence (cauda equina syndrome)

CLINICAL PEARLS
- Check medications for any that might cause parkinsonism or unsteadiness.
- Is there a family history of any gait disorders, suggestive of, for example, a hereditary cerebellar condition?
- Falling within 5 years of onset of a parkinsonian disorder indicates an atypical parkinsonian syndrome, not idiopathic Parkinson's disease.
- Idiopathic Parkinson's disease typically starts asymmetrically. Atypical Parkinson's disorders are more commonly symmetrical from onset.
- Is there lightheadedness on standing or walking? Orthostatic hypotension can be subtle in presentation and is a major cause of non-specific difficulty in walking.
- Dementia is a late symptom of normal pressure hydrocephalus and is more commonly due to Alzheimer's dementia.

Key elements of physical examination
- Weakness
- Hypo- or hyperreflexia
- Ataxia
- Sensory level or Brown-Séquard syndrome
- Gait apraxia
- Parkinsonism

Table of elements of physical examination by disease

Disease	Signs on examination
Stroke	Unilateral weakness, hyperreflexia; unilateral cerebellar signs; other localizing signs (e.g. sensory loss, cranial nerve findings)
Parkinsonian disorders	Generalized bradykinesia, stooped posture, shuffling gait, narrow base, freezing, festination, resting tremor, hypophonic monotonous voice
Parkinson's disease	Often asymmetric resting tremor of hand (leg, chin), increased tone, positive glabellar tap; activation of tremor with movements of another limb, e.g. repetitive hand movements
Progressive supranuclear palsy	Gaze paresis, especially downward gaze; difficulty descending stairs; surprised expression; retrocollis; frontal lobe signs – positive "clap" sign[a]
Multiple system atrophy	Autonomic or cerebellar signs; diplophonia
Corticobasal syndrome	Asymmetric parkinsonism, dystonia; asymmetric cortical signs related to most affected hemisphere, e.g. aphasia, limb apraxia, "alien" hand
Dementia with Lewy bodies	Cortical and subcortical cognitive impairment; parkinsonism
Vascular parkinsonism	May have other signs of stroke Unilateral weakness, hyperreflexia; unilateral cerebellar signs; other localizing signs, sensory loss, cranial nerve lesions
Cerebellar disease	Abnormalities of eye movements; dysarthria, limb ataxia; may have specific findings related to specific genetic diagnoses
Gait apraxia	May have frontal signs
Peripheral motor neuropathy	Hyporeflexia, distal weakness (may be subtle)
Peripheral sensory neuropathy	Sensory loss, especially vibration; balance worse with eyes closed (Romberg sign)
Myopathy	Proximal muscle weakness, neck flexor weakness, preserved reflexes
Psychogenic	Give-way weakness, leg-buckling, falling into examiner's arms or only when within reach of a support; inconsistent neurologic examination (Video 14.1 on the companion website)
Normal pressure hydrocephalus	Wide-based "magnetic" gait
Spinal cord lesion (structural or intrinsic myelopathy)	Evaluate for sensory or hemi-sensory level, motor level, bowel/bladder function
Cervical stenosis	Hyperreflexia, positive Babinski sign; may have focal weakness of upper limbs or dermatomal sensory loss related to cervical radiculopathy
Lumbar stenosis/ radiculopathy	Hyporeflexia; may have focal weakness of legs or dermatomal sensory loss related to lumbar radiculopathy

[a] The affected patient is instructed to copy the examiner in clapping their hands the correct number of times (e.g. two or three times). The patient performs extra claps as they are unable to inhibit the performance of repetitive movements.

CLINICAL PEARLS
- Atrophy of the small muscles of the hands can indicate cervical stenosis, especially when combined with leg hyperreflexia and a positive Babinski sign.
- Look for a generalized decrease in spontaneous movements, e.g. of hands or face, as a clue to the presence of parkinsonism. If the patient comes in with their partner of similar age, compare them. Advanced age alone does not result in decreased movements.
- Weakness of foot dorsiflexion may not be apparent on confrontation; ask patients to stand on their toes and observe them walking to determine if there is a foot-drop.
- Anxiety and fear of falling can compound a relatively minor neurologic problem. If the gait improves markedly when the examiner is holding the patient's hand this may be a significant factor. (This feature may also be seen in parkinsonian disorders.)
- Gait apraxia can be seen in patients with an otherwise normal examination.

Diagnostic tests

Disease	Test findings
Stroke	Abnormalites on brain imaging (MRI or CT)
Parkinsonian disorders	May consider DAT scan (decreased dopamine transporter uptake, although only supportive of diagnosis); diagnosis of PD rather than atypical parkinsonism is supported by the absence of "red flags,"[a] a typical disease course, and sustained and consistent response to L-dopa
Intracerebral lesion (tumor, multiple sclerosis)	Abnormalites on brain imaging (MRI or CT)
Cerebellar disease	MRI brain – cerebellar atrophy
Gait apraxia	MRI brain may be normal or show frontal lesions
Peripheral motor neuropathy	Electromyography/nerve conduction studies (EMG/NCS). See Chapter 3
Peripheral sensory neuropathy	EMG/NCS. See Chapter 3
Myopathy	EMG/NCV. Muscle enzymes, biopsy, see Chapter 3
Psychogenic	All testing negative or not consistent with presentation
Normal pressure hydrocephalus	CT/MRI brain – dilated ventricles, flow void in aqueduct; response to lumbar drainage
Cervical stenosis	MRI, CT, see Chapters 2 and 3
Lumbar stenosis/radiculopathy	EMG/NCS, MRI, CT, see Chapters 2 and 3

[a] "Red flags" include significant autonomic dysfunction; falls, hallucinations, or dementia within 5 years of disease onset; impaired downward gaze.

Recommended diagnostic strategy
See Algorithm 14.1

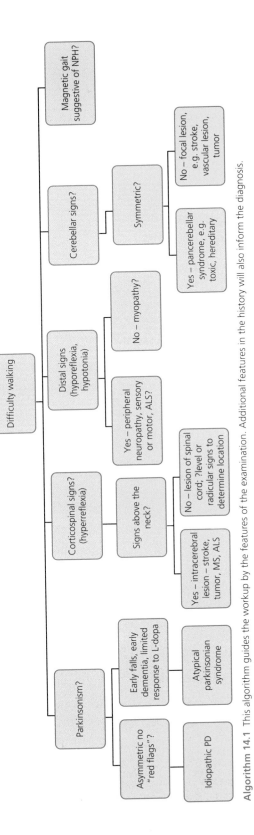

Algorithm 14.1 This algorithm guides the workup by the features of the examination. Additional features in the history will also inform the diagnosis.

BOTTOM LINE
- The initial priority in the differential diagnosis of difficulty walking is to identify causes that are treatable, have treatable risk factors, or have hereditary bases with potential screening implications.
- Structural lesions causing cord compression require urgent neurosurgical evaluation to avoid permanent loss of function, in particular of bowel and bladder.
- Risk of progression is a major consideration and should guide the urgency of the workup and the treatment.
- Fall prevention is paramount.

Reading list

Key reading sources for this chapter can be found online at www.mountsinaiexpertguides.com

Suggested websites

MedlinePlus: Walking abnormalities: http://www.nlm.nih.gov/medlineplus/ency/article/003199.htm

everyday health: Tips to help Parkinson's patients move through a freezing episode: http://www.everydayhealth.com/parkinsons-disease/freezing-episodes.aspx

The Foundation for Peripheral Neuropathy: https://www.foundationforpn.org

**Additional material for this chapter can be found online at:
www.mountsinaiexpertguides.com**

This includes advice for patients, a case study, multiple choice questions, a reading list, and Video 14.1.

CHAPTER 15

Muscle Weakness and Paralysis

Rajeev Motiwala
Icahn School of Medicine at Mount Sinai, New York, NY, USA

Background
Definition
Patients who develop muscle weakness can present with difficulty with ambulation, impairment of functional motor activities, or specific problems such as respiratory paralysis or bulbar weakness. A wide variety of neurologic and systemic diseases can present in this manner.

Approach to diagnosis
Getting your bearings
Patients presenting with acute muscle weakness require urgent assessment and efficient workup to identify life-threatening illnesses. Patient who have a more chronic course require a selective and sequential approach.
- Determine whether the problem is primarily neurologic or is related to a severe systemic illness.
- Localize the problem in the nervous system:
  - Upper motor neuron (UMN) or lower motor neuron (LMN)?
  - Where is the site within the neuromuscular pathway – anterior horn cell, root, plexus, peripheral nerve, neuromuscular junction, or muscle?
- Identify the cause.

Key elements of history
- Pre-existing neurologic disease: e.g. multiple sclerosis, previous stroke, known neuromuscular disorder.
- Duration of symptoms: acute, subacute, or chronic.
- Associated systemic features: fever, rash, other organ diseases, trauma, gastrointestinal disturbances.
- Other neurologic symptoms besides weakness: tingling or numbness, bladder-bowel involvement, respiratory compromise, slurred speech, hoarseness of voice, difficulty clearing secretions, double vision.
- Distribution of weakness: hemiparesis, paraparesis, proximal or distal, focal weakness restricted to muscle groups.

Mount Sinai Expert Guides: Neurology, First Edition. Edited by Stuart C. Sealfon, Rajeev Motiwala, and Charles B. Stacy.
© 2016 John Wiley & Sons, Ltd. Published 2016 by John Wiley & Sons, Ltd.
Companion website: www.mountsinaiexpertguides.com

Table of elements of history and diseases

Disease	Symptoms	Duration	Other key features
Stroke	Hemiparesis, facial weakness, double vision, slurred speech, hemisensory symptoms	Acute	History of a prior stroke Vascular risk factors: hypertension, diabetes, heart disease, smoking, hyperlipidemia
Brain tumor	Headache, seizures, progressive neurologic dysfunction	Subacute	History of systemic malignancy, history of previously treated tumor
Multiple sclerosis	Hemiparesis, paraparesis, sensory symptoms, symptoms suggesting cranial nerve involvement	Acute, subacute, or chronic	Known multiple sclerosis, relapsing and remitting course, classic symptoms such as visual impairment due to optic neuritis, positive Lhermitte sign
Cord compression	Quadriparesis (cervical) Paraparesis (thoracic) Localized spinal pain Sensory symptoms, band-like sensation Bladder-bowel involvement Flexor spasms	Acute, subacute, or acute exacerbation	Known systemic malignancy Fever or other infectious symptoms in epidural abscess Trauma
Acute transverse myelitis	Similar to "Cord compression" above	Acute	Preceding febrile illness, vaccination
Chronic non-compressive myelopathy	Weakness in extremities, sensory loss, ataxia	Chronic	Malabsorption, pernicious anemia, skeletal deformities in developmental or genetic disorders
Anterior horn cell disease	Weakness, muscle twitching	Acute or chronic	Fever – poliomyelitis, West Nile virus infection Progressive course with muscle wasting in motor neuron disease
Polyradiculopathy: multiple roots, lumbar roots as in cauda equina syndrome	Pain, weakness, paresthesia, numbness, bladder and bowel dysfunction	Acute, subacute, or chronic	Tick bite or skin rash in Lyme disease; underlying HIV infection in CMV radiculitis; dermatomal rash in herpes zoster; low back pain and radicular pain in compression of cauda equina
Acute inflammatory demyelinating polyneuropathy (Guillain–Barré syndrome)	Weakness, distal sensory symptoms, facial weakness, respiratory failure	Acute	History of preceding infectious illness, *Campylobacter jejuni* infection, history of Lyme disease, HIV infection, or prior vaccination
Other peripheral neuropathies	Symmetric distal weakness and numbness	Subacute or chronic	History of diabetes, alcohol use, chemotherapy, systemic illnesses

Disease	Symptoms	Duration	Other key features
Neuromuscular junction disorders	Ocular and bulbar symptoms, fatigable weakness, no sensory complaints	Acute, subacute, or chronic	History of ingestion of canned food and GI symptoms in botulism. History of suicidal or accidental ingestion of compounds, lacrimation, wheezing and diarrhea in organophosphate and carbamate ingestion. History of prior episodes of a similar nature in myasthenia gravis History of lung cancer in Lambert–Eaton syndrome History of tick exposure
Muscle diseases	Proximal extremity weakness, neck flexor weakness, no sensory complaints	Acute, subacute or chronic	Medications such as statins in toxic myopathy, skin rash in dermatomyositis, recurrent episodes and positive family history in periodic paralysis, family history in muscular dystrophies

CLINICAL PEARLS
- History of associated systemic illness is extremely important.
- Distribution of muscle weakness and other neurologic symptoms as reported by the patient help in determining possible site of localization.

Key elements of physical examination
- Look for findings on general examination that may provide a clue to the underlying systemic disease.
- Identify pattern of weakness.
- Grading of motor strength (Medical Research Council) 0–5:
  - Grade 5: Normal contraction against full resistance.
  - Grade 4: Muscle strength is reduced but can still move joint against resistance.
  - Grade 3: Muscle strength is further reduced such that the joint can be moved only against gravity with the examiner's resistance completely removed.
  - Grade 2: Muscle can move only if the resistance of gravity is eliminated.
  - Grade 1: Only a trace or flicker of movement is seen or felt in the muscle.
  - Grade 0: No movement is observed.
- Localize the site of the lesion along the neuraxis using findings on motor examination, reflexes, and sensory examination. Determine if there is primary involvement of:
  - Upper motor neuron: most commonly hemiparesis, quadriparesis, paraparesis, monoparesis; central not primary modality sensory loss, reflexes and muscle tone increased unless acute, pathologic reflexes (Babinski sign), associated CNS findings.
  - Anterior horn cell: muscle atrophy, fasciculations, normal sensory function, reflexes proportional to weakness.
  - Root, plexus, peripheral nerve: focal motor deficit, decreased tone, loss of deep tendon reflexes, peripheral pattern of sensory loss, may have pain.

- Neuromuscular junction: in myasthenia gravis – fatigability, such as on persistent upward gaze, normal sensory examination and reflexes; in myasthenic syndrome – increased power on repeated activity, sensory normal, reflexes absent.
- Muscle: symmetric proximal weakness, deep tendon reflexes normal or proportional to weakness, normal sensation.

Table of elements of physical examination by disease

Disease	Physical findings
Stroke	Aphasia, UMN facial weakness, hemiparesis, ataxia, extensor plantar response
Brain tumor	Focal neurologic deficits, papilledema, altered sensorium
Multiple sclerosis	Dysarthria, afferent pupillary defect, nystagmus, internuclear ophthalmoplegia, UMN signs in extremities with weakness, ataxia, sensory deficits
Cord compression	Fever may be present in epidural abscess, bony tenderness and deformity, quadriparesis in cervical cord compression, paraparesis in thoracic and lumbar cord (conus medullaris) lesions, UMN signs with hyperreflexia and spasticity below the level of the lesion, horizontal sensory level on the trunk
Spinal cord injury	Evidence of spine tenderness or deformity, recent surgical scar
Acute transverse myelitis	Usually severe or complete paralysis and sensory loss below the site of involvement
Other chronic non-compressive myelopathies	Variable weakness and sensory findings Syringomyelia: dissociated anesthesia with loss of pain and temperature and preserved light touch, vibration, and proprioception Subacute combined degeneration: predominant posterior column loss with absent distal reflexes in lower and brisk reflexes in upper extremities Friedreich's ataxia: associated cerebellar signs, kyphoscoliosis, pes cavus, absent distal reflexes
Acute anterior horn cell disorders	Flaccidity, weakness with absent deep tendon reflexes, flexor or mute plantar responses, normal sensation
Motor neuron disease	Combination of LMN signs – fasciculations, atrophy, and muscle weakness with UMN signs such as hyperreflexia often in the same anatomic segments and extensor plantar responses
Cauda equina syndrome	Asymmetric lower extremity weakness with depressed or absent reflexes, saddle anesthesia, impaired anal sphincter tone
Acute inflammatory demyelinating polyneuropathy	Symmetric or asymmetric motor weakness, hypoactive or absent deep tendon reflexes, associated bilateral facial weakness or other motor cranial nerve involvement, mild distal sensory deficits
Other peripheral neuropathies	Distal weakness, sensory loss in a glove-and-stocking distribution, hypoactive or absent distal reflexes
Myasthenia gravis	Ptosis, fatigable weakness of extraocular muscles with diplopia, bulbar weakness, muscle weakness with preserved reflexes, normal sensation
Lambert–Eaton syndrome	Proximal muscle weakness, absent deep tendon reflexes, improvement in muscle strength and reflexes after exercise
Botulism	Ptosis, extraocular muscle weakness, fixed and dilated pupils, flaccid weakness in extremities with absent reflexes
Organophosphate and carbamate poisoning	Miosis, excessive lacrimation, sialorrhea, wheezing, bradycardia, muscle weakness
Tick paralysis	Flaccid paralysis, nystagmus, lethargy, presence of a tick

Disease	Physical findings
Inflammatory myopathies	Proximal muscle weakness, neck muscle weakness, may have muscle tenderness, preserved reflexes and normal sensation Dermatomyositis: heliotrope discoloration, Gottron's nodules
Muscular dystrophies	Duchenne's: pseudohypertrophy of calves Myotonic dystrophy: temporal wasting, ptosis, sternocleidomastoid atrophy, distal weakness Limb girdle muscular dystrophy: proximal weakness
Metabolic myopathies and channelopathies	Symmetric weakness in periodic paralysis, myotonia in hyperkalemic variety, exercise-induced pain or cramps and rhabdomyolysis in certain metabolic varieties

CLINICAL PEARLS
- Sudden onset of hemiparesis – consider stroke syndrome.
- Ptosis, diplopia, fluctuating weakness in extremities, respiratory muscle weakness – consider myasthenia gravis.
- Subacute progressive proximal muscle weakness – consider inflammatory myopathy, drug-induced myopathy, or limb girdle muscular dystrophy.
- Combination of lower motor neuron and upper motor neuron findings without any sensory involvement or sphincter dysfunction – consider motor neuron disease.
- Acute onset of progressive motor weakness with distal sensory symptoms and absent reflexes – consider acute inflammatory demyelinating polyneuropathy.

Diagnostic tests

Stroke	Neuroimaging – CT, MRI, vascular studies
Brain tumor	Neuroimaging, systemic malignancy workup, biopsy
Multiple sclerosis	MRI brain and spine, CSF examination, evoked potentials
Cord compression	Urgent MRI, or CT myelogram if MRI is not possible; systemic evaluation for malignancy or source of infection
Spinal cord injury	CT, X-rays, and MRI depending on clinical context
Acute transverse myelitis	MRI of spine excludes cord compression and may show presence of cord swelling and signal abnormality CSF examination: elevated protein, pleocytosis, viral cultures, Lyme antibody

Other non-compressive myelopathies	MRI of spine:
	    Multiple sclerosis: patchy signal abnormalities
	    Neuromyelitis optica: longitudinally extensive signal abnormality
	    Subacute combined degeneration: posterior and lateral column signal abnormality
	MRI of brain:
	    May show presence of white matter lesions consistent with demyelinating disease
	Metabolic and serologic studies:
	    Neuromyelitis optica (NMO)-IgG (aquaporin) antibody, vitamin B12 level, copper level, Lyme disease serology, syphilis serology, HTLV1/2 antibody, tests for collagen vascular diseases – antinuclear antibody (ANA), Sjögren antibodies, angiotensin-converting enzyme (ACE) level
	CSF examination:
	    Elevated protein, pleocytosis, Lyme and syphilis tests, ACE level, oligoclonal bands and IgG synthesis rate, NMO-IgG antibody
	Genetic testing:
	    Hereditary spastic paraplegia, Friedreich's ataxia

(Continued)

Acute anterior horn cell diseases – polio-like illnesses	MRI of spine:
	   Rule out cord compression, signal abnormalities may be seen
	 CSF examination:
	   Increased protein, lymphocytic pleocytosis, may show polymorphonuclears in early stage, West Nile virus PCR and antibodies, polio virus PCR and antibodies, Coxsackie, ECHO, EV7, HSV, and VZV PCR and antibodies
	 Serologic studies:
	   Acute phase and convalescent antibody viral titers
	 EMG/NCV study:
	   Reduced amplitudes of compound muscle action potentials, normal sensory nerve conduction studies, acute neurogenic changes after 2–3 weeks

Motor neuron disease	EMG/NCV study:
	   Active and chronic neurogenic changes in at least three segments (bulbar, cervical, thoracic, and lumbar), normal sensory nerve conduction studies, absence of multifocal motor conduction block
	 Appropriate imaging studies:
	   MRI of brain and spine to rule out other causes of weakness
	 Serologic studies to exclude other conditions that can mimic:
	   Ganglioside monosialic acid 1 (GM-1) antibodies, Lyme serology, parathyroid hormone level, serum and urine immunofixation, paraneoplastic antibodies

Cauda equina syndrome and other polyradiculopathies	MRI of lumbosacral spine without and with contrast:
	   Disk herniation, mass lesion, thickening and enhancement of roots
	 CSF examination:
	   Elevated protein and pleocytosis in infections and meningeal neoplasia, Lyme antibody, viral studies – CMV, herpes zoster, ACE level, elevated protein without pleocytosis in chronic inflammatory demyelinating polyneuropathy

Acute inflammatory demyelinating polyneuropathy (Guillain–Barré syndrome)	CSF examination:
	   May be normal in the first week, typically shows elevated protein without pleocytosis (albuminocytologic dissociation)
	 EMG/NCV study:
	   Slow conduction velocities, prolonged distal latencies and late responses, relatively preserved amplitudes of motor potentials

Other peripheral neuropathies	See Chapter 32
Myasthenia gravis	Tensilon (edrophonium) test Serology to look for presence of acetylcholine receptor antibodies, anti-striated muscle antibody, muscle-specific kinase (MuSK) antibody EMG/NCV study: repetitive nerve stimulation and single fiber EMG CT/MRI chest: rule out presence of thymoma
Lambert–Eaton (myasthenic) syndrome	EMG/NCV study: paradoxical facilitation of motor response after brief exercise and after fast rates of repetitive stimulation Blood test for presence of voltage-gated calcium channel antibody Systemic search for underlying malignancy – commonest association is with lung cancer
Botulism	Botulinum toxin and spores in stool sample, serum analysis for toxin by bioassay, nerve conduction study shows reduced compound motor action potential (CMAP) amplitudes, 40–200% post-activation facilitation
Organophosphate and carbamate poisoning	Mainly a clinical diagnosis RBC acetylcholinesterase level not useful for immediate management Atropine challenge can confirm clinical suspicion

Inflammatory myopathies	Elevated muscle enzymes: creatine kinase and aldolase EMG: myopathic changes and evidence of increased insertional activity Muscle biopsy: typical inflammatory changes
Muscular dystrophies	Elevated muscle enzymes, myopathic changes in EMG with increased insertional activity or myotonic discharges, genetic testing, muscle biopsy in selected cases only
Metabolic myopathies and channelopathies	Serum electrolytes, serum biochemical markers – pyruvate, lactate, acylcarnitine panel, ammonia level, provocative tests, muscle biopsy

Table of frequency of each disease

Stroke	First stroke: 191/100,000 in Blacks 149/100,000 in Hispanics 88/100,000 in Whites Overall (first and recurrent stroke): 223/100,000 in Blacks 196/100,000 in Hispanics 93/100,000 in Whites
Brain tumor	19.9/100,000: 7.3/100,000 malignant tumors 12.6/100,000 benign tumors
Multiple sclerosis	85/100,000 in USA 47.2/100,000 in Texas study area 86.3/100,000 in Missouri study area 109.5/100,000 in Ohio study area
Cord compression	3.4% annualized incidence in hospitalized cancer patients (one US study) 2.54% of cancer patients with at least one episode in the last 5 years of their life
Spinal cord injury	12,000 new cases per year in USA 40 new cases per million
Acute transverse myelitis	1–8 new cases per million or approximately 1400 new cases per year
Other non-compressive myelopathies	Heterogeneous group of conditions – data not reliable
Acute anterior horn cell disease	No reliable data
Motor neuron disease	2 per 100,000
Cauda equina syndrome	No reliable data
Acute inflammatory demyelinating neuropathy	0.81–1.89 per 100,000 person years 20% increase with every 10-year increase in age
Peripheral neuropathies	Prevalence: 2400 per 100,000 >55 years: 8000 per 100,000
Myasthenia gravis	Incidence: 3–30 per 1,000,000 Prevalence: 14–20 per 100,000
Lambert–Eaton syndrome	Incidence: 0.48 per 1,000,000 Prevalence: 2.32 per 1,000,000
Botulism	Average 110 cases per year in USA
Organophosphate and carbamate poisoning	Accurate current data not available 2007: out of 96,307 calls to the poison centers (3.4% of all human exposures) related to pesticide exposure, many were related to organophosphate compounds

(Continued)

Inflammatory myopathies	Incidence: 5.8–7.9 cases per million per year Prevalence: 14–17.4 cases per million
Muscular dystrophies	Prevalence of Duchenne and Becker muscular dystrophy in males aged 5–24 years: 1.3–1.8 per 10,000
Metabolic myopathies and channelopathies	Heterogeneous group

Recommended diagnostic strategy

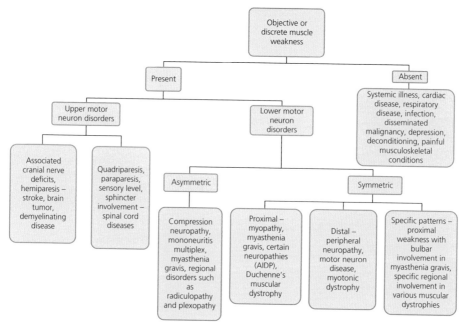

Algorithm 15.1 Differential diagnosis

Note: AIDP = acute inflammatory demyelinating polyneuropathy.

BOTTOM LINE
- Identify critical patients with respiratory muscle weakness – is ventilator support necessary?
- Identify patients who need emergent surgical consultation – spinal cord trauma, spinal cord compression.
- Identify intoxications or infections that require urgent intervention – e.g. atropine in organophosphate poisoning, removal of tick in tick paralysis.
- Localize the site of involvement along the neuraxis on examination, which will guide further investigations and management. Upper motor neuron disorders are likely to require imaging studies, lower motor neuron disorders may require electrodiagnostic studies, and a strong suspicion of a genetic disorder may prompt genetic testing.
- Patients with potentially serious conditions that are known to progress quickly require hospitalization and prompt investigations. Patients with more chronic or subacute presentations need more sequential testing and possibly a period of observation before considering invasive procedures.

Reading list

Key reading sources for this chapter can be found online at www.mountsinaiexpertguides.com

Suggested websites

Centers for Disease Control. Botulism Epidemiological Overview for Clinicians: emergency.cdc.gov/agent/Botulism/clinicians/epidemiology.asp

Spinal Cord Injury Facts and Figures at a Glance: https://www.nscisc.uab.edu

Additional material for this chapter can be found online at:
www.mountsinaiexpertguides.com

This includes a case study, multiple choice questions, and a reading list.

CHAPTER 16

Tingling and Loss of Sensation

Lan Zhou
Icahn School of Medicine at Mount Sinai, New York, NY, USA

Background
Definition

Tingling is a positive sensory symptom that is often described as a pins and needles sensation in the affected body area.

Loss of sensation is a negative sensory symptom that refers to an inability to feel sensory stimuli. Awareness of sensory loss is usually described by patients as numbness. It is important to distinguish sensory loss from weakness, which may also be reported as numbness by the patient.

Impact

• Seeking medical attention for tingling and numbness is common. These symptoms can be caused by many diverse neurologic diseases that affect the sensory pathways in the peripheral nervous system or the central nervous system. Therefore, it is difficult to estimate their annual incidence or social impact.

Approach to diagnosis
Getting your bearings

• Tingling and numbness indicate impairment of sensory pathways, which can be at the level of cutaneous nerves, peripheral sensory nerves, spinal cord, or brain.
• It is important to know the distribution of sensory symptoms: whether focal, patchy, diffuse, unilateral, bilateral, symmetric, asymmetric, deficit increasing with distance from the spinal cord (length-dependent), or non-length-dependent. It is also important to know whether there are other associated neurologic symptoms. This information will help to localize the lesion.
• It is important to know the tempo and progression of the sensory symptoms: whether acute, subacute, or chronic, and whether constant, intermittent, static, or progressive. It is also important to know whether there are any underlying medical or neurologic conditions, neurotoxic drug exposure, alcohol abuse, or a positive family history. The information will help to identify the etiology.

Key elements of history

• When and how did the tingling and numbness develop?
• How did the sensory symptoms progress?
• Are there any other symptoms?

Mount Sinai Expert Guides: Neurology, First Edition. Edited by Stuart C. Sealfon, Rajeev Motiwala, and Charles B. Stacy.
© 2016 John Wiley & Sons, Ltd. Published 2016 by John Wiley & Sons, Ltd.
Companion website: www.mountsinaiexpertguides.com

- Are there any medical or neurologic diseases?
- Does the patient take any medications or drink alcohol?
- Are there any family members who have or have had similar symptoms?

Table of elements of history and diseases

Disease	Symptoms	Duration/ tempo	Circumstances/other key features
Neuropathy			
Mononeuropathy	Tingling, numbness in one individual nerve distribution	Acute, subacute, or chronic	A common cause is entrapment affecting the median nerve at the wrist, the ulnar nerve at the elbow, the radial nerve at the spiral groove, or the peroneal nerve at the fibular head
Mononeuropathy multiplex	Tingling, numbness involving multiple individual nerves	Acute or subacute	Often caused by vasculitis
Polyneuropathy			
Axonal	Tingling, numbness in distal limbs, often symmetric	Acute, subacute, or chronic	Associated with diabetes, connective tissue diseases, paraproteinemia, B12 deficiency, thyroid dysfunction, HIV, HCV, or Lyme infections, cryoglobulinemia, neurotoxic drug exposure, alcohol abuse, and paraneoplastic syndrome. It can be hereditary (Charcot–Marie–Tooth, CMT)
Demyelinating: • AIDP (acute inflammatory demyelinating polyneuropathy, Guillain–Barré syndrome)	Ascending tingling, numbness. May have limb, bilateral facial, or respiratory muscle weakness	Acute	Often idiopathic May develop after infection, vaccination, or surgery
• CIDP (chronic inflammatory demyelinating neuropathy)	Tingling, numbness, and weakness in limbs	Chronic	Associated with diabetes, connective tissue diseases, lymphoma, monoclonal gammopathy, HIV infection, chronic hepatitis, and drug therapy
• CMT (Charcot–Marie–Tooth)	Early onset and slowly progressive distal limb tingling, numbness, and weakness	Chronic	Caused by genetic defects. A positive family history is common
Other diseases			
Plexopathy	Patchy pain, tingling, numbness, and weakness affecting one limb or asymmetrically affecting bilateral upper or lower limbs	Acute, subacute, or chronic	Acute idiopathic brachial plexitis can be post-infectious or post-surgical. Plexopathy can also be caused by tumor infiltration, compression, or prior radiotherapy

(Continued)

Disease	Symptoms	Duration/ tempo	Circumstances/other key features
Radiculopathy	Shooting pain from spine to limb(s). Tingling and/or numbness in root distribution	Acute, subacute, or chronic	Often due to disk herniation or degenerative spine disease. Rarely results from inflammation, infection, or tumors
Sensory ganglionopathy	Numbness and imbalance	Subacute or chronic	Can be caused by Sjögren's syndrome, vitamin B6 toxicity, paraneoplastic syndrome, etc.
Myelopathy	May have a sensory level (e.g. numbness from chest down). Limb stiffness and weakness and bowel/ bladder incontinence may also be present	Acute, subacute, or chronic	Can be caused by cord compression, intrinsic cord lesions, or metabolic abnormalities
Stroke	Hemi-body numbness. May also have hemi-body weakness, language abnormality, double vision, slurred speech, trouble swallowing, or dizziness depending on the location of the stroke	Acute	Risk factors include: prior stroke, hypertension, hyperlipidemia, diabetes, cigarette smoking, or heart disease
Multiple sclerosis	May have visual, bulbar, motor or coordination symptoms depending on lesion locations	Acute, subacute, or chronic	Often has known history of multiple sclerosis or history of multiple episodes having different localization

---

CLINICAL PEARLS
- Acute hemi-body loss of sensation suggests a CNS vascular event (stroke).
- Acute onset and rapid progression (patchy or ascending) of tingling or loss of sensation can be the early presentation of Guillain–Barré syndrome.
- Rapid and stepwise progression of sensory and motor symptoms involving multiple individual nerves suggests mononeuritis multiplex.
- Loss of sensation with a sensory level suggests a myelopathy.
- Tingling or loss of sensation in a limb with shooting pain from the spine suggests a radiculopathy.
- Tingling or loss of sensation symmetrically in distal limbs suggests a peripheral neuropathy.
- Early-onset and slowly progressive numbness, tingling, and weakness or skeletal abnormalities suggest a hereditary neuropathy (CMT), especially if there is a positive family history.
- Tingling or loss of sensation with or without weakness in individual nerve distribution suggests a mononeuropathy.

Key elements of physical examination
- Positive sensory signs include allodynia, hyperalgesia, and hyperesthesia. Negative sensory signs include impaired pinprick, light touch, thermal, vibratory, and proprioceptive sensation. Pinprick and thermal sensation are the functions of small sensory fibers, while vibratory sensation and proprioception are the functions of large sensory fibers.
- The key point of the physical examination is to characterize the pattern of sensory abnormalities to localize the lesion(s) to brain, spinal cord, nerve roots, plexus, or peripheral nerve(s).

- A thorough neurologic examination is essential because other neurologic findings, such as cortical signs, brainstem signs, motor deficit, abnormal deep tendon reflexes, and the presence of pathologic reflexes, will also help to localize the lesion(s).
- It is also important to dissect which sensory modalities are impaired to determine whether the disease process affects small sensory fibers, large sensory fibers, or both.

Table of elements of physical examination by disease

Disease	Physical findings
Neuropathy	
Mononeuropathy	Sensory deficit is in one nerve distribution, such as median nerve, ulnar nerve, peroneal nerve, radial nerve, or trigeminal nerve
Mononeuropathy multiplex	Sensory deficits correspond to multiple individual nerves. Motor deficits are also present in the same distribution
Polyneuropathy Axonal polyneuropathy	Sensory deficit is usually length-dependent with a stocking-glove pattern. If motor weakness is present, it involves distal limb muscles. Ankle jerks are often reduced or absent
Demyelinating polyneuropathy	Sensory deficit can be in a stocking-glove pattern or patchy. Weakness is often detected in both distal and proximal limb muscles. Deep tendon reflexes are characteristically reduced or absent
Small fiber sensory neuropathy	Only pinprick, light touch, and thermal sensation are impaired. Proprioception, motor strength, and deep tendon reflexes are well preserved
Other diseases	
Plexopathy	Sensory and motor deficits are detected in the distribution of brachial plexus or lumbosacral plexus, that do not correspond to individual roots or nerves
Radiculopathy	Sensory deficit is in a root distribution. Motor weakness and reflex changes may also be found in the same root distribution
Sensory ganglionopathy	Sensory deficits are patchy and non-length-dependent. Sensory ataxia is often prominent. Motor weakness is absent
Myelopathy	A sensory level to pinprick or light touch is common. Motor weakness and brisk or pathologic reflexes are often detected
Stroke	Unilateral sensory deficit involving face and limbs, or sensory deficit in one side of face and the opposite side of limbs. Motor weakness, cortical signs, or brainstem signs may also be detected
Multiple sclerosis	Sensory deficit in face, limbs. Visual impairment, limb spasticity, weakness, and brisk and pathologic reflexes are often present

CLINICAL PEARLS
- Hemi-body sensory deficit indicates a brain lesion, which can be seen with stroke, multiple sclerosis, and other CNS disorders.
- A sensory level indicates a lesion in the spinal cord, which can be caused by cord compression, inflammation, infection, infarction, or tumor.
- Sensory deficit in a root distribution indicates a radiculopathy.
- Sensory deficit in multiple areas in one limb along with motor weakness of lower motor neuron nature may represent a plexopathy.

- Sensory deficit in an individual nerve distribution may represent a mononeuropathy, such as median neuropathy at the wrist, ulnar neuropathy at the elbow, radial nerve at the spiral groove, and peroneal neuropathy at the fibular head.
- If multiple individual nerves are affected with both sensory and motor deficits, mononeuritis multiplex should be considered.
- Sensory deficit in a stocking-glove pattern indicates a peripheral neuropathy.
- Impairment of pinprick and thermal sensation with preservation of proprioception, motor strength, and deep tendon reflexes, is typical for small fiber sensory neuropathy.
- Foot deformities, such as pes cavus and hammer toes, indicate chronic denervation and are commonly seen in Charcot–Marie–Tooth disease.

Diagnostic tests

Disease	Diagnostic test(s)
Neuropathy	Nerve conduction studies (NCS) will show reduced sensory ± motor nerve action potential amplitudes in affected nerve(s) In demyelinating neuropathy, the conduction velocities are significantly reduced, and the distal latencies and F-wave latencies are prolonged. Conduction block(s) may also be present NCS in small-fiber neuropathy are typically normal, but skin biopsy shows reduced intraepidermal C-fiber densities Nerve biopsy may be utilized to confirm the clinical suspicion for vasculitis, amyloidosis, or inflammatory demyelinating neuropathy
Plexopathy	NCS/EMG show reduced conduction responses and motor denervation in the distribution of brachial plexus or lumbosacral plexus. MRI of affected plexus may show enhancement or compressive lesion. Ultrasound increasingly useful in evaluation
Radiculopathy	Sensory NCS are normal. Motor NCS may show reduced compound muscle action potential amplitudes if the disease is severe. EMG will show muscle denervation in the distribution of nerve root(s). Spine MRI may show root compression
Sensory ganglionopathy	NCS will show reduced or absent sensory conduction responses in a non-length-dependent manner. Motor NCS are normal
Myelopathy	Spine MRI may show cord compression, cord edema, cord tumor, or spinal dural arteriovenous fistula. CSF studies may show pleocytosis, elevated protein, increased IgG synthesis or index, or positive microbial PCR, cultures, or antibodies depending on the cause. Serum B12 and copper levels may be low; rheumatologic markers and paraneoplastic antibodies may be positive; RPR, HIV, HTLV-1, or Lyme serology may be positive
Stroke	Brain MRI with DWI most sensitive; non-contrast CT may show subtle signs of acute stroke
Multiple sclerosis	Brain and spine MRI will show demyelinating lesions in the white matter of brain and spinal cord. CSF study may show pleocytosis, elevated protein, increased IgG synthesis and index, positive myelin basic protein, and the presence of oligoclonal bands

Table of frequency of each disease

Condition	Frequency
Peripheral neuropathy	2–3% in general population 8% in people >55 years
Plexopathy	Uncommon
Radiculopathy	Common
Sensory ganglionopathy	Rare
Myelopathy	Common
Stroke	100–200/100,000
Multiple sclerosis	85/100,000 in USA

BOTTOM LINE
- Tingling and loss of sensation are non-specific neurologic symptoms that can be caused by a variety of neurologic diseases affecting different parts of sensory pathways.
- A thorough history and physical examination, the recognition of typical or characteristic patterns, and diagnostic testing are essential to localize lesions, determine etiologies, and treat patients appropriately.
- Acute onset and rapid progression of tingling and loss of sensation may indicate neurologic emergencies, such as acute stroke, spinal cord compression, acute transverse myelitis, Guillain–Barré syndrome, and vasculitic neuropathy. It is critical to recognize and treat these conditions without delay.

Reading list
Key reading sources for this chapter can be found online at www.mountsinaiexpertguides.com

Suggested websites
Charcot-Marie-Tooth Association: www.cmtausa.org
Foundation for Peripheral Neuropathy: www.neuropathy.org

Additional material for this chapter can be found online at:
www.mountsinaiexpertguides.com

This includes advice for patients, a case study, multiple choice questions, and a reading list.

CHAPTER 17

Low Back Pain and Neck Pain

Charles B. Stacy
Icahn School of Medicine at Mount Sinai, New York, NY, USA

Background
Definition

Low back pain and neck pain are very common complaints of patients with a wide variety of pathologies connected to the mobile areas of the spine. Yet, the association of these regional complaints with the spine does not always indicate true spinal pathology, and even less often involvement of nerve roots. Therefore, the approach initially must be the analysis of axial mechanics and only in certain cases relies on the evidence of specific neurologic deficits.

Since most causes of low back and neck pain do not threaten life or neurologic function, it is important to distinguish the signs and symptoms that merit immediate investigation, and in the remainder focus on the reduction in pain and disability.

Impact

- Low back pain is the most common complaint bringing patients to a doctor. It carries a lifetime prevalence of 58–84% and a 1-year incidence of 18–50%. Fortunately, only 5–10% of acute low back pain evolves into chronic pain.
- The annual economic burden of chronic low back pain for the USA is estimated around $86 billion.
- For neck pain, the annual incidence is around 15%, with 0.6% new cases.
- In its social impact, chronic low back pain is notorious for disrupting both productive and recreational life patterns, as well as for its destructive behavioral and psychological consequences. In fact, chronic low back pain has become the paradigm for pain as illness behavior.

Approach to diagnosis
Getting your bearings

- Establish by history and examination the relationship of the pain to movement, posture, and weight bearing.
- Determine the presence or absence of neurologic deficits.
- Assess the likelihood of serious underlying illness and prioritize the sequence of tests.

Key elements of history

- Onset – abrupt, following trauma or particular activity; or insidious, or with antecedents?
- Pain site and radiation; pain character?
- Mechanical factors: what worsens or relieves the pain; what is avoided; what functions are prohibited by pain?

Mount Sinai Expert Guides: Neurology, First Edition. Edited by Stuart C. Sealfon, Rajeev Motiwala, and Charles B. Stacy.
© 2016 John Wiley & Sons, Ltd. Published 2016 by John Wiley & Sons, Ltd.
Companion website: www.mountsinaiexpertguides.com

Table of elements of history and diseases

Disease	Features of history
Disk herniation:	
Cervical	Acute pain in neck, one or both sides, with radicular radiation, and immobility, focal or generalized weakness or numbness
Lumbar	Acute pain in low back, or buttocks, thigh, or distal; immobility; weakness, urinary symptoms
Spinal stenosis:	
Cervical	Often painless; weakness or clumsiness in hands, numbness; may have changes in gait, typically increased tripping
Lumbar	Claudication symptoms, including buttocks, usually bilateral, on standing or walking, with variable weakness and numbness
Spinal degeneration:	
Osteophyte	Recurrent bouts of pain, radicular in case of osteophyte
Facet	Facet pain local, very postural specific
Listhesis	Listhesis may cause variable stenosis symptoms, movement dependent
Trauma:	
Whiplash	Intense pain in neck, including anterior, and tremendous spasm; may have radiation
Compression fracture	Localized pain with marked postural sensitivity, may have bi-radicular pain
Instability	High sensitivity to motion; careful attention to myelopathic and caudal symptoms
Rheumatologic:	Single or multiple sites; ligaments, joints, epidural masses; also involvement of extraspinal sources of pain
Infection:	
Discitis/osteomyelitis	Escalating pain, initially local, then radicular, even at rest; may have symptoms of cord or cauda equina involvement; thoracic common as well
Meningitis	Pain may be felt first in neck, or diffuse in back, body
Malignancy: vertebral, meningeal	Back pain most common symptom in systemic cancer; escalating and unrelieved; ask about cord and cauda features; thoracic common
Plexus: brachial, lumbosacral	Lack of spinal mechanical or postural dependence; prominent sensory and motor symptoms, wider than root alone
Muscular:	
Myositis	Ache, generally broad distribution; depends on use, variable interference with function, may be associated weakness
Strain	Follows unusual or repetitive use; may be hard to localize
Myofascial pain	Referred from site, which may be unnoticed; interferes with function
Fibromyalgia	Widespread ache with many constitutional complaints
Radiculitis	Radiating pain and sensory symptoms; may be multiple; less mechanical
Joint: hip, shoulder	Usually worse on movement of joint. Joint motion may be limited and may erroneously suggest muscle weakness from radicular involvement
Visceral	Radiating regional pain with poor localization, such as from pleura or mediastinum, or pelvic organs
Malingering	Intense complaints, intractability; but the diagnosis depends on examination

---

CLINICAL PEARLS
- Triage potentially serious scenarios by mode of onset and symptoms of neurologic dysfunction.
- Focus on mechanical features as much as on deficits.

Key elements of physical examination
- Determine by specific manipulations which structures are involved.
- Test for deficits taking into account the effects of pain.
- Keep a high index of suspicion for dangerous patterns, such as cord, cauda, root, or plexus.

Table of elements of physical examination by disease
(see also Table 17.1)

Disease	Examination
Disk herniation: cervical, lumbar	Reflex, motor, or sensory deficits (the entire trio occurs in a small percentage) Signs related to nerve compression or traction (cervical tilt and rotation, straight leg raising [SLR], reverse SLR, crossed SLR) Signs of spinal segment sensitivity (palpation, torsion, flexion, extension)
Spinal stenosis: Cervical	Atrophy of intrinsic hand muscles; clumsiness; bilateral posterior cervical and occipital tenderness; Lhermitte's sign; leg spasticity; mixed hypo- and hyperreflexia in arms
Lumbar	Weakness, atrophy, sensory loss in various combinations, bilateral but asymmetric; may simulate distal neuropathy; mechanical lumbar signs

Spinal degeneration:
  Osteophyte
  Facet
  Listhesis
	Radicular deficits and mechanical signs; less spasm than acute disk
	Elicited by segmental spinal manipulation, may have radicular signs
	Varying deficits, bilateral; strongly elicited by truncal manipulation

Trauma: Whiplash	Tremendous spasm and sensitivity to motion in all axes; unrelated to presence of deficits
Instability (caused by ligamentous injury without bone damage)	Spasm, sensitivity to motion; variable deficits
Compression fracture	Lumbar and thoracic load-bearing sites; point tenderness and sensitivity to manipulation; may have radicular or cord, caudal deficits
Rheumatologic	Rheumatoid arthritis (RA) – cervical apophyseal joints and odontoid ligament signs Ankylosing spondylitis – multiple levels Psoriatic arthritis, gout, SLE – more often mechanical than radicular
Infection: Discitis or osteomyelitis	Escalating segmental tenderness and mechanical sensitivity; evolving cord or cauda equina deficits; with fever
Meningitis	May present as polyradiculitis
Malignancy: Vertebral	Marked segmental mechanical sensitivity; escalating deficits in biradicular cord or cauda equina pattern; often thoracic as compared to degenerative causes
Meningeal	Polyradicular deficits, may have encephalopathy
Plexus: brachial, lumbosacral	Absence of spinal mechanical signs; deficits beyond single radicular territory; rarely bilateral

Disease	Examination
Muscular: Myositis	Muscle tenderness and weakness, but no spinal mechanical signs; not confined to standard radicular (myotomal) patterns
Strain	Single muscle with spasm and tenderness, often palpable
Myofascial pain	Characteristic patterns of periaxial muscular tender points whose palpation elicits pain at a predictable nearby site
Fibromyalgia	Generalized distribution of tender points at standard sites; may be confused with chronic cervical and lumbar spinal disorders
Radiculitis	Single or multiple roots with signs of sensitization and deficits in sensory or motor function; rash in herpes zoster virus, target lesions in Lyme disease
Joint: hip, shoulder	Pain on movement of joint and limitation of joint motion
Visceral (thoracic or abdominal pathology)	Limited sensitivity to spinal manipulation; local tenderness or guarding, absence of radicular signs unless nerves directly invaded by disease process
Malingering	Exaggerated pain behavior; inconsistencies of deficit depending on the task tested; Hoover's sign (absence of heel pressure on attempt to lift opposite leg)

Table 17.1 Specific features of cervical and lumbosacral radiculopathies.

Root	Pain	Sensory	Motor	Reflex
C5	Scapula, lateral arm	Lateral arm and elbow	Supraspinatus and infraspinatus, deltoid, biceps	Biceps
C6	Radial hand, forearm	Thumb, index, radial forearm	Biceps, pronator	Biceps
C7	Posterior arm, dorsal forearm and hand	Middle fingers dorsal	Triceps, wrist and finger extensors	Triceps
C8	Ulnar hand and forearm	Fifth finger and ulnar forearm	Abduction thumb, index, and fifth fingers	Finger flexor
T1	Inner arm, axilla	Medial arm	Abduction thumb, index, and fifth fingers	Finger flexor
L2	Anterior thigh	Upper anterior thigh	Hip flexion	Hip flexor
L3	Anterior knee	Low anterior thigh, knee	Hip flexion	Adductor
L4	Anterolateral thigh; medial shin	Medial shin	Knee extension, thigh adduction, foot dorsiflexion	Quadriceps
L5	Posterior or lateral thigh; shin; foot dorsal	Dorsal foot	Toe and foot dorsiflexion, foot eversion	Medial hamstring[a]
S1	Posterior thigh; calf; sole	Lateral foot, sole	Foot plantarflex, hip extensors	Achilles

[a]Note: the hamstrings span four myotomes, medial L4-5, lateral L5-S1.

Diagnostic tests

Disease	Tests
Disk herniation: cervical, lumbar	MRI superior to CT but complementary; contrast if prior surgery at level; myelogram and CT if ambiguous. Flexion/extension films in certain cases to see impingement. EMG may clarify site or nature of weakness (Utility of discogram uncertain)
Spinal stenosis: cervical, lumbar	All the above

Spinal degeneration:
  Osteophyte
  Facet
  Listhesis
	
	May be visualized on plain films
	Diagnostic posterior branch blocks
	Requires flexion and extension studies
	Nuclear bone scan indicates site of activity

Trauma:
  Whiplash
  Compression fracture
  Instability
	
	Often nothing visible on radiological testing
	Plain X-rays show presence; MRI shows acuity and pathology
	Flexion/extension studies

Rheumatologic	Serologies; CRP, HLA B27 Odontoid ligament and pannus in RA

Infection:
  Discitis/osteomyelitis
  Meningitis
	MRI with contrast most sensitive; serial studies
	Needle aspiration
	Lumbar puncture

Malignancy:
  Vertebral
  Meningeal
	
	MRI with contrast; PET scan; skeletal survey; nuclear scan
	Lumbar puncture, contrast MRI, sometimes CT myelogram

Plexus: brachial, lumbosacral	MRI with contrast; EMG may localize

Muscular:
  Myositis
  Strain
  Myofascial pain
  Fibromyalgia
	
	EMG, CPK, ESR
	No specific test results
	Trigger point injection relieves pain
	Careful palpation; no laboratory findings

Radiculitis	CSF examination
Joint: hip, shoulder	Radiology of joint; diagnostic block
Visceral	MRI or CT of chest, abdomen, or pelvis, according to the region of pain origin
Malingering	Often have radiologic findings

BOTTOM LINE

The question is always when to defer or perform tests. Acute neck and low back pain are so common and generally self-limited that symptomatic treatment alone may fairly be administered in the absence of neurologic deficits or underlying diseases. If symptoms escalate or deficits accrue, then studies should commence.

- In 90% of cases of low back pain, no specific causes can be identified.
- In cases of neck pain, roughly one-third resolve, one-third improve, and one-third persist or recur.
- Intractable pain forces investigation even in the absence of neurologic deficits, but the majority of cases still resolve.
- The issue of surgery or other invasive therapies will not be considered here.

Reading list
Key reading sources for this chapter can be found online at www.mountsinaiexpertguides.com

Suggested websites
Cochrane Back and Neck: back.cochrane.org
International Association for the Study of Pain: www.iasp-pain.org/
American Pain Society: americanpainsociety.org

Additional material for this chapter can be found online at:
www.mountsinaiexpertguides.com

This includes a case study, multiple choice questions, and
a reading list.

CHAPTER 18

Suspected Spinal Cord Dysfunction

Aaron Miller

Icahn School of Medicine at Mount Sinai, New York, NY, USA

Background
Definition

The spinal cord is a very compact structure composed of gray matter containing the anterior horn cells or primary motor neurons, autonomic cells, sensory processing neurons, and white matter, which contains a variety of ascending and descending tracts. Because of the complexity of this nervous system organ, the definition of "spinal cord dysfunction" involves the occurrence of motor, sensory, or autonomic symptoms resulting from damage of any type to either the neurons or the ascending or descending tracts. The impairment may result from either intrinsic disease of the spinal cord or extrinsic compression. Because the pathologic processes affecting the spinal cord are so numerous and diverse, this chapter can only highlight those that are most frequent or representative of a spectrum of disorders of a particular type.

Presenting complaints

The specific presenting complaints related to spinal cord dysfunction depend on the level and precise location of the pathology, the nature of the pathologic process, and the chronology of the disorder. In general, spinal cord dysfunction is likely to be bilateral and more likely to involve the legs (or both the legs and the arms) than the arms alone. Often a particular locus of spinal cord dysfunction is implied by the presence of a "sensory level," particularly the impairment of pain and temperature sensation, below the level of the lesion. Bladder and bowel symptoms are common. Many exceptions to these general rules occur, however, especially with diseases selectively involving anterior horn cells or tracts that are selectively vulnerable to a particular disease process.

Impact

It is impossible reliably to estimate the incidence of new cases of spinal cord dysfunction each year. Although some causes of spinal cord dysfunction are uncommon, suffice it to say that the typical primary care physician is likely to encounter at least several cases involving spinal cord symptoms each year from among the more prevalent conditions. These include cervical stenosis, multiple sclerosis, metastatic spinal cord compression, and trauma. Because many spinal cord disorders significantly impair ambulation, the social impact is great. Many patients with severe mobility problems are unable to work and those conditions that affect both upper and lower extremity function frequently render the patient unable to manage self-care. Thus, the consequences, in both physical and emotional terms for the patient and family and in economic costs to society, are great.

Mount Sinai Expert Guides: Neurology, First Edition. Edited by Stuart C. Sealfon, Rajeev Motiwala, and Charles B. Stacy.
© 2016 John Wiley & Sons, Ltd. Published 2016 by John Wiley & Sons, Ltd.
Companion website: www.mountsinaiexpertguides.com

Approach to diagnosis
Getting your bearings
The following points should especially raise the possibility of spinal cord dysfunction:
- A sensory level to pain and temperature.
- Bilateral involvement of the lower extremities or both the lower and upper extremities.
- Sensory or motor symptoms that spare the face.
- Symptoms of bladder, bowel, or sexual dysfunction.
- A pattern of motor loss on one side of the body and sensory symptoms (impairment of pain and temperature) on the other (the Brown-Séquard syndrome).
- Focal back pain.

Key elements of history
- Is there any weakness?
- Is there any numbness or decreased sensation?
- Are there any problems with urination, moving your bowels, or sexual function?
- Is there any back pain?
- When were symptoms first noticed and how have they changed over time?

Disorders to consider
- Acute (minutes to days):
  - Trauma
  - Vascular disease
  - Acute idiopathic transverse myelitis
  - Multiple sclerosis
  - Neuromyelitis optica
- Subacute (days to weeks):
  - Cord compression due to metastases
  - Intrinsic tumors of the cord
  - Epidural abscess
  - Other infections
- Chronic (months to years):
  - Hereditary spastic paraplegia
  - Metabolic (subacute combined degeneration; copper deficiency)
  - Cervical spondylotic myelopathy
  - Extramedullary tumors (meningiomas, schwannomas)
  - Syringomyelia

Table of elements of history and diseases

Condition	Symptoms	Duration/tempo	Circumstances/other key features
Trauma	Variable severity from mild sensory or motor loss to picture of complete cord transection May have Brown-Séquard syndrome of cord hemi-section Initial picture may be of "spinal shock" with flaccid paralysis and autonomic dysfunction, evolving to spastic paraparesis	The lesion occurs acutely with the injury In mild cases, especially with contusion where the integrity of the cord is preserved, improvement or even full resolution of function may occur In severe cases in which the cord is transected or its architecture destroyed, the condition is permanent, although the clinical picture may evolve from a flaccid motor state to spasticity	The nature of the injury, as well as the severity, varies from blunt trauma to penetrating injuries Often the injury to the spinal cord results from damage produced as a result of injury to the bony spine
Spinal cord infarction	Unusual event in anterior spinal artery territory; spares posterior column function producing pain, temperature, and motor loss below lesion	Very acute onset Deficit generally permanent	Often occurs in setting of hypotension, either due to illness or iatrogenic (e.g. after cardiopulmonary bypass, aortic dissections, and aortic stenting)
Acute idiopathic transverse myelitis	Inflammatory lesion typically producing severe impairment of spinal cord function at and below the lesion Clinical picture of severe spinal cord trauma May be accompanied by local pain	Acute onset, typically over hours to days Nadir generally reached within 10 days (but up to 21 days) Prognosis variable, but many patients are left with moderate to severe disability	May follow viral infection Etiology uncertain, suspected autoimmune Generally a monophasic event
Multiple sclerosis (MS)	Extremely variable, mono- or multi-focal manifestations Cervical cord most often affected Numbness, tingling, or corticospinal tract symptoms common acutely Spastic paraparesis, as well as bladder and bowel symptoms, frequent in more chronic cases	Acute relapses or exacerbations occur over hours to a few days, then plateau, and usually improve Full recovery frequent, especially early in illness Often a later progressive course About 10–15% of patients have primary progressive MS, worsening from onset, usually with spastic paraparesis	Availability of numerous disease-modifying treatments to significantly reduce frequency of attacks

Condition	Symptoms	Duration/tempo	Circumstances/other key features
Neuromyelitis optica (NMO; Devic's disease)	Episodes vary but often more severe than those of typical MS	Similar to MS, but progression almost invariably results from recurrent attacks, rather than insidious progression	Classic NMO involves myelopathy plus episodes of optic neuritis, characterized by pain on eye movement and monocular visual impairment Cord lesions typically extend more than three levels Serum antibody to aquaporin-4 often present
Cord compression due to metastases	Initial symptom is almost always localized back pain, followed by progressive motor or sensory loss below the level of the lesion	Localized pain typically days to weeks before focal neurologic deficits Motor deficit may progress over days Sudden severe loss of sensory, motor, and autonomic function can occur because of spinal cord infarction Urgent diagnosis is critical	Most common tumor types resulting in epidural spinal cord compression are: • Lung • Breast • Prostate carcinoma • Lymphoma
Intramedullary spinal cord tumors (ependymoma, glioma)	Variable; pain often present in areas overlying tumor Gait difficulties often present In children, orthopedic conditions such as kyphoscoliosis may be present	With benign or low-grade malignancy, course may be very indolent Course shorter with more malignant tumors Occasionally hemorrhage causes acute presentation	Ependymoma most common and often presents with central cord syndrome characterized by dissociated sensory loss (loss of pain and temperature in shawl-like pattern with relative preservation of light touch, position and vibration sense)
Intrinsic spinal cord infection	HIV-associated myelopathy resembles subacute combined degeneration, with leg weakness, gait imbalance, numbness HTLV-1/2: progressive spastic leg weakness and bladder dysfunction Enteroviruses, especially polio, and West Nile virus, cause acute lower motor neuron picture Variable symptoms with other bacteria, fungal, or parasitic infections	Variable; dependent on specific organism	Important to know specific predilection of organism, e.g.: • HIV for posterior and lateral column involvement • Enteroviruses, including poliomyelitis, for ventral horns

(*Continued*)

Condition	Symptoms	Duration/tempo	Circumstances/other key features
Epidural abscess	Local pain and tenderness; progressive motor or sensory loss below lesion	Typically days, but sometimes more indolent	Usually due to hematogenous dissemination from remote suppurative focus May result from spread from local osteomyelitis *Staphylococcus aureus* responsible for more than 50% Back trauma, often minor, may be reported in as many as 1/3 High degree of suspicion when IV drug abuse history present
Hereditary spastic paraplegia	Pure form with progressive stiffness and weakness of lower extremities with gait impairment Complex forms have variable neurologic abnormalities Urinary disturbances in up to 50%	Insidiously progressive Age of onset extremely variable from early childhood to eighth decade, but most typically in second to fourth decade	Great genetic heterogeneity Each phenotype can have either autosomal dominant, autosomal recessive, or X-linked form of inheritance About 25% of carriers are clinically unaffected because of reduced penetrance
Metabolic myelopathy (subacute combined degeneration most common)	Fatigue and generalized weakness may precede more specific symptoms Progressive stiffness, weakness, and gait disturbance Sometimes cognitive change, psychiatric symptoms, or autonomic symptoms	Usually slowly progressive	Most cases of subacute combined degeneration are due to vitamin B12 deficiency Chronic nitrous oxide intoxication and HIV-associated vacuolar myelopathy mimic B12 deficiency Copper deficiency may cause similar clinical picture
Cervical spondylotic myelopathy	Stiffness and weakness of lower extremities May be accompanied by pain, numbness, or weakness in arms, especially if cervical radiculopathy is also present Bladder or bowel dysfunction may occur	Usually insidiously progressive but acute worsening may occur	Corticospinal tract features are usually much more prominent in the legs Bladder and bowel symptoms are important A variety of pathologic changes in the cervical spine may be associated with the progressive myelopathy Lower motor neuron features may be present in arms
Benign extramedullary spinal cord tumors (typically meningiomas or schwannomas)	Progressive weakness and stiffness of one or both legs Local pain often present, but typically less severe than with metastatic cord compression	Clinical presentation typically over months	Radicular symptoms of pain and numbness may be present, more often with schwannomas

Condition	Symptoms	Duration/tempo	Circumstances/other key features
Syringomyelia	Often segmental lower motor neuron weakness and atrophy, but spastic weakness very common Loss of deep pain sensation common Segmental sensory symptoms (loss of pain and temperature)	Insidiously progressive, but may have more rapid course initially	Clinical picture extremely variable Most often associated with Chiari 1 malformation Kyphoscoliosis common

---

CLINICAL PEARLS
- Involvement of both lower extremities should always suggest spinal cord disease.
- Symptoms often suggest a spinal cord level, e.g. sensory loss below a particular level.
- Combination of atrophy and weakness may suggest intrinsic spinal cord disease.
- Pain is an important early symptom of spinal cord compression (particularly for extrinsic lesions) and has localizing value.

Key elements of physical examination
- Spastic paraparesis and other features of corticospinal tract dysfunction, including hyperreflexia and Babinski signs.
- Sensory loss to pain and temperature below the level of the lesion.
- Look for hemisensory loss and contralateral motor weakness (hemicord syndrome, Brown-Séquard).
- Posterior column signs such as loss of position and vibration sense.
- Signs of anterior horn cell disease include focal motor weakness, atrophy, and fasciculations.

Table of elements of physical examination by disease

Condition	Signs
Trauma	Varying severity of motor and sensory impairment below lesion. Initially "spinal shock" with severe cases, manifest by flaccid para- or quadriplegia and urinary retention
Spinal cord infarction (anterior spinal artery syndrome)	Loss of motor function and pain and temperature below level of lesion. Eventually signs of lower motor neuron lesion (atrophy, fasciculations) at affected level. Spares joint position and vibratory sensation
Acute idiopathic transverse myelitis	Varying degrees of sensory and motor loss below lesion. Typically includes impairment of all sensory modalities
Multiple sclerosis	Often mild, asymmetric signs. Sensory may predominate, but corticospinal tract signs common (weakness, spasticity, hyperreflexia). Signs of involvement of other neurologic sites common
Neuromyelitis optica	Full-blown syndrome includes optic neuropathy and spinal cord signs, which are variable in severity but often more severe than in MS
Cord compression due to metastases	Local tenderness. Corticospinal tract signs and loss of pain and temperature below lesion. May have Brown-Séquard syndrome

(Continued)

Condition	Signs
Intrinsic spinal cord tumors	Variable sensory and motor signs
Intrinsic infections	Lower motor neuron signs with poliomyelitis, other enteroviruses, and West Nile virus HIV: posterior and lateral column signs HTLV-1/2: spastic paraparesis
Epidural abscess	Local tenderness. Corticospinal tract signs and loss of pain and temperature below lesion
Hereditary spastic paraplegia	Spastic paraparesis and abnormal gait. Sensory usually spared, but may have distal vibratory sense impairment
Metabolic myelopathy	Most often picture of subacute combined degeneration (posterior and lateral columns) with spastic paraparesis and impairment of position and vibration sense
Cervical spondylotic myelopathy	Spastic paraparesis, usually spares sensory function. Vibratory loss may be present. Often associated with atrophic intrinsic hand muscles
Benign extramedullary tumor	May have local tenderness. Weakness, spasticity, and sensory loss below level of pathology
Syringomyelia	Variable findings involving lower motor neuron signs and corticospinal tract signs. Usually segmental loss of pain and temperature sensation

CLINICAL PEARLS
- Prominent local tenderness suggests bony involvement, especially metastatic cord compression.
- Presence of lower motor neuron signs usually indicates intrinsic spinal cord pathology.
- Sensory level usually at or a little below level of pathology.
- Combination of posterior column signs (loss of proprioception and vibration) and corticospinal tract signs suggests metabolic abnormality such as B12 deficiency.

Diagnostic tests

Condition	Test findings
Acute trauma	Plain spine films; CT; MRI; look for bony disruption, fragments, hematoma
Spinal cord infarction	MRI – intrinsic cord lesion, sparing posterior columns
Acute transverse myelitis	MRI – intrinsic cord lesion, may be longitudinally extensive; gadolinium enhancement; often with CSF pleocytosis and elevated protein; oligoclonal bands (OCB) absent
Multiple sclerosis	Spinal cord MRI with one or more lesions, usually less than 1–2 segments long; may enhance with gadolinium if acute; brain MRI with multiple T2 hyperintense lesions; CSF usually positive for OCB or elevated IgG index
Neuromyelitis optica (NMO)	Longitudinally extensive spinal cord lesion on MRI; brain MRI not characteristic of MS; CSF often with pleocytosis, but usually negative for oligoclonal bands; NMO-Ig antibody (anti-aquaporin 4) positive in about 70% of classic NMO and in about 50% of NMO spectrum disorders (e.g. longitudinally extensive myelitis without optic nerve involvement)

Condition	Test findings
Cord compression due to metastases	Plain spine films show bony involvement; often multifocal bony lesions. Spine MRI usually shows gadolinium enhancing epidural mass
Intrinsic spinal cord tumors	Spine MRI shows intrinsic lesion, often with variable gadolinium enhancement. Cord width often expanded, indicating mass
Intrinsic spinal cord infection	Findings vary with specific infection. MRI may show focal pathology or suggest leptomeningeal involvement (gadolinium enhancement); CSF may be helpful by demonstrating pleocytosis; PCR or specific antibody determination helpful with some viral infections
Epidural abscess	Spinal MRI will show local epidural collection and discitis; may be gadolinium enhancement. Depending on pathology, bony lesion may be seen; organism usually not present in CSF
Hereditary spastic paraplegia (HSP)	Spinal cord imaging generally normal, helps to rule out other conditions. Brain MRI may be abnormal in complex cases. CSF usually normal. Genetic testing may detect about 50% of autosomal dominant HSP and most X-linked HSP, but should only be done in conjunction with genetic counseling
Metabolic myelopathies	Spinal cord imaging may show abnormalities in affected tracts. Check complete blood count for macrocytic anemia. Serum vitamin B12 usually low in B12 deficiency; should be accompanied by elevated methyl malonic acid and homocysteine. Check serum copper, ceruloplasmin, and zinc. Adrenomyeloneuropathy diagnosed by elevated very-long-chain fatty acids
Cervical spondylotic myelopathy	Cervical spine X-rays and MRI show various types of degenerative pathology. Spinal canal generally <11 mm
Benign extramedullary tumors	Spine MRI should demonstrate the tumor, as T2 hyperintense mass, usually with gadolinium enhancement
Syringomyelia	May be demonstrated on spinal cord MRI as lesion within cord having same signal characteristics as CSF. MRI will demonstrate longitudinal extent of lesion

Table of frequency of each disease

Condition	Frequency
Acute spinal cord trauma	12,000 new cases per year in USA; 270,000 prevalence with injury (source: National Spinal Cord Injury Statistical Center); >80% males
Spinal cord infarction	Uncertain; incidence could be as high as 12/100,000
Acute transverse myelitis	Idiopathic or post-infectious transverse myelitis rare; incidence 1–8/million/year
Multiple sclerosis	Incidence about 10,000 new cases/year in USA; estimated prevalence about 400,000 in USA
Neuromyelitis optica	Rare; estimated US prevalence 4000 cases; more common in non-Whites
Metastatic cord compression	About 20,000 cases/year in USA; about 5% of people who die of cancer
Intrinsic spinal cord tumors	Incidence of 1.1/100,000 per year
Intrinsic spinal cord infection	Extremely variable, depending on type and geography; intramedullary abscess extremely rare

(Continued)

Condition	Frequency
Epidural abscess	2.5–3.0/10,000 hospital admissions
Hereditary spastic paraplegia	Rare; worldwide prevalence estimated at 2–6/100,000
Metabolic myelopathies	Subacute combined degeneration uncommon (usually from vitamin B12 deficiency), though B12 deficiency may affect between 300,000 and 3 million in USA; other metabolic myelopathies rare
Cervical spondylotic myelopathy	250,000 to 500,000 in USA with symptoms of spinal stenosis (this may include lumbar and cervical)
Benign extramedullary tumors	Rare
Syringomyelia	Rare

BOTTOM LINE
- While highly variable, spinal cord disease is often bilateral, more commonly involves the legs, and may show a sensory level to pain and temperature as well as bowel and bladder involvement.
- Cervical stenosis, multiple sclerosis, metastatic spinal cord compression, and trauma are the most common causes of dysfunction of the spinal cord.
- Due to its potential for rapid deterioration, spinal cord compression must be diagnosed urgently; localized pain is an important clue.
- The specific pattern of symptoms and signs guides the differential diagnosis, the location for imaging studies, and the laboratory tests.
- High-resolution MRI imaging with and without contrast is important for evaluating most spinal cord disorders.

Reading list

Key reading sources for this chapter can be found online at www.mountsinaiexpertguides.com

Additional material for this chapter can be found online at: www.mountsinaiexpertguides.com

This includes a case study, multiple choice questions, and a reading list.

CHAPTER 19

Bladder and Sexual Dysfunction

Steven J. Weissbart and Jonathan M. Vapnek
Icahn School of Medicine at Mount Sinai, New York, NY, USA

Disorders of bladder and sexual function are commonly seen in neurologic patients. In the first section of this chapter we address bladder dysfunction and in the second section, sexual dysfunction.

Section 1: Bladder dysfunction
Background
Definition
Urinary incontinence is any involuntary leakage of urine. Urinary incontinence may be the presenting symptom of a neurologic lesion or may be a later sequela of neurologic disease. *Urinary retention*, on the other hand, is present when there is incomplete emptying of the bladder. Urinary retention can be acute or chronic, and may or may not cause pain.

Impact
Bladder dysfunction has a profound impact on quality of life. Although data are available on the prevalence of urinary incontinence (UI) in the general population, the overall prevalence of UI caused by neurologic disease in the general population is unclear.

Approach to diagnosis
Getting your bearings
Patients with urinary incontinence rarely require an urgent in-hospital workup except when the incontinence is associated with an acute neurologic deficit. The workup of a patient with a complaint of urinary incontinence, like most other medical complaints, includes a detailed history, physical examination, and appropriately selected diagnostics tests. We will primarily present the workup and treatment of urinary incontinence in a patient with neurologic disease, keeping in mind that patients with neurologic disease may also suffer from incontinence from non-neurogenic etiologies. These will be briefly described.

  Urinary retention, conversely, is more likely to result in hospitalization, as this may result in acute renal failure. In men, the vast majority of cases are caused by benign prostatic hyperplasia (BPH) causing bladder outlet obstruction. In women, on the other hand, neurologic etiologies are a far more common cause, as mechanical obstruction is extremely rare.

- Try to determine whether the urologic presentation is primarily a failure of the bladder to *store* urine, a failure of the bladder to *empty* urine, or both, through history, bladder palpation, sonography, and post-void residual volume.

Mount Sinai Expert Guides: Neurology, First Edition. Edited by Stuart C. Sealfon, Rajeev Motiwala, and Charles B. Stacy.
© 2016 John Wiley & Sons, Ltd. Published 2016 by John Wiley & Sons, Ltd.
Companion website: www.mountsinaiexpertguides.com

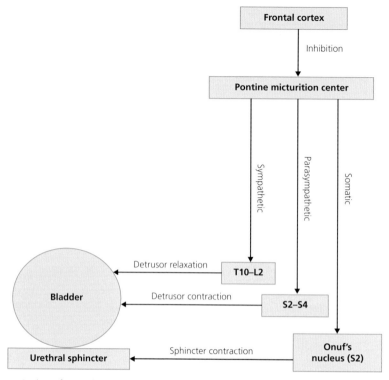

Figure 19.1 Review of normal voiding neurophysiology.

- Normal voluntary micturition requires an advanced intact neurologic network with coordination at the level of the pons. Therefore any disruption in this network may result in urinary incontinence or retention.
- Because the neurophysiologic network required for normal voluntary micturition is well mapped (Figure 19.1), it may be possible to determine if the urologic complaint is due to a suprapontine, suprasacral spinal cord, or peripheral lesion.

Key elements of history

The history of a patient with urinary complaints, either incontinence or retention, is important and often provides insight into whether the problem is primarily neurologic. Important aspects of the history include the following key elements:

- Does the patient have a prior history of neurologic disease? Urologic disease?
- Onset of urinary complaints: before, with, or after other neurologic symptoms?
- Are there associated symptoms such as urinary urgency, frequency, hematuria, dysuria, or nocturia?
- For incontinence, are the symptoms primarily those of urge incontinence, stress incontinence, or unaware incontinence?
- For retention, is there a prior history or is this the initial presentation?
- Medication history: have there been any recent changes in medication or dosage? Was there pre-existing incontinence that was improved by an anticholinergic drug?

Table of elements of history and diseases

Disease	Symptoms	Duration	Other key features
CNS disease	Urgency Frequency Urinary urge incontinence Detrusor overactivity (DO) on urodynamics	Acute, subacute, or chronic	Patient may report a severe urge to void prior to incontinent episode. Neurogenic patients with DO may have involuntary loss of urine without urgency if a sensory deficit is present
Suprasacral spinal cord disease	Urinary urge incontinence with incomplete bladder emptying from detrusor-sphincter dyssynergia (DSD)	Acute, subacute, or chronic	Acutely, during spinal shock, retention is often present After spinal shock has resolved, patients often have both incontinence and incomplete bladder emptying
Sacral spinal cord/ peripheral nervous system disease/ muscle disease	Urinary stress incontinence – leakage of urine with increases in abdominal pressure Incomplete bladder emptying Urinary retention	Acute, subacute, or chronic	Usual presentation is acute retention Overflow incontinence, in which the patient has frequent leakage, with or without sensation, can present in a similar fashion to bladder overactivity

---

CLINICAL PEARLS
- Neurogenic patients with urge incontinence (UUI)/detrusor overactivity (DO) may not have the classic symptom of urgency secondary to a sensory defect. Thus, while history is important and may lead the clinician to the correct classification of incontinence, physical examination and correctly selected diagnostic tests are paramount.
- The type of incontinence may change according to history of their neurologic disease. For example, a patient with multiple sclerosis who has UUI/DO from a CNS lesion may later develop incomplete bladder emptying secondary to detrusor-sphincter dyssynergia (DSD) from a thoracic cord lesion.
- It has been said that the bladder is an unreliable witness, with only a limited range of presentations. Therefore, given the well-mapped neurophysiology of voiding, the location of a patient's neurologic lesion may help determine the type of incontinence.

Key elements of physical examination
- Suprapubic palpation may detect an overly distended bladder, as seen in patients with overflow urinary incontinence.
- A rectal examination is important to assess anal sphincter tone as well as sacral sensation. Patients with overflow incontinence from neurologic disease often demonstrate lax anal sphincter tone.
- A bulbo-cavernosus reflex is performed by pinching the glans penis in men or the labia or clitoris in women while the index finger of the opposite hand assesses the response of the anal sphincter.

- To assess for stress incontinence, ask the patient to cough with a full bladder. If possible, to improve sensitivity, this test should be performed in the standing position.
- In men, a prostate examination is important to assess for BPH (smooth large prostate) or prostate cancer (nodular prostate). A patient may have urinary obstruction and overflow incontinence from prostatic disease.
- In women, a pelvic examination is important to assess for prolapse, such as a cystocele or uterine prolapse, which may be associated with stress incontinence. In rare cases, severe prolapse can "kink" the urethra and cause urinary obstruction and resulting retention.
- Motor function is assessed by asking the patient to "squeeze" the examining finger by contracting the pelvic floor muscles. The absence of a voluntary contraction, unfortunately, is common in neurologically intact individuals and is not always indicative of disease.

Table of elements of physical examination by disease

Disease	Physical findings
CNS disease	Normal to increased anal tone, brisk bulbo-cavernosus (B-C) reflex, adequate bladder emptying
Suprasacral spinal cord disease	Normal to increased anal tone, brisk B-C reflex, elevated residual urine volumes
Sacral spinal cord/peripheral nervous system disease/muscle disease	Normal to reduced anal tone, absent B-C reflex, demonstrable stress incontinence, elevated residual urine volumes

---

CLINICAL PEARLS
- There are very few physical examination findings that are "classic" for a specific neurologic diagnosis. However, there are still clues that can be gleaned from the examination.
- In patients with stress incontinence, it is not always possible to demonstrate incontinence via the stress test. The history and voiding diary become much more important.
- An absent bulbo-cavernosus reflex is almost always pathologic in men.
- Women without a neurogenic lesion may lack this reflex, reducing its utility in the workup of incontinence in women.
- If anal sphincter tone is severely decreased in patients presenting with retention, think cord compression.

Diagnostic tests
- A voiding diary is a commonly used tool to obtain a detailed history of a patient's urinary symptoms. The patient records (usually over a 2–3-day period) his/her fluid intake, incontinence episodes, activity associated with incontinence episodes (moving, coughing, etc.) and level or urgency to urinate preceding these episodes.
- Measuring post-void residual volume (PVR) – the amount of urine remaining in the bladder after voiding – is the most important diagnostic test for the workup of all urinary symptoms.
- A normal PVR (<100 mL) rules out overflow urinary incontinence.

- The PVR can be determined by inserting a catheter after voiding or by non-invasive bladder ultrasound (bladder scan).
- Urine analysis and culture are paramount to diagnose a urinary tract infection, which may cause urge incontinence and detrusor overactivity.
- Imaging studies such as CT and MRI of the CNS should be considered if there are associated abnormalities on physical examination. Imaging studies of the urinary tract are rarely helpful if the physical examination and labs are normal.
- Urodynamic testing plays an important role in evaluating incontinence and retention when the etiology is unclear, but the findings can be non-specific.
- In a patient with a neurologic lesion and urinary symptoms, a baseline urodynamic evaluation is recommended to measure baseline bladder compliance and rule out DSD.
- Urine cytology is rarely indicated but can be helpful if gross or microscopic hematuria is present, or if the patient has other risk factors for urothelial cancer.
- Cystoscopy is rarely useful unless the patient has new-onset urinary symptoms with gross or microscopic hematuria and is at elevated risk for bladder cancer. Cystoscopy may also be useful in a patient at risk for urethral stricture (history of pelvic trauma, venereal disease, difficulty placing urethral catheter).

Differential diagnosis

Disease/lesion	Presenting symptoms/type of bladder dysfunction	Diagnostic test findings
CNS lesion above the pontine micturition center (PMC)	Upper motor neuron dysfunction Suprapontine lesion leaves coordination intact Urge incontinence/overactive bladder	Normal PVR Urodynamics: detrusor overactivity (DO) without DSD
Suprasacral spinal cord lesion	Upper motor neuron dysfunction Infrapontine lesion disrupts coordination and causes dyssynergia Urge incontinence/retention	Elevated PVR Urodynamics: detrusor overactivity (DO) with DSD Autonomic dysreflexia may result from lesions above T6
Sacral spinal cord lesion Peripheral nervous system disease Neuromuscular disease	Lower motor neuron dysfunction Overflow incontinence/retention	Elevated PVR/retention Urodynamics: detrusor underactivity, often with flaccid sphincter
Parkinson's disease (PD)	Upper motor neuron dysfunction Urge incontinence ± bradykinesia of external urethral sphincter Men with PD are the same age group as men with bladder obstruction from BPH	PVR often elevated Urodynamics: DO with bradykinesia of relaxing urethral sphincter may resemble DSD and is sometimes referred to as pseudo-DSD Urodynamics do not easily distinguish between PD and BPH
Multiple sclerosis	Upper motor neuron dysfunction most commonly About 10% of patients present with voiding symptoms	PVR normal in CNS disease Urodynamics: DO without DSD If PVR elevated, may indicate MS of suprasacral spinal cord – urodynamics show DO with DSD

(Continued)

Disease/lesion	Presenting symptoms/type of bladder dysfunction	Diagnostic test findings
Multiple system atrophy	Upper motor neuron dysfunction Urge incontinence most common but presentation quite variable Urinary symptoms more prevalent and severe than PD Similar to PD except also involves Onuf's nucleus, which is responsible for sphincter control	PVR often elevated Urodynamics: similar to PD – DO with bradykinesia of relaxing urethral sphincter (pseudo-DSD) Urodynamics do not easily distinguish between MSA, PD, and BPH
Normal pressure hydrocephalus (NPH)	Upper motor neuron dysfunction Urge incontinence Although patients with NPH often have voiding complaints, incontinence is usually seen late in the disease process	PVR low or normal Urodynamics: DO without DSD
Diabetic cystopathy	Sensory and lower motor neuron dysfunction results from microvascular damage Overflow incontinence/urinary retention Classic diabetic cystopathy rare – seen with end-stage renal and retinal disease The vast majority of diabetic patients with urinary symptoms have overactive bladder	PVR significantly elevated Urodynamics: detrusor underactivity or acontractility Diabetic cystopathy is a late complication of diabetes Overflow incontinence is a late manifestation of diabetic cystopathy
Alzheimer's disease	Upper motor neuron dysfunction Urge incontinence or overflow incontinence May develop incontinence from loss of matter in cerebrum or develop overflow incontinence from lacking desire to void	PVR variable Urodynamics: DO without DSD, or detrusor underactivity in some cases

CLINICAL PEARLS

- Although a PVR <100 mL is generally considered normal, it is not uncommon for elderly men to have an asymptomatic PVR of 200 or 300 mL from BPH.
- Urodynamics are rarely useful in the acute setting.
- Be careful of treating urinary tract infections in patients with indwelling Foley catheters or on an intermittent bladder catheterization regimen. In general, these patients will have "dirty" urine analyses (UAs) and positive cultures related to the catheter. Antibiotics should be reserved for those patients with symptoms of a urinary tract infection (UTI) such as fever, chills, spasticity, and so forth. Overzealous use of antibiotics will select for resistant organisms in these patients.
- Rarely is imaging useful for evaluating incontinence in a patient with a normal physical examination.
- A baseline urodynamic test is recommended for patients with incontinence related to neurologic disease to assess the resting compliance of their bladder. Patients with poorly compliant bladders are at risk of vesicoureteral reflux, renal scarring, and renal failure.
- Patients with high bladder pressures may benefit from periodic urodynamics to reassess compliance and emptying function.
- Cystoscopy and cytology are commonly performed yearly for patients with indwelling catheters since they are at elevated risk of developing bladder cancer.

Recommended diagnostic strategy

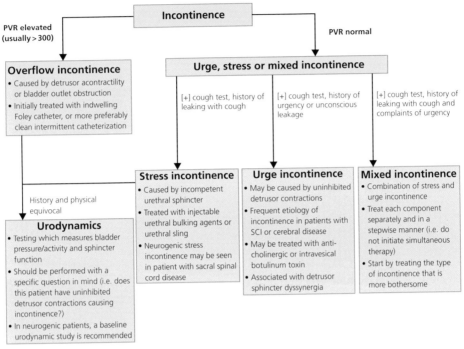

Algorithm 19.1 Approach to determine type of incontinence.

BOTTOM LINE
- A history and focused neuro-urologic examination is sufficient in most cases to make a presumptive diagnosis.
- Measuring the post-void residual urine volume (PVR) is the next and most important step in evaluating the incontinent patient after history and physical examination.
- The majority of patients with neurologic disease will have urge incontinence/detrusor overactivity, with urinary retention being less common.
- Urodynamic studies are useful when the type of incontinence is equivocal, and for all patients who have spinal cord disease with incontinence to measure their bladder pressures.

Section 2: Sexual dysfunction
Background
Definition
Sexual dysfunction is the failure of normal sexual experience and may result from a variety of conditions. Under the umbrella of sexual dysfunction disorders, the most common subset is erectile dysfunction (ED) – the pathophysiologic condition in which a male lacks the ability to maintain an erection satisfactory for intercourse. Less commonly seen is ejaculatory dysfunction. In this chapter, we will primarily focus on ED given its high incidence in patients with neurologic illness. While ejaculatory disorders are relatively common, their treatment is more sophisticated and typically requires urologic referral.

Impact

Sexual dysfunction is extremely prevalent and is especially common in patients with neurologic disease. Studies reporting the rates of ED and ejaculatory disorders in men with neurologic illness show large differences depending on the lesion site as well as the disease process. Sexual dysfunction also impacts women with neurologic disease, with studies showing that almost half of women with spinal cord injury (SCI) report decreased interest in sexual activity. In general, however, sexual dysfunction is less well studied in females because of the difficulties defining and measuring it.

Approach to diagnosis

Getting your bearings

As sexual satisfaction is clearly subjective, the diagnosis of sexual dysfunction is often made by history alone. The neurologic examination is used to detect possible causes of the patient's complaint. Laboratory testing or imaging are rarely required to detect the presence of sexual dysfunction, but studies may be indicated to evaluate an underlying cause.

A review of normal male erection and ejaculation is provided below. Understanding the physiology of erection in a healthy male is important, as erectile function is dependent upon an intact nervous system. Additionally, understanding the blueprint for a normal erection has led to the development of therapies that possess distinctive physiologic targets to treat ED.

Review of normal male erection and ejaculation

- In the normal state, stimulation of parasympathetic fibers from the sacral spinal cord causes release of nitric oxide into the vascular corpora cavernosa, causing smooth muscle relaxation, which in turn leads to increased penile blood flow and penile erection.
- On a molecular level, nitric oxide causes smooth muscle relaxation via an increase in cyclic guanosine monophosphate (cGMP).
- The mechanism of action of the commonly used phosphodiesterase inhibitors (sildenafil, tadalafil, vardenafil) is to increase the levels of cGMP by inhibiting phosphodiesterase type-5 (PDE-5), the enzyme responsible for the breakdown cGMP.
- Erections are mediated by the parasympathetic nervous system, but normal ejaculation is a sympathetic nervous system phenomenon.
- Ejaculation occurs secondary to thoracolumbar sympathetic neuronal discharge, causing emission of semen into the urethra as well as pudendal nerve stimulation of nicotinic receptors in the bulbospongiosus muscle, causing rhythmic muscular contraction and expulsion of semen.
- The commonly used mnemonic "Point and Shoot" is a convenient way to remember that erection is parasympathetically mediated while ejaculation is sympathetically mediated.

Key elements of history

The first task in taking a history of a man complaining of a sexual disorder is to decipher whether the patient has a problem with sexual desire, an issue with erection, or a problem with ejaculation. The table below can be used to classify the exact type of sexual disorder.

- The differential diagnosis for ED is considerable, but a common classification scheme divides ED into vascular, neurogenic, and psychological etiologies.
- A patient's history may suggest multiple causes for his ED (e.g. depression, diabetes, hypertension, neuropathy, medication side effect). Therefore, by history and physical examination alone, it is often difficult to discern the etiology of a patient's ED.
- Approximately 75% of men with SCI will have complaints of ED, which in most cases is purely neurogenic.
- Patients with SCI experience two "types" of erections: reflexogenic or psychogenic. Both can be present in the same patient. Men with complete SCI above T6 have an intact sacral cord and therefore can often develop involuntary reflexogenic erections from local stimuli. Less commonly,

men with sacral cord damage may experience psychogenic erections in the absence of genital sensation – in which erections are mediated from the brain through the thoracolumbar pathway.

- For patients complaining of ejaculatory disorder, it is imperative to discuss their interest in paternity. Because the treatment of ejaculation issues is so difficult, patients who are not interested in paternity should know that they may not benefit from an involved workup.
- A medication history is important when assessing both ED and ejaculatory disorders. Common medications that may contribute to both include: sedatives, antihypertensives, anticholinergics, opioids, and antidepressants. In addition, alpha-receptor antagonists may cause either retrograde ejaculation or failure of emission.
- There are numerous disorders that fall under the umbrella of sexual dysfunction. While erectile and ejaculatory dysfunction are most pertinent to patients with neurologic disease, clinicians should be aware of other disorders, which are listed and briefly described in the table below.

Table of elements of history and diseases

Disease	Historical complaint	Commonly related to neurologic disease
Hypoactive sexual desire disorder (low testosterone/hypogonadism)	Poor desire for sex	No
Erectile dysfunction	Cannot achieve or maintain erection sufficient for intercourse	Yes
Anejaculation	Absent ejaculate	Yes
Premature ejaculation	Ejaculation sooner than desired	No
Orgasm disorder	Failure to achieve orgasm during sex	No
Dyspareunia/sexual pain disorder	Sensation of pain during sex	No
Priapism	Painful erection lasting more than 4 hours	Can be seen early after SCI
Peyronie's disease	Curvature of penis and penile plaque development	No

CLINICAL PEARLS
- Erectile dysfunction (ED) is multifactorial in most patients and it is often difficult to determine the exact etiology of a patient's ED. One exception would be the young male with SCI, where neurogenic ED is the likely source.
- Ejaculatory complaints are commonly obtained when taking a sexual history of a patient with neurologic disease, specifically SCI. Workup and further investigation are often dictated by the desire to achieve paternity.
- Medication history is important. For example, alpha-receptor antagonists may cause retrograde ejaculation and/or failure of emission. In both cases, semen is not released even when orgasm is present.
- While less obvious than in men, women can also experience sexual dysfunction from neurologic disease. After SCI women have a decreased interest in sexual activity and may suffer from disorders of sexual arousal and sexual interest. Taking a sexual history on a female patient with neurologic disease is important.

Key elements of history and diagnostic tests
- Physical examination and diagnostic tests play a limited role in the workup of sexual dysfunction itself.
- There is no pathognomonic finding on examination that points to a diagnosis of ED. Neurologic examination findings consistent with pelvic nerve or spinal cord damage can confirm the diagnosis of neurogenic ED.
- Diagnostic tests are rarely employed or needed in the workup of ED. A serum morning testosterone may be checked to assess for hypogonadism in the evaluation of a patient with poor libido but is otherwise rarely helpful in the workup of ED.
- On rare occasions, the use of nocturnal penile tumescence testing can be helpful in distinguishing psychogenic from neurogenic ED. Duplex ultrasound evaluation of the cavernosal arteries can also be used to quantify blood flow. Once again, these tests rarely change the treatment algorithm.
- A urine analysis with microscopy can confirm retrograde ejaculation by demonstrating sperm in the urine after orgasm.

Recommended diagnostic/treatment strategy
- For the chief complaint of male ED, regardless of the etiology, the first-line treatment is frequently the trial of a phosphodiesterase inhibitor. Therefore, with a few exceptions, deciphering the exact cause of ED becomes less important.
- For patients with SCI, PDE-5 inhibitors are often efficacious and well tolerated. They should be started at a lower dose than in men with other etiologies for their ED because of potential for exaggerated cardiovascular autonomic dysfunction. The dose may then be titrated upwards as needed (see Algorithm 19.2).

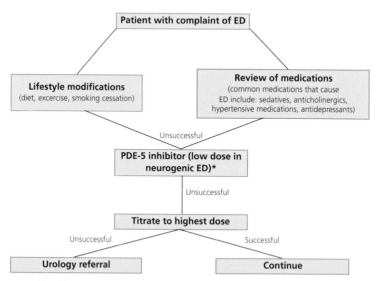

Algorithm 19.2 Algorithm to manage erectile dysfunction (ED).*Note doses of PDE-5 inhibitors: sildenafil 25 mg, vardenafil 2.5–5 mg, tadalafil 2.5–5 mg. Prescribing physicians should review with patients the complete side-effect profile of these medications before prescribing. PDE-5 inhibitors are contraindicated in patients who are on a nitrate medication as concomitant use may cause severe hypotension. There have been rare reports of priapism, a persistently painful penile erection. These cases require immediate medical attention. Also, all patients should undergo cardiovascular risk assessment before starting ED pharmacotherapy to ensure cardiac safety during sexual activity (see Kostis et al. in Reading list).

- Ejaculatory disorders are extremely common in patients with neurologic disease owing to the complex neurophysiology involved. When a patient complains of a "dry ejaculate" (no semen after orgasm), a urologic referral is advised if the patient is interested in paternity. There are sophisticated fertility treatments that urologists use to assist patients with ejaculatory dysfunction. The first step that should be taken for a patient with ejaculatory dysfunction is stopping any alpha-receptor antagonist (commonly used for BPH/voiding dysfunction). Patients with a known neurologic injury who report a "dry ejaculate" should be reassured that it is not harmful, and this usually does not require further evaluation.

BOTTOM LINE

- Sexual disorders (specifically ED and ejaculatory malfunction) are common in patients with neurologic disease.
- With the exception of young otherwise healthy men with SCI, most patients have multiple contributing etiologies for their ED.
- Regardless of the specific cause, PDE-5 inhibitors are considered first-line therapy. Primary care physicians, neurologists, and physiatrists should feel comfortable prescribing oral PDE-5 inhibitors to their patients with ED.
- In patients who do not respond to this therapy, urologic evaluation should be conducted. This may include more sophisticated testing, prescribing more advanced pharmacotherapy including intracavernosal injections, or surgery.
- Anejaculation, which is common in men with SCI, requires urologic referral if the patient is interested in paternity.
- Women also suffer from sexual dysfunction from neurologic disease. Unfortunately, the pathophysiology of sexual dysfunction in women with neurologic disease is less clear than in men and there are few approved treatment options.

Reading list

Key reading sources for this chapter can be found online at www.mountsinaiexpertguides.com

---

Additional material for this chapter can be found online at:
www.mountsinaiexpertguides.com

**This includes a case study, multiple choice questions, and
a reading list.**

PART 3

NEUROLOGIC DISEASES AND THERAPEUTICS

Vascular Diseases: Ischemic Stroke, Intracerebral and Subarachnoid Hemorrhage, Cerebral Venous Thrombosis, Arterio-Venous Malformations

Stanley Tuhrim
Icahn School of Medicine at Mount Sinai, New York, NY, USA

OVERALL BOTTOM LINE

- There are three subtypes of stroke: ischemic (IS) accounts for 85%; intracerebral hemorrhage (ICH) for 10%; and subarachnoid hemorrhage (SAH) for 5%.
- IS and ICH present with the abrupt onset of focal neurologic symptoms and signs while SAH presents with sudden, severe headache and stiff neck but infrequently with focal deficits.
- Acutely, CT scanning usually distinguishes among the three types of stroke, with subtle parenchymal findings in IS and intraparenchymal hyperdensity in ICH and in the subarachnoid space in SAH.
- Prompt thrombolytic treatment in appropriate patients can markedly improve the outcome in IS, while in ICH and SAH attention must be focused on reducing the amount of bleeding and the risk of recurrent hemorrhage or other complications (hydrocephalus, vasospasm).
- Control of risk factors, especially hypertension, can significantly reduce the risk of initial and recurrent stroke.

Section 1: Background
Definition of disease
Stroke occurs when the blood supply to part of the brain is blocked (ischemic stroke, IS) or when a blood vessel in (intracerebral hemorrhage, ICH) or around (subarachnoid hemorrhage, SAH) the brain bursts. In each case, part of the brain is damaged or dies.

Disease classification
- IS is classified as due to the following:
  - large artery atherosclerotic disease;
  - small vessel disease (affecting the penetrating arteries within the brain substance, typically causing lacunar infarctions);
  - cardioembolic disease, stroke of unknown etiology, and stroke of unusual etiology (e.g. cerebral venous thrombosis).

Mount Sinai Expert Guides: Neurology, First Edition. Edited by Stuart C. Sealfon, Rajeev Motiwala, and Charles B. Stacy.
© 2016 John Wiley & Sons, Ltd. Published 2016 by John Wiley & Sons, Ltd.
Companion website: www.mountsinaiexpertguides.com

- ICH is categorized as primary (typically associated with longstanding hypertension) or secondary, when an underlying vascular anomaly such as an arteriovenous malformation (AVM) is identified.
- SAH is categorized as aneurysmal or non-aneurysmal.

Incidence/prevalence

- There are an estimated 780,000 strokes in the USA annually; 180,000 are recurrent events in patients who have previously suffered a stroke. IS accounts for 85% of all strokes, ICH for 10%, and SAH for 5%.

Economic impact

The economic impact of stroke has been estimated at over $73 billion dollars annually (in the USA alone) in direct costs for acute treatment and indirect costs such as chronic care and lost productivity.

Etiology

- IS results from three main causes:
  - Cardioembolic infarcts occur when material, usually clot that has formed in a dilated, hypo-contractile left atrium, or less frequently clot or debris from an infected or degenerating heart valve, dislodges and travels downstream to obstruct a cerebral artery.
  - Large artery atherosclerotic infarction results from hemodynamic compromise of the circulation distal to the segment of artery narrowed by atherosclerotic plaque, or from embolism of platelet-rich thrombi that tend to form at the site of ruptured atherosclerotic plaque (artery-to-artery emboli).
  - Lacunar infarctions result from occlusion of the small, penetrating arteries narrowed by lipohyalinosis or obstructed by atherosclerotic plaque in the wall of their parent vessels.
  - Ischemic strokes can also result from arterial dissection or hypercoagulable states, including those associated with antiphospholipid antibody syndrome, adenocarcinoma, hyperhomocystinemia, factor V Leiden, and deficiencies in protein S, protein C, and antithrombim III.
- Primary ICH results from the rupture of the small penetrating arteries that originate from the major arteries providing blood to the brain. Degenerative changes in the vessel wall induced by chronic hypertension reduce compliance and increase the likelihood of spontaneous rupture.
- Secondary ICH results from rupture of underlying vascular anomalies, such as AVMs or cavernous angiomas, as well as trauma, coagulopathy, and bleeding into a mass. Amyloid angiopathy, occurring in the elderly, results in weakened arteries predisposing to repeated hemorrhages.
- SAH occurs when an aneurysm, typically formed at the branch point of major arteries at the base or on the surface of the brain, ruptures. The etiology of non-aneurysmal SAH is not known definitively, but is thought to arise from rupture of venous structures on the surface of the brain in some instances.

Pathology/pathogenesis

- IS results from marked or prolonged reduction in cerebral blood flow (ischemia) depriving neurons and their supporting cells (the neurovascular unit) of the oxygen and glucose needed for cellular metabolism. Because neurons do not store alternative energy sources, this hemodynamic compromise results in reduction of required metabolites, producing metabolic stress, energy failure, ionic perturbations, and ultimately cellular injury and death, primarily from necrosis.
- ICH initially causes mechanical compression of the adjacent structures, disrupting the normal architecture and initiating cerebral edema and neuronal damage in the surrounding

parenchyma. This edema results from the release of osmotically active proteins from the clot and usually persists for 1 to 2 weeks. Disruption of the blood–brain barrier contributes to edema formation (vasogenic edema) and cytotoxic edema follows, resulting from failure of the sodium pump, and the death of neurons. Cerebral ischemia in the region surrounding the hematoma was thought to result from mechanical compression, but recent studies have failed to confirm this. Neuronal death in the region around the hematoma is predominantly necrotic, although recent evidence suggests apoptosis also plays a role.

- SAH produces an immediate, dramatic decrease in cerebral blood flow (often resulting in a brief loss of consciousness) that can have devastating consequences. Toxic breakdown products of extravasated blood mediate the delayed development of vasospasm and, secondarily, ischemic injury.

Predictive/risk factors

Hypertension increases the risk of all types of stroke. Excessive alcohol consumption, particularly binge drinking, increases the risk of all types of stroke, especially hemorrhagic stroke, while moderate amounts of alcohol, especially red wine, are thought to reduce the risk of IS.

Disease: risk factor	Odds ratio
IS: hypertension	3–4:1
ICH: hypertension	8:1
SAH: cigarette smoking	2:1

Section 2: Prevention and screening

> **BOTTOM LINE/CLINICAL PEARLS**
> - Control of hypertension and cessation of cigarette smoking are the most important interventions to decrease the risk of initial and recurrent cerebrovascular events.
> - Treatments of coagulation status (antiplatelets, anticoagulation), hypercholesterolemia, and other metabolic conditions are important preventive measures in specific patients.

Screening

- Reducing hypertension is indicated for the prevention of several disease states; all adults should have their blood pressure checked. No other screening is recommended for the primary prevention of stroke, except in special populations (e.g. adults with more than one first-degree relative with an aneurysmal SAH or a relative with multiple aneurysms should have intracranial arterial imaging – see Guidelines below).

Primary prevention

- Control of hypertension reduces the risk of all types of stroke.
- Smoking cessation reduces the risk of ischemic and hemorrhagic stroke.
- An active lifestyle and Mediterranean diet lower the risk of IS.

Secondary prevention

- Control of hypertension reduces the risk of all types of stroke or stroke recurrences.
- Smoking cessation reduces the risk of recurrent ischemic and hemorrhagic stroke.
- Use of "statins" reduces the risk of recurrent IS.
- Use of antithrombotic medication reduces the risk of recurrent IS.
- Carotid endarterectomy or stenting reduces the risk of IS in patients with symptomatic carotid stenosis.

Section 3: Diagnosis

BOTTOM LINE/CLINICAL PEARLS
- IS and ICH present with the acute onset of focal neurologic deficits.
- SAH presents with sudden severe headache, usually without focal deficits.
- Neuroimaging, usually CT scan, is needed to distinguish ICH from IS.
- SAH is usually evident on CT scan done within 48 hours of onset.

Differential diagnosis

Differential diagnosis	Features
ICH or IS:	
• Subdural hematoma	Headache, waxing and waning signs
• Metabolic encephalopathy	Low serum glucose or other metabolic abnormality
• Drug overdose	Change in medication, hx of drug abuse
• Post-ictal state	Hx of seizure disorder, lesion on imaging
• Cerebritis	Fever, prodromal illness, CSF leukocytosis
SAH:	
• Migraine, thunderclap headache	
• Infectious meningitis	Fever, prodromal illness, CSF leukocytosis
• Pituitary apoplexy	Visual field deficits

Typical presentation

The salient characteristic of acute stroke presentation is its abrupt onset. Symptoms typically stay the same, or worsen in a smooth or stepwise manner, but IS symptoms may improve over the next several hours, or even rapidly resolve (hence the term transient ischemic attack, or TIA). The symptoms of IS will be referable to the distribution of a single vascular territory, so patients will present with signs and symptoms in the anterior, middle, or posterior cerebral territories, a penetrating artery (lacune), or the vertebral or basilar artery. ICH presents similarly, except that there is more likely to be headache, nausea, vomiting, and decreased level of consciousness initially. SAH typically presents with sudden, severe headache, often accompanied by a stiff neck, nausea, vomiting, and loss of consciousness. Focal neurologic signs are usually absent; if present, they are due to compression of a cranial nerve or signify bleeding into the adjacent brain parenchyma.

Clinical diagnosis

History

Clinicians should enquire about the time of onset of symptoms, as this may determine the course of initial therapy, especially in IS. Often the onset of symptoms is not witnessed, so it is important to establish when the patient was last known to be normal, or at their baseline. If the patient awoke with symptoms, it is important to ask when they went to bed and if they awoke during the night (e.g. to use the bathroom). If the patient or observer is unclear about the time of onset, asking about if television was on and what program was being viewed may pinpoint the time. Excluding stroke mimics is crucial, so a history of recent head trauma or seizure, as well as causes of metabolic derangement, such as change in antidiabetic medication or use of sedative-hypnotics or other medications that may alter consciousness, should be sought. A history of recreational drug use should be sought, as some commonly used drugs are associated with stroke, especially ICH. A history of prior stroke or TIA, cardiac arrhythmia, hypertension, diabetes, hypercholesterolemia, or cigarette smoking will help establish that the patient is at risk for stroke.

Physical examination

The general physical examination in the stroke patient should focus on establishing the adequacy of respiration and circulation. Hypotension or an irregular heartbeat, in addition to requiring immediate intervention, may be a clue to the etiology of the stroke. Meningismus should be excluded. Funduscopic examination may reveal papilledema or hemorrhage. The neurologic examination should include the seven basic categories: mental status (including an assessment of language function), cranial nerve, motor, coordination, reflexes, sensation, and gait (when feasible). An attempt must be made to place the lesion in a single vascular distribution. In IS the NIH Stroke Scale (NIHSS) should be performed. It is also helpful in describing the severity of illness in the awake ICH patient. The Glasgow Coma Scale Score is similarly helpful in the less alert patient.

Disease severity classification

- The NIH stroke scale (NIHSS) has become the de facto standard for determining the initial severity of an IS. It has proven to be reliable and reproducible when performed by trained personnel (not limited to neurologists). Online training and competency evaluations are available (www.strokeassociation.org). Performing this evaluation in a standardized manner allows rapid communication of the severity of the patient's condition among personnel caring for the patient, especially in the initial phases of treatment.
- The Glasgow Coma Scale (GCS) score is useful in the ICH patient whose level of consciousness does not permit cooperation with a detailed neurologic assessment. When coupled with knowledge of the size of the hemorrhage it can provide important information regarding prognosis, as well as an easily reproducible measure of the patient's status:
  - A GCS <9 and ICH volume >60 mL is associated with a 90% 30-day mortality.
  - A GCS ≥9 and ICH volume <30 mL carries a 17% 30-day mortality.
- The ICH Score, which, in addition to GCS and size, includes the presence of intraventricular hemorrhage (IVH), brainstem location, and age, provides a 6-point scale that correlates well with outcome.
- The Hunt and Hess Scale is a 5-point scale that correlates well with SAH outcome and is often used to guide early management:
  - Grade I (asymptomatic, mild headache or nuchal rigidity) and II (moderate to severe headache but no neurologic deficit except cranial nerve palsy) patients have less than a 25% chance of a poor outcome (death or severe neurologic deficit).

- Grade III patients (drowsy, confused, mild focal deficit) have a 50% chance of poor outcome.
- Grade IV (stupor, hemiparesis) and V (coma) patients have >90% chance of a poor outcome.

Laboratory diagnosis

List of diagnostic tests

A CT scan should be performed in a suspected acute IS to rule out ICH and other possible causes of acute neurologic deficits, assess for prior strokes, and detect early signs of acute ischemia. An electro-cardiogram, serum glucose and electrolytes, renal function tests, complete blood count, and prothrombin time (INR) and activated partial thromboplastin time should be obtained in all patients.

The following diagnostic tests may be useful, but the performance of additional studies in acute IS depends upon the clinical situation, resource availability, and time constraints.

- MRI with diffusion-weighted imaging will demonstrate an acute stroke, usually within minutes of onset, and precisely localize the area of ischemia.
- Magnetic resonance angiography (MRA) will aid in understanding the mechanism of the infarct by showing the artery affected. MR venography should be performed in suspected cases of cortical vein or sinus thrombosis.
- CT angiography (CTA) can demonstrate similar findings in patients unable to have an MRA or where the MRA is technically suboptimal.
- Echocardiography can detect embolic sources such as a damaged valve, an akinetic segment, a patent foramen ovale (PFO) (if done with a "bubble study"), or decreased cardiac ejection fraction.
- Transesophageal echocardiography can assess embolic sources not easily seen on transthoracic echo, such as a PFO with atrial septal aneurysm, left atrial appendage thrombus or spontaneous echo contrast ("smoke"), or aortic arch atheroma.
- Carotid ultrasound assesses the internal carotid for hemodynamically significant stenosis or emboligenic plaque.
- In suspected SAH a lumbar puncture (LP) should be performed to determine the presence of blood in the CSF if the CT scan or MRI fails to detect hemorrhage.
- In ICH or SAH vascular imaging (MRA, CTA, or catheter angiography) will help determine the source of bleeding.

Diagnostic algorithm

There is no precise paradigm for the evaluation of the IS patient, beyond obtaining the initial CT scan to exclude other causes. The goal of the acute diagnostic evaluation is to determine the best acute treatment option, if applicable, and then to determine how best to prevent a recurrence. The etiology of the bleeding in a hemorrhagic stroke should be evaluated by one of the above methods with the method and timing determined by the clinical situation.

Potential pitfalls/common errors made regarding diagnosis of disease

- Subdural hematoma may mimic an IS or TIA and may not be preceded by recognized head trauma, especially in the elderly.
- The post-ictal state may include focal neurologic deficits identical to those seen in stroke. If no seizure was witnessed it may be impossible to distinguish from an acute IS.
- Migraine aura may be indistinguishable from an IS, especially in a patient without a known migraine history.

- Metabolic derangements, most commonly hypoglycemia, may produce focal neurologic deficits identical to acute stroke, especially in patients with prior neurologic damage. Drug overdose or infection may act similarly.
- Subarachnoid hemorrhage may be missed on brain imaging studies, especially if it occurred more than 24 hours prior to imaging or the patient is severely anemic.
- Illicit drugs, especially cocaine, MDMA, and amphetamine, are associated with ICH. Note, however, that 50% of drug-associated ICH patients have an underlying vascular anomaly.

Section 4: Treatment (Algorithm 20.1)
Treatment rationale
Ischemic stroke

Intravenous administration of tissue plasminogen activator (tPA) is the only FDA-approved treatment for acute stroke and should be given to an IS patient aged 18 years or older with a measurable neurologic deficit less than 3 hours in duration who meets the published criteria.

- Exclusion criteria include:
  - symptoms minimal (NIHSS <4) or rapidly improving;
  - symptoms suggestive of SAH;
  - any bleeding, significant hypodensity, or mass effect on pretreatment CT;
  - history of intracranial hemorrhage;
  - intracranial neoplasm, AVM, or aneurysm at risk of bleeding;
  - stroke, intracranial surgery, or significant head trauma in the previous 3 months;
  - major surgery within the past 14 days;
  - GI or urinary tract hemorrhage within the past 21 days;
  - arterial puncture at a non-compressible site or LP within the past week;

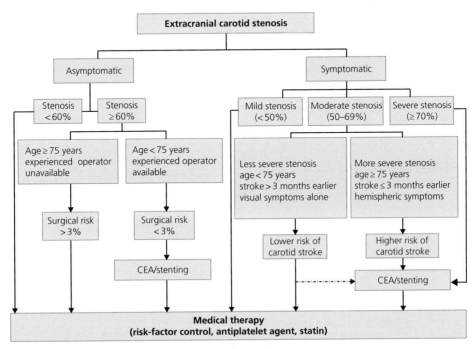

Algorithm 20.1 Management of extracranial carotid stenosis.

- platelet count <100,000 or INR >1.7, or known bleeding diathesis;
  - heparin administration within 48 hours and elevated PTT;
  - blood pressure above 185/110, despite treatment.
- Relative contraindications include:
  - blood glucose <50 or >400 mg/dL (if patient remains symptomatic after normalization then may be considered candidates);
  - myocardial infarction within the past 6 weeks (especially if transmural).

Consideration should be given to administering i.v. tPA between 3 and 4.5 hours after symptom onset if the patient meets the criteria above and is less than 80 years of age, has not received any anticoagulant in the past 48 hours, and does not have a history of prior stroke *and* diabetes.

Intra-arterial thrombolysis and mechanical clot extraction are promising new therapies for patients suffering from large vessel occlusions. They are available at comprehensive stroke centers and have recently been demonstrated to be efficacious. Criteria for administration vary by center, but the available evidence suggests benefit if treatment has been initiated within 6 hours of symptom onset. All stroke patients should be admitted to an acute stroke unit or neuro-intensive care unit, if available.

Intracerebral hemorrhage
- The acute management of ICH is directed at limiting the bleeding.
- Because elevated blood pressure is associated with hematoma expansion (which is associated with poorer outcome), blood pressure should be lowered if markedly elevated. Recent data suggest that a target of 140/90 is safe and may limit expansion.
- Coagulopathies should be corrected. Most commonly, this is related to warfarin administration; fresh frozen plasma and vitamin K should be administered. Protamine is used to counteract heparin. No specific antidote yet exists for the new oral anticoagulants. Patients who have been taking antiplatelet agents are treated with platelet transfusion (and desmopressin in some centers), although evidence for the effectiveness of this approach is limited. In most patients, hematoma growth is limited to the first 6 hours after onset, but in those with a coagulopathy this window is extended to 24 hours or more. Activated Factor VII has not been demonstrated to be of benefit in unselected ICH patients, but may be used in selected coagulopathic patients.
- There is no evidence that clot evacuation is of overall benefit in supratentorial hemorrhage, but it may be indicated in carefully selected cases.
- Cerebellar ICH >3 cm in diameter is a neurosurgical emergency requiring immediate evacuation. Deterioration can be sudden and prognosis for recovery is excellent in cases operated upon before stupor or coma develops.
- Evacuation of superficial hemorrhages and placement of a ventriculostomy in patients with IVH and hydrocephalus (sometimes with the instillation of tPA through the ventriculostomy catheter) are commonly undertaken and are the subject of ongoing investigation.

Subarachnoid hemorrhage
- When due to a ruptured aneurysm the main focus of treatment is securing the bleeding aneurysm. This should be accomplished as quickly as feasible and may be achieved by coiling or clipping. Severely ill patients may be supported until stabilized but increasingly coiling is being utilized even in grade V patients.
- Ventriculostomy may be lifesaving in a patient with acute hydrocephalus and may result in rapid improvement in neurologic status in apparently moribund patients.

- Vasospasm, commonly associated with large SAH, and its ischemic consequences, can be treated prophylactically with nimodipine. If vasospasm develops after the aneurysm is secured, it can be treated with endovascular angioplasty and administration of other intra-arterial calcium channel blockers. Vasospasm is also treated with hypervolemia, hemodilution, and induced hypertension ("triple H" therapy).

When to hospitalize

All patients with acute IS, ICH, or SAH should be hospitalized. Patients with subacute (>48 hours old) IS or TIA may be evaluated as outpatients if this can be done expeditiously. The greatest risk for recurrent events is in the first 2 weeks after the initial one, so instituting appropriate prophylactic measures efficiently is crucial. Many hospitals are developing special observation areas to accomplish rapid evaluation of these patients without the need for hospital admission.

Managing the hospitalized patient

- Preventing complications is essential to the recovery of all stroke patients.
- Swallowing evaluations should be done prior to administering oral medication or food to prevent aspiration.
- Prophylactic anti-seizure medication is often administered to hemorrhagic but not ischemic stroke patients, but seizures remain a risk in all types of stroke and should be recognized and treated promptly.
- Neurologic deterioration may occur in all stroke patients; it must be recognized promptly and its etiology determined. Common causes in addition to those discussed above include the development of cerebral edema, decreased perfusion pressure, metabolic disturbance, and fever.
- Early rehabilitation efforts aid recovery; patients should be evaluated for the appropriate form of therapy as soon as feasible.

Table of treatment

Medical therapy for ischemic stroke prevention • Aspirin 60–650 mg daily (most commonly 81–325 mg) • Clopidogrel 75 mg daily • Aspirin/extended release dipyridamole 25/200 mg b.i.d. • Warfarin (dosed by INR) • Dabigatran 150 mg b.i.d. • Rivaroxaban 20 mg daily • Apixaban 5 mg b.i.d.	• In patients without atrial fibrillation or a specific clotting disorder antiplatelet agents are preferred. All can cause bleeding; aspirin is the most likely to cause gastric irritation • In patients with atrial fibrillation, antithrombotic therapy is preferred. These drugs can cause bleeding. Warfarin must be monitored by checking the INR, while the newer agents are a fixed dose for all patients with normal renal function
Surgical ischemic stroke prevention • Carotid endarterectomy (CEA) • Carotid stenting	Appropriate for symptomatic high-grade (>70% and selected 50–69%) carotid stenosis. May be considered in asymptomatic patients with high-grade stenosis (>60%). Efficacy of the approaches similar. Stenting associated with slightly more perioperative strokes. Endarterectomy associated with more Myocardial infarctions and cranial neuropathies but may be preferable in older patients

Prevention/management of complications

- Intracranial hemorrhage occurs in about 6% of IS patients treated with i.v. tPA, so all patients receiving thrombolysis should be monitored for signs and symptoms of CNS hemorrhage, including neurologic deterioration, development of severe headache, sudden elevation of blood pressure, and onset of nausea and vomiting. If hemorrhage is suspected, tPA infusion should be stopped and a head CT obtained.
- Aspiration is a common problem in stroke patients, who may have difficulty protecting their airway because of a decreased level of consciousness or focal neurologic dysfunction. A water swallow test should be performed in all patients prior to administering anything by mouth. This can be accomplished by having the patient take sips of water from a cup filled with approximately 90 mL of water, without interruption. For one minute after drinking monitor for signs of aspiration including coughing with water intake, absent swallowing or pocketing of water in cheeks, wet or dysphonic voice, audibly "wet" respirations, drooling or pooling of saliva, or throat clearing.
- Increased intracranial pressure can occur in each type of stroke. Patients should be monitored for signs of its development, including decreased level of consciousness, increased blood pressure with widening of pulse pressure and decreased heart rate, and clinical signs of brainstem or cranial nerve (especially CN III) compression. Common causes include mass effect from hematoma expansion or edema, which sometimes requires decompressive hemicraniectomy, and acute hydrocephalus, usually best treated by ventriculostomy.
- Seizures complicate about 10% of strokes and are usually easily recognized if they include repetitive tonic posturing or clonic movements, but non-convulsive seizures (or non-convulsive status epilepticus) should be suspected in unexplained, decreased consciousness, and an EEG (or continuous EEG monitoring, when available) obtained.

CLINICAL PEARLS
- Ischemic stroke risk is greatest in the 2 weeks after a transient ischemic attack.
- Asymptomatic carotid disease may be managed conservatively; the decision to intervene should involve shared decision-making between patient and physician.
- There is no clear superiority between CEA and stenting. Choices should be based upon individual patient characteristics, local expertise, and patient preference.

Section 5: Special populations (Figures 20.1, 20.2, and 20.3)

Pregnancy

- The peripartum period is associated with increased risk of stroke. Eclampsia can result in cerebral edema and ICH but rarely infarction. Cerebral vein and sinus occlusion is the most common stroke type in the peripartum period. Once the child is delivered, anticoagulation is usually instituted and additional hypercoagulant markers are sought.

Children

- Ischemic stroke in children is rare, and is most commonly due to cardioembolism. Children with sickle-cell disease are also at increased stroke risk; periodic exchange transfusion reduces this risk substantially. Although not approved for use in children under 18 years of age, anecdotally, i.v. tPA has been used successfully. Hemorrhagic stroke is most commonly due to vascular malformations with treatment directed at correction if possible.

Elderly

- Stroke occurs primarily in those over 60, but the very elderly experience a greater proportion of ICH than the general population, primarily due to amyloid angiopathy. The same acute treatment and prevention strategies are effective in the very elderly, including the use of i.v. tPA.

Section 6: Prognosis

> **BOTTOM LINE/CLINICAL PEARLS**
> - Prognosis in IS is determined primarily by the severity of the initial deficit.
> - Approximately 20% of IS patients progress after hospital admission, but no accurate means for predicting progression exists.
> - The most important determinant of thrombolysis efficacy is time from onset to treatment.
> - ICH mortality is predicted by initial GCS score, hemorrhage size, and presence of IVH.
> - SAH mortality can be predicted by the Hunt and Hess Scale, but some grade IV and V patients can respond to aggressive intervention.

Follow-up tests and monitoring
- IS patients with evidence of atherosclerotic disease should have periodic (initially annual) follow-up with carotid ultrasound to monitor progressive stenosis.
- Patients who have had coiling of intracranial aneurysms need a follow-up catheter angiogram, generally at 6–12 months, to ensure that the aneurysm has been eliminated.
- All stroke patients need to have their blood pressure controlled and checked regularly. Hypertension is the single most important modifiable stroke risk factor.

Section 7: Reading list
Key reading sources for this chapter can be found online at www.mountsinaiexpertguides.com

Suggested websites
American Heart Association: www.heart.org
American Stroke Association: www.strokeassociation.org
National Institute of Neurological Disorders and Stroke: www.ninds.nih.gov/disorders/stroke/stroke.htm
National Stroke Association: www.stroke.org
stroke-site: www.stroke-site.org

Section 8: Guidelines
American Heart Association/American Stroke Association (AHA/ASA) guidelines

Title	Source	Weblink
Guidelines for the Early Management of Patients With Acute Ischemic Stroke	American Heart Association/ American Stroke Association (AHA/ASA), 2013	http://stroke.ahajournals.org/content/44/3/870
Guidelines for the Management of Aneurysmal Subarachnoid Hemorrhage	American Heart Association/ American Stroke Association (AHA/ASA), 2012	https://stroke.ahajournals.org/content/early/2012/05/03/STR.0b013e3182587839.full.pdf+html
Guidelines for the Management of Spontaneous Intracerebral Hemorrhage	American Heart Association/ American Stroke Association (AHA/ASA), 2015	http://stroke.ahajournals.org/content/early/2015/05/28/STR.0000000000000069
Guidelines for the Prevention of Stroke in Patients with Stroke or Transient Ischemic Attack	American Heart Association/ American Stroke Association (AHA/ASA), 2014	http://stroke.ahajournals.org/content/early/2014/04/30/STR.0000000000000024

Mount Sinai guidelines

Title	Source	Weblink
Protocol for the Initial Evaluation and Management of Patients with Ischemic or Hemorrhagic Stroke	Mount Sinai, 2012 Step-by-step guide for the emergent management of stroke and its complications	
Policy for IA/Catheter-Based Reperfusion Therapy and Procedure for Pre-, Intra-, and Post-Intervention Nursing Care	Mount Sinai, 2012 Criteria and procedures for the administration of endovascular therapy for acute IS at Mount Sinai	

Section 9: Evidence

Type of evidence	Title and comment	Weblink
Randomized controlled trial (RCT, 1996)	Tissue plasminogen activator for acute ischemic stroke **Comment**: Demonstrated that i.v. rt-PA was effective in improving outcome in acute IS patients treated up to 3 hours from symptom onset	http://www.ncbi.nlm.nih.gov/pubmed/7477192
RCT, 2000	Early stroke treatment associated with better outcome **Comment**: This analysis demonstrated that the sooner patients are treated with i.v. tPA the more likely they are to benefit	http://www.ncbi.nlm.nih.gov/pubmed/11113218
RCT, 2008	Thrombolysis with alteplase 3 to 4.5 hours after acute ischemic stroke **Comment**: Demonstrated benefit of i.v. tPa extends to 4.5 hours from stroke onset	http://www.ncbi.nlm.nih.gov/pubmed/18815396

Section 10: Images

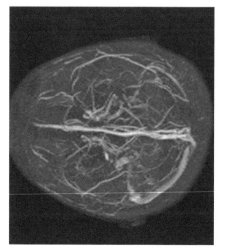

Figure 20.1 Venogram demonstrating lateral sinus thrombosis. *Source*: author's personal collection.

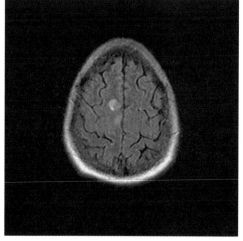

Figure 20.2 Parasagittal cortical hemorrhage in a young post-partum woman with lateral sinus thrombosis. *Source*: author's personal collection.

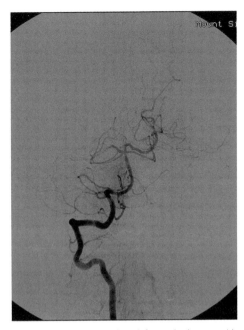

Figure 20.3 Occlusion of the left vertebral artery with vasospasm (secondary to dissection [see, specifically, Case study 20.1]) evident in the basilar and right posterior cerebral arteries. *Source*: author's personal collection.

Additional material for this chapter can be found online at:
www.mountsinaiexpertguides.com

This includes advice for patients, a case study, multiple choice questions, and a reading list.

CHAPTER 21

Neurologic Complications of Systemic Disease

Michelle T. Fabian

Icahn School of Medicine at Mount Sinai, New York, NY, USA

OVERALL BOTTOM LINE

- When the neurologist consults on other services for neurologic symptoms or signs, often this evaluation leads to the discovery of a previously unsuspected medical condition.
- There is a multitude of systemic diseases that directly or indirectly cause neurologic dysfunction or damage.
- The new appearance of a focal neurologic deficit in the presence of systemic disease does not always mean a new neurologic event has occurred. Instead this may be unmasking by systemic disease of subclinical residual damage to the nervous system from a previous neurologic event such as a stroke or MS.
- There are many neurologic syndromes that point toward certain possible underlying medical conditions.
- In order to identify a potential relationship between a systemic disease and the neurologic presentation, it is crucial to obtain a detailed history of present illness, to get a complete review of systems, to consider the entire past medical history, and to review all available laboratory and imaging tests during a neurologic consultation.
- The evaluation must include a general medical examination with careful attention to systems in which suspicions are raised from the history.
- The therapeutic plan is best formulated taking into account input from all relevant specialists.

Section 1: Background
Definition of disease
A neurologic complication of systemic disease refers to any neurologic disorder caused by a condition with an origin outside of the nervous system. The diagnosis of the systemic disease may be well established or may be unknown when the neurologic complications develop.

Disease classification
The best way to consider and to classify the neurologic manifestations of systemic disease is by the causative system, for example neurologic complication of cardiac disease, neurologic complications of hepatic disease, and so forth.

Mount Sinai Expert Guides: Neurology, First Edition. Edited by Stuart C. Sealfon, Rajeev Motiwala, and Charles B. Stacy.
© 2016 John Wiley & Sons, Ltd. Published 2016 by John Wiley & Sons, Ltd.
Companion website: www.mountsinaiexpertguides.com

Pathology/pathogenesis

The pathogeneses for the neurologic complications of systemic disease are wide ranging. The systemic disease may either cause a complication in the nervous system through the same mechanisms as it does in other organs (e.g. inflammation from temporal arteritis involving intracranial vasculature), or the effect on the nervous system may be entirely different from the pathogenesis of the systemic disease (e.g. malabsorption from a GI disorder causing the development of a peripheral neuropathy).

Section 2: Prevention and screening

Not applicable for this topic.

Section 3: Diagnosis

> **BOTTOM LINE/CLINICAL PEARLS**
> - Careful attention should be paid to all past medical history and current medications.
> - The initial examination of the patient must include a general medical examination, that is, heart, skin, and joint examination to evaluate for signs of disease outside of the nervous system.
> - Imaging or laboratory tests should be ordered to evaluate the neurologic manifestations but also to allow for diagnosis or further evaluation of the systemic disease as well.

Differential diagnosis

Typical presentation

As there are many neurologic complications caused by various systemic diseases, the presentation depends on the underlying disease and specific complication.

Clinical diagnosis

History

The aim of the history should be to query the patient in a focused manner that will result in accurate localization and diagnosis, as discussed elsewhere in this book. Careful attention must be paid not only to the known medical diagnoses, but also to the timing of onset of neurologic symptoms in relation to any worsening of one of these conditions. Surgical history, including complications of the surgery, should be noted. Because the systemic disease may not be diagnosed at the time of presentation, a general review of systems should never be overlooked. The medication record needs to be fully explored for any possible relationship to the patient's symptoms. It is especially important to inquire about medications that were recently started, recently adjusted, or given on an as-needed basis.

Physical examination

The mental status examination may be of key importance and should be comprehensive. Asterixis or myoclonus can be seen in toxic-metabolic syndromes. Ophthalmologic examination should include the iris and retina, in addition to the optic nerve. The cardiovascular examination should be performed looking for arrhythmia, murmur, bruit, and presence of pulses in the extremities. Pulmonary examination should look for signs of obstructive airway disease or

Differential diagnosis	Presentation	Diagnostic features
Cardiac and aortic disease		
Cardiac arrhythmia, cardiomyopathy, recent myocardial infarction, infectious or aseptic endocarditis, aortic aneurysm, aortic dissection, and aortic thrombus all can cause neurologic vascular sequelae	Sudden onset of focal neurologic symptoms or decreased responsiveness	Neurologic examination may show focal deficit or decreased level of consciousness. Cardiac examination may reveal rhythm disturbance or murmur. There may also be signs of embolism in other areas such as the distal limbs or kidneys. Brain MRI or MRA may show changes such as infarction consistent with embolism, and echocardiography or Holter monitoring may reveal the underlying cardiac etiology. Chest CT and CTA can detect aortic abnormalities
Pulmonary disease		
Hypercapnea or hypoxia	Subacute or acute presentation may include headache, confusion, or altered level of consciousness	Tremor, myoclonus, brisk reflexes, and encephalopathy can be seen on neurologic examination. General examination may reveal clubbing or cyanosis of the extremities. Arterial blood gas analysis for CO_2, O_2, acid–base status
Hepatic disease		
Hepatic encephalopathy	Most commonly there is history of confusion and somnolence. There also may be periods of agitation	Examination most commonly reveals fluctuating level of consciousness. There may be asterixis and hyperreflexia. EEG may show triphasic waves or slowing Liver function tests may be abnormal and arterial ammonia is often high
Wilson's disease	Patients with Wilson's disease may present with cognitive dysfunction, psychosis, and tremor	The key finding is the Kayser–Fleischer ring, a brown- or gray-colored ring encircling the iris, on slit-lamp examination. Brain MRI may show abnormal signal in the basal ganglia and rarely may reveal the pathognomonic "double panda sign." Decreased serum ceruloplasmin level, elevated urinary copper, and copper deposition on liver biopsy are typically present

Renal disease

Uremic encephalopathy	The presentation is similar to other metabolic encephalopathies with fluctuating level of consciousness. Patients may also present with seizures	Commonly there will be myoclonus and asterixis on examination. EEG may show triphasic waves and slowing. BUN and creatinine will be elevated, though these may not correlate with severity

Hematologic disease

Antiphospholipid antibody syndrome (APS)	APS may occur in patients with rheumatologic conditions such as lupus or also may exist in isolation Presentations vary and could be focal, consistent with CNS venous or arterial occlusion, or global, most commonly resulting in cognitive dysfunction caused by a vasculopathy	In addition to cognitive changes and focal neurologic deficit, examination may reveal livedo reticularis or evidence of distal ischemia in the limbs. Neuroimaging in APS may show evidence for infarct or white matter lesions similar to those seen in multiple sclerosis. Diagnosis of APS hinges on blood serologies. As elevated antibodies may represent false positives, they should be repeated for confirmation
Polycythemia vera (PCV)	The hyperviscosity caused by PCV can cause arterial thrombosis and also leads to accelerated atherosclerosis with resultant infarct. Patients may also present with headache, dizziness, and cognitive complaints	Neurologic examination may reveal a focal neurologic deficit. Rarely chorea may occur. Systemically, patients may have flushing of the face and limbs. Brain MRI is used to evaluate for infarct. Diagnosis of PCV is suggested by CBC and confirmed by bone marrow biopsy
Sickle-cell anemia	Patients can encounter a multitude of neurologic complications including infarct (1/4 of all sickle-cell patients have a stroke before age 45), hemorrhage (either subarachnoid or intraparenchymal), meningitis, and epilepsy	Patients presenting with focal neurologic signs should have imaging of the brain with MRI or CT. If infection is suspected LP should be performed. DNA-based testing can confirm a diagnosis of sickle-cell anemia in the prenatal period. Otherwise diagnosis is usually made after newborn screening detects an abnormality that is then confirmed by DNA testing
Thrombotic thrombocytopenic purpura (TTP)	Patients with TTP may present with altered mental status, headache, seizures, and possibly focal deficit from stroke in addition to the other systemic features: fever, thrombocytopenia, hemolytic anemia, and renal involvement	Neurologic symptoms may warrant an MRI. EEG may also be done to exclude non-convulsive status epilepticus or more obvious seizure activity. A blood smear showing microangiopathic hemolytic anemia and thrombocytopenia is diagnostic for TTP
Multiple myeloma	Multiple myeloma can affect the nervous system in a myriad of ways. Myelopathic symptoms are secondary to cord compression that occurs either as direct extension of a vertebral plasmacytoma or because of vertebral collapse after bony involvement. Rarely a patient may present withw focal symptoms relating to a plasmacytoma infiltrating the brain. Rarely, patients may develop a peripheral neuropathy	Neurologic evaluation can be performed using CT or MRI for spinal cord and brain symptoms, and EMG for peripheral symptoms Diagnosis of multiple myeloma is confirmed on bone marrow biopsy

(Continued)

Differential diagnosis	Presentation	Diagnostic features
Endocrine/metabolic		
Sodium disturbance	Hyponatremia and hypernatremia often cause encephalopathy. Seizures can occur in both as well, though more commonly with hyponatremia	On examination there may be waxing and waning of consciousness, myoclonus, or asterixis. CT or MRI may show alterations in brain volume. Electrolyte panel will lead to diagnosis. Underlying cause for the derangement should also be worked up including dehydration, SIADH, and adrenal insufficiency
Hyperkalemia	Severe hyperkalemia may cause an acute flaccid paraplegia	Serum potassium is elevated. In severe cases changes may be apparent on EKG
Hypocalcemia	Severe hypocalcemia may cause paresthesias, muscle cramping, myalgias, and tetany	Chvostek's sign (spasm of the ipsilateral face with tapping of the facial nerve anterior to the ear) and Trousseau's sign (carpopedal spasm with inflation of a blood pressure cuff) may be apparent on examination. Hypocalcemia is confirmed through serum calcium testing. Variation in albumin may lead to abnormally high or low total calcium. Therefore ionized calcium is the most accurate test for the true calcium level
Hypercalcemia	Hypercalcemic patients may experience both psychiatric and neurologic symptoms including cognitive dysfunction, anxiety, depression, altered mental status, and, if acute, alteration in consciousness including coma	Hypercalcemia is diagnosed in a similar fashion to hypocalcemia, through ionized calcium levels
Hypoglycemia	Hypoglycemia often causes anxiety, tremor, somnolence, and cognitive dysfunction. Severe hypoglycemia may lead to obtundation, coma, or seizure	Diagnosis is most rapidly made through fingerstick glucose testing. Brain imaging with CT, MRI to evaluate for cerebral edema may be performed if recovery is delayed
Hyperglycemia	Neurologic dysfunction most commonly occurs in patients with plasma osmolality >330 mosmol/kg. Patients will typically develop cognitive dysfunction, which may progress to coma. They may also develop seizures, most classically continuous simple partial seizures (usually termed epilepsia partialis continua)	Diagnosis of hyperglycemia is most often made through fingerstick glucose testing. Osmolality may be calculated using basic metabolic profile
Hyperthyroidism	Hyperthyroidism, most often a consequence of Graves' disease or an adenoma, may cause neuropsychiatric manifestations such as inability to focus, anxiety, agitation, and psychosis. Patients may have a tremor, and develop myopathy, neuropathy, and eye movement abnormalities	General physical examination can reveal a thin, tachycardic, and hypertensive patient. There may be tremor and increased sweating. Exophthalmos may be present. Neurologic examination may reveal inattention and anxious affect. Eye movements may be dysconjugate. There may be proximal muscle weakness and hyperreflexia. Diagnosis is confirmed by presence of low TSH and elevated thyroid T_3 or T_4 hormones

Hypothyroidism	Neurologic symptoms present in hypothyroidism can be wide-ranging, from fatigue, depression, and mild mental slowing to coma. As in hyperthyroidism, patients may also experience myopathy or neuropathy	General systemic examination may show an overweight or obese patient who is bradycardic and hypertensive. There may be dryness to the skin and also evidence of hair thinning. Neurologic examination may reveal cognitive slowing and depressed affect. There may be proximal muscle weakness, and reflexes may be absent or show slow relaxation. There may also be distal sensory changes. Diagnosis is confirmed by presence of elevated TSH and depressed thyroid T_3 or T_4 hormones. Thyroperoxidase antibodies may also be elevated
Hypoadrenalism	Patients with hypoadrenalism will often present with headaches, cognitive dysfunction, behavioral disturbances, and rarely psychosis, in addition to the systemic symptoms of fatigue, hyperpigmentation, hypotension, and weight loss	Hyponatremia and hyperkalemia may be the first clues toward diagnosis. Diagnosis in primary adrenal failure is confirmed by finding low plasma levels of cortisol in conjunction with elevated ACTH levels and also failure of response with ACTH stimulation testing
Hyperadrenalism	Hyperadrenalism can most commonly impact the nervous system by causing cognitive changes and muscle weakness	Measurement of serum cortisol, urinary cortisol, and ACTH can determine if hyperadrenalism exists. Low- and high-dose dexamethasone suppression test can help localize the abnormally functioning area
Hypopituitarism	Hypopituitarism may be the result of many etiologies including non-functioning pituitary adenomas, invasive tumors, inflammatory processes, infarction or hemorrhage. Patients can present with headaches, visual loss, cranial neuropathies. Hormonal deficiencies result in amenorrhea in women, in addition to hypothyroidism and hypoadrenalism	Neurologic examination may reveal chiasmal visual deficits (such as bitemporal) as well as other cranial neuropathies if the cavernous sinus is involved (cranial nerves V1, III, IV, VI). Systemic examination may show findings consistent with hypoadrenalism, hypothyroidism, hypogonadism, or hyperprolactinemia depending on what deficiencies are most prominent. Brain MRI with attention to the pituitary and surrounding structures is used to evaluate for structural causes. Serum testing of individual hormonal levels can identify deficiencies
Functional pituitary tumors	The two most common hypersecretion syndromes are caused by increased prolactin and increased growth hormone. Prolactinomas can cause amenorrhea and galactorrhea in women, and impotence, infertility, and rarely galactorrhea in men. Acromegaly, caused by overproduction of growth hormone, causes excessive growth in addition to impaired glucose metabolism. Headaches, fatigue, myopathy, and neuropathy occur	Focused MRI is best for pituitary imaging. As in pituitary deficiency, serum abnormalities in pituitary hormones will lead to diagnosis

(Continued)

Differential diagnosis	Presentation	Diagnostic features
Neoplastic disease		
Metastasis	Presentation depends on the location of metastasis. Brain metastases may present with headache, seizures, or contralateral motor or sensory deficits. Masses compressing the spinal cord will often manifest as weakness and sensory disturbance with pain at the level of compression. Leptomeningeal carcinomatosis can cause headaches, cognitive dysfunction, alterations in consciousness, and cranial neuropathies	Examination will show corresponding focal deficits. MRI of brain or spinal cord is most useful for defining the extent of the involvement. Where there is suspicion for leptomeningeal disease, LP is used to obtain cytology
Paraneoplastic syndromes	Paraneoplastic syndromes can present in a patient with known cancer and can also be the presenting complaint in a patient before cancer is suspected. There are multiple paraneoplastic syndromes that can affect the central and peripheral nervous systems. Paraneoplastic syndromes may result in an encephalitis, a pancerebellar syndrome, opsoclonus, myoclonus, myelitis, neuromuscular junction disorder, or myopathy	Neurologic symptoms can be further evaluated with MRI, and EMG and nerve conduction studies. Serum, and sometimes CSF, testing for paraneoplastic antibodies should be done. When a paraneoplastic syndrome is confirmed in the absence of a known cancer, a thorough investigation to find an underlying malignancy should be pursued. This can include body CT, mammogram, and colonoscopy. PET scan can increase the yield
Nutritional deficiency		
Inflammatory bowel disease, celiac disease, history of gastric or intestinal resection, gastric bypass, and pernicious anemia all may lead to neurologic complications	Presentation may reflect peripheral or central nervous system pathology depending on the deficient vitamin(s). Patient may develop cognitive dysfunction, paresthesias in the extremities, gait dysfunction, or limb weakness	General medical examination may show skin rash. Neurologic examination may show signs of dementia, myelopathy, and peripheral neuropathy. Laboratory studies may show deficiencies in vitamin B12, thiamine, niacin, and copper, among others. Methylmalonic acid may be elevated and reveal a metabolic B12 deficiency even when B12 is low normal
Rheumatologic/inflammatory disease		
Systemic lupus erythematosus (SLE)	50–75% of SLE patients have neurologic manifestations, most commonly cognitive or psychiatric symptoms including psychosis. Patients may also present with a Guillain–Barré-like syndrome or symptoms consistent with peripheral neuropathy	General examination findings may include a malar rash and arthritis. Rheumatologic panel would be consistent with lupus. Brain MRI and MRA may be abnormal in cases of lupus vasculopathy

Rheumatoid arthritis (RA)	Patients with RA may present with high cervical cord compression as a result of pannus formation at the atlanto-axial joint. They also may develop vasculitic neuropathies	MRI reveals the site of compression of the pannus. Muscle and nerve biopsy will confirm a diagnosis of vasculitic neuropathy
Sjögren's syndrome	Multiple neurologic complications have been reported including trigeminal sensory neuropathy, other cranial neuropathies, myelitis, peripheral neuropathy, and autonomic neuropathy	MRI can identify spinal cord disease, EMG can diagnose peripheral neuropathy, tilt-table test will detect autonomic neuropathy. Schirmer's test is positive for decreased tear production. Many patients have positive ANA and positive Sjögren's antibodies
Behçet's disease	Patients may present with symptoms resulting from increased intracranial pressure from a venous sinus thrombosis, focal deficits secondary to arterial or venous thrombosis, or as a result of focal parenchymal lesions from a vasculitic process. Other presentations can include seizure, encephalitis, and aseptic meningitis	Diagnosis of Behçet's, especially in the absence of systemic disease, is notoriously difficult. On systemic examination there may be oral or genital ulcers. The skin may also be affected with a variety of dermatologic appearances. Ophthalmologic exam may show evidence for uveitis. Also there may be sign of deep venous thrombosis. Neurologic evaluation should include MRI, MRV (magnetic resonance venogram), and LP where applicable. Pathergy test (skin lesions or ulcers from pinprick or mild trauma) is pathognomonic when positive
Sarcoidosis	Neurosarcoidosis can affect every aspect of the nervous system, including: cognitive syndrome, focal deficits secondary to parenchymal lesions, aseptic meningitis, cranial neuropathies from basal leptomeningeal disease, myelopathic presentations from cord lesions, peripheral neuropathies, and myopathies	Diagnosis of neurosarcoidosis can be challenging. Presence of sarcoidosis in another body system should alert the clinician to this possibility. If there is no evidence for sarcoidosis on ophthalmologic, dermatologic, or pulmonary examinations, a gallium scan may reveal areas of activity that could provide a site for biopsy. ACE level in blood or CSF is often elevated in sarcoidosis, but this test is not especially sensitive or specific. MRI, LP, and EMG may be used depending on presentation

Infection

	Systemic infections can cause profound neurologic dysfunction. Altered mental status can occur in the setting of sepsis especially in a patient who has baseline cognitive dysfunction. Commonly, sepsis unmasks a deficit due to a previous neurologic event, such as stroke or multiple sclerosis. Direct extension of the infection into the CNS, e.g. meningitis caused by a bacteremia or extension from a parameningeal abscess, is uncommon but should always be considered	Examination for any sign of active infection, including presence of fever, rigors, and leukocytosis, is important. Less obvious sources for infection, such as pressure ulcers, should also be considered. Neuroimaging with CT or MRI may rule out a new event causing the deficit, but will be less helpful when the neurologic symptoms are residual

infection. The skin should be examined for rashes, bruising, or ulcerations. The joints should be examined for erythema or swelling. The extremities must be assessed for signs of vascular compromise or edema.

Laboratory diagnosis

List of diagnostic tests

- Neurologic tests may include brain or spine CT scan or MRI, lumbar puncture, EMG, or EEG, depending on presentation.
- Systemic testing may include a metabolic panel, rheumatologic panel, CBC, coagulation parameters, ACE level, electrocardiogram, echocardiogram, chest/abdomen/pelvis CT, and skin biopsy.

Potential pitfalls or common errors made regarding diagnosis of disease

- The role of known systemic diseases may be overlooked as a potential cause for a neurologic process due to incomplete history taking or failure to identify an association between the two conditions.
- Conversely, a medical condition may be erroneously assumed to be the cause of a neurologic process, when in fact the two disease processes are distinct. Symptom and sign emergence from an old neurologic event such as stroke in the setting of systemic disease can be mistaken for an acute neurologic event.

Section 4: Treatment

Treatment rationale

Treatments are widely varied and dictated by the primary medical problem and the neurologic complication.

Managing the hospitalized patient

- It is crucial to involve all relevant subspecialists whenever indicated, as this will greatly aid in efficient diagnosis and parsimonious treatment strategies.

Table of treatments for selected disorders

Systemic disorder/ neurologic complication	Treatment
Cardiac arrest or severe global circulatory dysfunction (cardiac arrest, ventricular fibrillation, or pulseless tachycardia)	Unresponsive patients following arrest should be treated with therapeutic hypothermia. Optimally cooling should begin within 6 hours of the arrest and be maintained for at least 24 hours. Cooling may be achieved by infusion of cold saline or use of a cooling vest
Thromboembolic disease from a cardiac source	Patients with atrial fibrillation or a known cardiac thrombus should be treated with anticoagulation to prevent further stroke. Size of infarct will determine point of initiation – if an infarct is large anticoagulation may be deferred up to a few weeks to decrease risk of hemorrhage into the stroke. In acute stroke, tPA or thrombus extractions are used when appropriate

Systemic disorder/ neurologic complication	Treatment
Hepatic encephalopathy	Lactulose is a common first line of treatment. Rifaximin may be added
Uremic encephalopathy	Treatment of significant uremic encephalopathy is urgent dialysis. Improvement may lag behind treatment by a period of days
Hyponatremic encephalopathy	Slow correction of hyponatremia with infusion of hyperosmotic saline; too rapid a correction puts the patient at risk for central pontine myelinolysis, a potentially devastating condition
Metastatic disease	Symptomatic treatment with steroids may be indicated to decrease symptoms caused by mass effect. Solitary masses in accessible areas of the brain or spinal column may be surgically removed for improved prognosis. Radiation therapy may also be a palliative option. Pretreatment function is best predictor of post-treatment function and thus those with worsening neurologic deficit should be treated quickly
Autoimmune disease	In general treatment of neurologic complications from autoimmune disease will parallel treatment of the disease itself and will typically involve an immunosuppressant agent, treatment with steroids, IVIG, and plasmapheresis

Section 5: Special populations

Pregnancy

- Pre-eclamptic patients are at risk for PRES (posterior reversible encephalopathy syndrome) as well as for encephalopathy and seizures. Embolic stroke may occur because of hypercoagulability or amniotic embolus. Sheehan's syndrome (post-partum pituitary hemorrhage) presents as headache, visual loss, or third nerve lesion. Venous sinus thrombosis presenting with headache, seizures, or altered mental status is seen in the peripartum period.
- Peripheral nervous system complications including sciatica, meralgia paresthetica, and carpal tunnel syndrome are extremely common and can be attributed to the accumulation of interstitial fluid and structural changes that occur in the pregnant state.

Elderly

- Elderly patients are more prone than younger patients to develop nervous system dysfunction from metabolic derangements or infections. Mild metabolic disturbances and infections without any specific symptoms or signs, especially bladder, should always be considered and addressed as they often cause reversible global or focal neurologic deficits in the elderly.

Section 6: Prognosis

BOTTOM LINE/CLINICAL PEARLS
- Accurate prognosis is often difficult in a systemically ill patient with neurologic complications.
- Because prognosis is so difficult, communication among all consultants and caregivers to provide a consistent message to the patient and family is essential.
- After a devastating neurologic complication (e.g. anoxic injury during cardiac arrest) the overall prognosis may be dictated by neurologic status alone.

Section 7: Reading list

Key reading sources for this chapter can be found online at www.mountsinaiexpertguides.com

---

Additional material for this chapter can be found online at:
www.mountsinaiexpertguides.com

This includes advice for patients, a case study, multiple choice questions, a reading list.

CHAPTER 22

Neuro-Oncology

Isabelle M. Germano
Icahn School of Medicine at Mount Sinai, New York, NY, USA

OVERALL BOTTOM LINE
- Neuro-oncology is the discipline treating neoplasms of the brain and spine, primary and metastatic.
- The presenting symptoms depend on tumor size and location. Diagnostic steps include neurologic examination, imaging, CSF testing when applicable, and ultimately tissue diagnosis.
- Treatments are best carried out in a multidisciplinary fashion. The treatment is specific to the tumor type, its location, its molecular characteristics, and whether first presentation or recurrence.
- It is strongly encouraged to offer patients the option to participate in a clinical trial.
- Quality of life is one of the highest priorities in neuro-oncological care and should be heavily weighted in finalizing the best treatment option.

Section 1: Background
Definition of disease
Brain and spine tumors can be primary or metastatic.
- *Primary brain tumors* include any tumor that originates in the brain; they can arise from the meninges or Schwann cells (meningiomas, schwannomas), the nerve cells (gliomas, neurocytoma), embryonal tissue (medulloblastoma, primitive neuroectodermal tumor (PNET), teratoma, dermoid, epidermoid), or the glands (pituitary, pineal).
- *Metastatic brain tumors* are the most common intracranial neoplasms in the adult. They originate from a cancer located elsewhere in the body, with the majority being from one of three primary malignancies: lung cancer (40–50%), breast cancer (15–25%), and melanoma (5–20%).
- *Spine tumors* can be classified by their locations as intramedullary (e.g. ependymoma, glioma), intradural extramedullary (e.g. meningioma, schwannoma), or extradural (e.g. bony metastases).
- Other disorders encountered in neuro-oncology include: leptomeningeal carcinomatosis, paraneoplastic syndromes, and neurologic manifestations related to cancer treatments.
  - Leptomeningeal carcinomatosis occurs when cancer cells invade the subarachnoid space.
  - Paraneoplastic syndromes are idiopathic or known to result from autoimmune responses.

Treatment-related syndromes result from toxicity secondary to radiation, chemotherapy, surgery, or other treatments.

Mount Sinai Expert Guides: Neurology, First Edition. Edited by Stuart C. Sealfon, Rajeev Motiwala, and Charles B. Stacy.
© 2016 John Wiley & Sons, Ltd. Published 2016 by John Wiley & Sons, Ltd.
Companion website: www.mountsinaiexpertguides.com

Table 22.1 WHO histologic classification of glial brain tumors.

Grade	Nomenclature	Histologic feature
I	Juvenile pilocytic astrocytoma (JPA)	Bipolar cells with pilocytic processes Rosenthal fibers
II	Astrocytoma Oligodendroglioma Ependymoma Pleomorphic xanthoastrocytoma	Well-differentiated glial cells, moderately increased cellularity, occasional nuclear atypia
III	Anaplastic astrocytoma Anaplastic oligodendroglioma Anaplastic oligo-astrocytoma Anaplastic ependymoma	Increased cellularity, nuclear atypia, and mitotic activity compared to grade II
IV[a]	Glioblastoma	As in grade III, plus microvascular proliferation and pseudopalisading necrosis

[a] Only astrocytomas can be grade IV.

Disease classification

Gliomas are classified according to the predominant cell population of the tumor: astrocytomas, oligodendrogliomas, or ependymomas. The World Health Organization (WHO) further classifies primary brain tumors into grades depending on their histologic features (Table 22.1).

Incidence/prevalence

- The incidence rate of primary brain and CNS tumors is 21/100,000. Their estimated prevalence is 222/100,000, with more than 680,000 people in the USA living with a diagnosis of brain tumor in 2010.
- Malignant primary brain tumors have a lower incidence than non-malignant (7/100,000 vs 14/100,000) and lower prevalence (62 vs 160/100,000).
- The exact prevalence of CNS metastases is unknown, with an incidence of approximately 170,000 new cases per year in the USA, which is increasing.
- Primary spine tumors comprise approximately 5% of all CNS primary tumors.
- Metastatic spine tumors occur in 30–70% of all patients with cancer.

Economic impact

- According to the American Cancer Society, primary brain tumors are among the top 10 causes of death in women and 11th in men.
- Brain tumors are the second most common malignancy in children.
- Neurologic sequelae of cancer have a significant economic impact as many patients will require full-time life-long assistance.

Etiology

- Approximately 40% of people with cancer will develop brain or spine metastasis.
- Specific causes for primary brain tumors are identified in approximately 5% of patients and include:
  - previous radiation to the head;
  - genetic syndromes such as tuberous sclerosis, von Hippel–Lindau disease, neurofibromatosis, Li–Fraumeni syndrome, and Turcot's syndrome;

Table 22.2 Chromosomal/signaling alteration in CNS tumors.

Risk factor/syndrome/diseases	Alteration
Previous radiation to head	DNA methylation
Neurofibromatosis (NF)	NF1: 17q; NF2: 22q autosomal dominant
Tuberous sclerosis (TSC)	TSC1: 9q34; TSC2: 16p13
Low-grade glioma	Single nucleotide polymorphism in 8q24.21
Secondary glioblastoma multiforme (GBM)[a]	p53, PTEN, EGFR amp; LOH 10q; p16 deletion, PDGF, IDH
De novo GBM[a]	p53; PTEN, EGFR amp, LOH 10q; p16 deletion

[a] Percentages of signaling alteration vary between de novo and secondary GBM as follows: p53 28% vs 65%; PTEN 28% vs 4%; p16 31% vs 19%; LOH 10q 70% vs 63%; EGFR 35% vs 8%.
Abbreviations: EGFR, epidermal growth factor receptor; IDH, isocitrate dehydrogenase; LOH, loss of heterozygosity; p53, tumor suppressor protein 53; PDGFR, platelet-derived growth factor receptor; PTEN, phosphate and tensin homolog.

- exposure to chemicals such as N-nitroso compounds;
  - changes in hormonal balance (e.g. pregnancy).
- Although for 95% of primary brain tumor cases the etiology remains unclear, it is known that these tumor cells have mutations in their signaling pathways inducing cell proliferation. The discovery of such mutations is important as they can be targeted for patient-specific therapeutic treatments.
- The basis of metastatic disease is systemic cancer. Although the exact mechanisms leading to the formation of CNS metastatic tumors are still being investigated, in principle cells must escape from the primary tumor, enter the arterial blood, extravasate, and "grow" within the CNS.

Pathology/pathogenesis

In genetic syndromes, chromosomal alterations can be found. In the vast majority of primary tumors, the pathogenesis revolves around alterations of signaling pathways as described below. The role of brain tumor cancer stem cells has also emerged and is supported by a large body of literature. Oncogenic transformation of neural stem cells (NSC) residing in the subventricular zone (SVZ) would then result in CNS tumor formation. Dedifferentiation is the other proposed mechanism. Approximately 74% of low-grade gliomas can progress to a higher grade due to alteration of their signaling pathways. De novo glioblastoma multiforme (GBM) is the most common and occurs in older patients. Secondary and de novo GBMs have different alterations of signaling pathways (Table 22.2).

The Cancer Genome Atlas recently classified GBM in at least four subtypes – proneural, classical, neural, and mesenchymal GBM – based on their genetic differences.

Section 2: Prevention and screening

> **BOTTOM LINE/CLINICAL PEARLS**
> - Since the etiologies of primary brain tumors are not clear, there is no screening or prevention.
> - There is no universal indication for screening cancer patients by brain MRI except as needed for staging of certain cancers or in the presence of neurologic symptoms.

Section 3: Diagnosis

BOTTOM LINE/CLINICAL PEARLS
- Seizures are the presenting symptoms in up to 60% of brain tumor patients independent of tumor size or location.
- Other presenting symptoms depend on size and location. Large tumors tend to present with symptoms secondary to mass effect. Small brain tumors present with focal signs depending on their location.
- Symptoms secondary to mass effect include:
  - headache
  - nausea/vomiting
  - altered level of consciousness
  - cognitive changes
- Localizing symptoms include:
  - speech difficulty (speaking or understanding)
  - sensory disturbance (vision, hearing, sensation)
  - motor deficit (face or limbs)
  - posture abnormality (gait, balance, coordination)
  - cognitive changes (personality, memory, calculation)
- Symptoms secondary to adjuvant treatment used for primary or metastatic CNS cancer include peripheral neuropathies (chemotherapy) and cognitive decline (whole brain radiotherapy).

Clinical diagnosis

History

It is important to note the following information: patient's hemispheric dominance (right-, left-handed, or ambidextrous), exact onset, duration, frequency, and factors ameliorating/worsening symptoms; detailed review of system as a systemic disease might mimic or worsen a neurologic problem. Family history is important to rule out genetic syndromes. Social history must be reviewed with attention to smoking and previous exposure to chemicals/radiation.

Physical examination

The neurologic examination should be detailed and cover all aspects.

Useful clinical decision rules

In preparing to decide best treatment options, the patient's Karnofsky Performance Status (KPS) must be assessed and scored (see Table 22.3).

Laboratory diagnosis

List of diagnostic tests

- Routine blood tests should include CBC with differential, chemistry panel, endocrine panel (if pituitary or skull base tumor suspected), ESR, angiotensin-converting enzyme (ACE; if sarcoidosis is suspected).
- Brain MRI without and with contrast is the preferred diagnostic test when a brain tumor is clinically suspected. Diffusion-weighted images (DWI) obtained with routine brain MRI are helpful in making a differential diagnosis between tumor and primary CNS lymphoma (PCNSL)

Table 22.3 Karnofsky Performance Status (KPS) scale.

100	Normal, no complaints, no evidence of disease
90	Able to carry on normal activity, minor signs or symptoms
80	Normal activity with effort, some signs or symptoms of disease
70	Cares for self. Unable to carry on normal activity or do active work
60	Requires occasional assistance, but is able to care for most of own needs
50	Requires considerable assistance and frequent medical care
40	Disabled, requires special care and assistance
30	Severely disabled, hospitalization is indicated although death is not imminent
20	Hospitalization necessary, very sick. Active supportive treatment necessary
10	Moribund, fatal processes progressing rapidly
0	Dead

or abscess. FLAIR (fluid-attenuated inversion recovery) sequences are helpful in the diagnosis of low-grade gliomas.

- Advanced MR images, including arterial spin labeling (ASL), perfusion, permeability, and MR spectroscopy should be ordered when MR images are compatible with a brain tumor. These sequences are helpful in finalizing the brain tumor diagnosis and providing additional information on its metabolic characteristics.
- Diffusion tensor imaging (DTI) and brain functional MRI (fMRI) should be ordered for surgery or radiation planning when necessary to establish the location of the tumor in relationship to eloquent cortex or white matter pathways.
- In cases of recurrent lesions, brain FDG-PET assesses the tumor metabolism and might be used to differentiate between tumor and treatment effects (radiation necrosis). Accuracy of interpretation and radiolabeled tracers limit its utilization.
- CSF cytology by lumbar puncture (if not clinically contraindicated) should be used for the diagnosis of PCNSL, leptomeningeal carcinomatosis, and pineal tumors.
- CSF analysis should include opening pressure, cell count, chemistry, microbiology, cytology, and flow cytometry. If a paraneoplastic syndrome is suspected, CSF should be tested for anti-neuronal antibodies. For pineal tumors, CSF markers should be ordered.
- Brain biopsy provides tissue diagnosis, molecular correlates, and chromosomal analysis to guide adjuvant therapy. It is indicated if surgical resection is not feasible or if PCNSL is suspected.

Diagnostic algorithm
- CNS tumor suspected clinically → brain or spine MRI
  - Brain MRI: images suggestive of brain tumor → advanced MR images
    - Positive DWI → LP (for PCNSL)
  - For surgery of lesions located near eloquent area → DTI, fMRI

Potential pitfalls/common errors made regarding diagnosis of disease
- A single brain or spine lesion on MRI can be a primary or metastatic brain tumor; however, the following differential diagnoses should be considered: hamartoma, vascular etiology (hemorrhage, AVM [arterovenous malformation], cavernous angioma), infection (abscess, PML [progressive multifocal leukoencephalopathy]), inflammatory (lupus, sarcoidosis, MS), trauma, developmental (benign congenital cyst).

- Multiple brain or spine lesions can be metastatic tumors; however, the following differential diagnoses should be ruled out: PCNSL, multifocal glioma, vascular etiology (as above), inflammatory (as above), infection (as above plus TB, toxoplasmosis), trauma, developmental.

Section 4: Treatment
Treatment rationale

- The treatment plans for CNS tumors require a multidisciplinary approach combining neurology, neurosurgery, oncology, and radiation oncology expertise.
- Options for CNS tumors vary depending on tumor burden, location, Karnofsky Performance Scale, goals of care (family and patient), WHO grade (primary tumors), histology, and systemic involvement (for metastatic disease).
- Surgery is typically recommended when radiographic progression is documented or the patient is symptomatic, except when PCNSL is suspected (see above) and for leptomeningeal carcinomatosis. A curative surgical resection can be obtained for most meningiomas, schwannomas, JPA, and pituitary adenomas. A true curative resection cannot be achieved for glial tumors due to their infiltrative pattern. In these tumors, however, the role of surgery is fundamental to obtain tissue diagnosis and for cytoreduction. When performed by an experienced oncological neurosurgeon, the latter alleviates mass effect, reducing the symptoms and allowing for the most effective adjuvant therapy.
- For metastases, surgery or radiosurgery can be offered depending on location, number, and size.
- For all patients undergoing surgery, a postoperative brain MRI before and after contrast should be obtained within 24–72 hours to document the extent of resected disease and plan adjuvant treatment.
- Tissue must be reviewed by an experienced neuropathologist.
- Adjuvant treatment is necessary for WHO grade III, IV, and metastatic tumors. External beam radiation (XRT) to tumor cavity plus margins (1.8–2 Gy per fraction for a total of 28–30 fractions) with concomitant temozolomide (TMZ) is the standard-of-care for GBM. Methylation of the promoter for the O^6-methylguanine-DNA methyltranspherase (MGMT) gene is a positive prognostic factor. Anaplastic oligodendrogliomas or oligoastrocytomas with a 1p19q chromosomal deletion have a much higher response rate to chemotherapy (procarbazine, carmustine, vincristine [PCV]) compared to a response rate of 23–31% without deletion, and therefore are treated with XRT and chemotherapy. Anaplastic astrocytomas and those without co-deletion are treated with XRT alone or in combination with TMZ, albeit this is still being tested in prospective trials.
- Chemotherapy can be delivered in situ at the time of surgery for GBM (carmustine wafers) or systemically: orally (TMZ), intravenously (carmustine, lomustine, PCV, bevacizumab), or intrathecally (methotrexate). Leptomeningeal carcinomatosis can be treated with intrathecal chemotherapy (methotrexate, cytarabine) or high-dose i.v. methotrexate.
- WBXRT is used for multiple metastases and PCNSL, craniospinal radiotherapy is used for ependymomas.
- Alternating electrical fields or tumor treating fields, causes tumor cell demise by interfering with the mitotic anaphase and is an FDA-approved treatment for newly diagnosed and recurrent GBM.
- Paraneoplastic syndromes are treated with immunotherapy and resection of primary tumor.

When to hospitalize

- Patients may require hospitalization to manage sudden worsening of neurologic status due to increased mass effect, intractable seizures, and secondary medical complications such as sepsis or pneumonia.

Managing the hospitalized patient

- Many neuro-oncology patients, especially those with metastatic cancer, have complicated medical and neurologic issues that require close coordination of multiple specialists for their care.

Table of treatment

Treatment	Comments
Conservative • Serial MRI • Physical, occupational, and speech therapy • Support groups • Nutritional support	Patients with low-grade gliomas when asymptomatic can be followed with serial MRIs Patients with a poor Karnofsky score and appropriate patient and family goals of care can be treated conservatively Physical, occupational, and speech therapy are very helpful Support group meetings organized by hospital and/or not-for-profit organizations serve as an excellent frame to help patients coping with financial, legal, and personal aspects of the disease Nutritional support is very important to avoid cachexia

Medical
• Corticosteroids
• Antiepileptic drugs
• Chemotherapy (with or without XRT), including:
  ◦ cytotoxic – interferes with DNA replication (temozolomide)
  ◦ adduct-forming agents – modify nitrogenous DNA bases leading to apoptosis (carmustine, locomustine)
  ◦ antimetabolites – inhibit the enzymes involved in DNA synthesis (methotrexate)
  ◦ topoisomerase inhibitors – relieve torsional DNA strain (topotecan, irinotecan)
  ◦ antimicrotubule agents – cause cell death by disrupting microtubule assembly (vincristine)
  ◦ vascular endothelial growth factor therapy – interferes with tumor vascularization (VEFG) (bevacizumab)
• Management of endocrinopathies and venous thromboembolism
• Palliative care and hospice care
	Corticosteroids should be used only if patient is symptomatic; they temporarily ameliorate symptoms secondary to mass effect
	Antiepileptic drugs (AEDs) are not recommended for asymptomatic patients except perioperatively. Many AEDs induce cytochrome P450 therefore interfering with the efficacy of chemotherapy; non-enzyme-inducing AEDs (such as valproic acid, lamotrigine, and levetiracetam) may be preferable when AEDs are needed
	The blood–brain barrier (BBB) poses a challenge for the delivery of chemotherapy for CNS tumors. It is therefore rarely used as the first-line therapy, often in combination with XRT. In situ chemotherapy can be used at the time of surgery (carmustine wafers)
	Endocrinopathies associated with pituitary adenomas, steroid intake, or hypothalamic tumors should be corrected and managed in conjunction with an endocrinologist
	Venous thromboembolism (VTE) is common in patients with brain and spine neoplasms and should be managed following VTE guidelines
	Palliative care and hospice care services are important elements in the care of patients with CNS tumors

(Continued)

Treatment	Comments
Surgical • Cytoreduction with maximal tumor resection • Stereotactic radiosurgery (SRS) • Biopsy • In situ chemotherapy	Surgical cure can be achieved for WHO grade I tumors Cytoreduction with maximal tumor resection when appropriate and feasible should be performed using minimally invasive techniques for high-grade tumors and metastases. There is growing evidence that this strategy is also applicable to low-grade tumors Intraoperative navigation, image guidance, brain mapping, and awake craniotomies help in performing aggressive tumor resection while decreasing morbidity Radiosurgery is an excellent option for patients with brain and spine metastasis or selected patients with recurrent disease if surgery is not indicated. Tissue diagnosis is obtained by a stereotactic biopsy allowing histologic and molecular correlates necessary to guide targeted therapy Chemotherapy can be delivered in situ at the time of surgery (carmustine wafers)
Radiation therapy (XRT) • X-rays, gamma rays • Radiation delivered as three-dimensional conformal (3D), intensity modulated radiation therapy (IMRT), stereotactic radiosurgery (SRS), or stereotactic radiotherapy (SRT)	Sources of ionizing radiation used in neuro-oncology are photons (X-ray, gamma ray) and protons. Photons can originate from a linear accelerator (LINAC, X-ray) or atomic nuclei (gamma ray) WBXRT can be used for multiple brain metastases, CNS lymphoma, and ependymoma (cranio-axial), leptomeningeal carcinomatosis Focal XRT usually encompassing the tumor cavity plus margins is used for high-grade gliomas (WHO III/IV), medulloblastoma, PNET, some low-grade gliomas SRS with or without WBXRT with or without surgery is used for brain metastases. SRS with or without EBXRT, with or without surgery is used for spine metastases
Psychological • Acknowledgement and support • Psychotropic medications	Fatigue is commonly experienced by brain and spine tumor patients and benefits from acknowledgment and support Depression is common in brain and spine tumor patients. This responds to psychotropic medications and/or family support and/or therapy
Complementary medicine • Acupuncture	Acupuncture might be effective in reducing pain in advanced peripheral CNS cancer. Central CNS cancer rarely is associated with pain syndrome Natural supplements might not be beneficial as they might be hepatotoxic (interfere with chemotherapy) and/or antioxidants (interfere with radiation therapy)
Therapies on the horizon • Tyrosine kinase receptor inhibitors • Immunotherapy (vaccine against EGFRvIII) • Cell-based gene therapy	Tyrosine kinase receptor inhibitors induce activation of the kinase domain with resulting phosphorylation of tyrosine residues that activate downstream signal transduction pathways leading to apoptosis

Prevention/management of complications

• Neurotoxicity is a common dose-limiting factor for chemotherapy and radiation therapy.
• If possible, the drug causing the symptoms should be removed from the therapy.
• Additional medical supportive therapy is necessary.

CLINICAL PEARLS
- Patients with brain tumors benefit from multi-disciplinary treatment.
- Tissue diagnosis is necessary to target best treatment.
- Minimally invasive surgery and/or radiosurgery are commonly used treatments.
- Radiation therapy and chemotherapy are important adjuvant treatments for brain tumor patients.

Section 5: Special populations

Pregnancy
- Brain and spinal tumors in pregnancy are rare, except for enlargement of pituitary tumors and meningiomas.
- Contrast media should not be used. MR sequences with non-contrast ASL are an excellent alternative.
- If possible, delivery is recommended in the third semester prior to surgery and adjuvant therapy.
- Brain and spine surgery can be performed on the pregnant patient. Chemotherapy and XRT should not be administered during pregnancy.

Children
- A gross-total resection of JPA provides a cure in >95% cases. Total or near total resection of medulloblastoma is associated with 90% progression-free survival at 5 years.
- To protect cognitive function of the developing brain, XRT is postponed when medically appropriate. Children treated with XRT may develop cognitive, endocrine, or cerebrovascular sequelae many years later.
- Toxicity is frequently dose limiting for chemotherapy in children (e.g. vincristine ototoxicity).

Elderly
- For patients of advanced age with high-grade gliomas, radiation alone without concomitant chemotherapy and with fewer fractions is recommended.
- Patient's age >65 is associated with lower survival rates independent of treatment for both primary and metastatic tumors.

Section 6: Prognosis

BOTTOM LINE/CLINICAL PEARLS
- Primary brain and spine tumors can be cured with surgical excision, e.g. JPA, meningiomas, and schwannomas.
- Gliomas are infiltrative tumors and tend to recur after surgical resection and adjuvant therapy (radiation and chemotherapy) is necessary. The best prognosis is associated with upfront aggressive surgical resection for high-grade gliomas. For brain and spine metastasis, radiosurgery provides a prognosis similar to surgical resection without the need to hospitalise.
- Higher KPS and younger age are associated with better prognosis regardless of the histologic grade.

Natural history of untreated disease
Duration of survival with symptomatic untreated metastasis of brain or spine is 4–8 weeks and for GBM 8–12 weeks.

Prognosis for treated patients

- Metastatic disease: best prognosis (KPS ≥70, age <65) after WBXRT is 7.1 months. Surgery and radiosurgery in combination with XRT significantly increase quality of life and survival.
- For GBM treated with surgery, XRT, and TMZ, the median survival is 15 months and a 26% 2-year survival, compared to 12 months and 10% for patients not treated with TMZ. For patients with methylated MGMT promoter the median survival was 22 months. In situ delivery of carmustine wafer in newly diagnosed GBM improves median survival from 12 months to 14 months.
- Anaplastic oligo- and strocytomas with the 1p10q deletion have prolonged median survival when treated with combined XRT and chemotherapy.

Follow-up tests and monitoring

- Follow-up brain MRI with advanced sequences is necessary for all patients with treated CNS tumors. For brain tumor differentiating between progression and pseudo-progression (temporary enlargement due to tumor edema/necrosis) is very important. Advanced MR images are helpful.
- Monitoring response to therapy of brain tumor is not just based on contrast enhancement images. MacDonald and Response Assessment in Neuro-oncology (RANO) criteria allow a more precise evaluation.

Section 7: Reading list

Key reading sources for this chapter can be found online at www.mountsinaiexpertguides.com

Suggested websites

American Association of Neurological Surgeons: www.aans.org
National Brain Tumor Society: www.braintumor.org

Additional material for this chapter can be found online at:
www.mountsinaiexpertguides.com

This includes a reading list.

CHAPTER 23

Multiple Sclerosis and Other Inflammatory Diseases

Fred D. Lublin
Icahn School of Medicine at Mount Sinai, New York, NY, USA

OVERALL BOTTOM LINE
- Multiple sclerosis (MS) is an inflammatory demyelinating disease.
- The underlying pathogenesis of MS involves both inflammatory demyelination and neurodegeneration.
- Guidelines exist that assist in the challenging diagnosis of MS.
- MS treatment consists of disease-modifying agents, treatment of acute exacerbations, and symptom management.

Section 1: Background
Definition of disease
Multiple sclerosis (MS) is the commonest of the central nervous system inflammatory demyelinating disorders and is identified by disseminated lesions in space and time. Related diseases are acute disseminated encephalomyelitis (ADEM) and neuromyelitis optica (NMO).

Disease classification
The diagnosis and differentiation of the various clinical multiple sclerosis syndromes are described below. The major clinical subtypes include:
- Clinically isolated syndrome (CIS)
- Relapsing-remitting MS (RRMS)
- Secondary progressive MS (SPMS)
- Primary progressive MS (PPMS)
- Progressive relapsing MS (PRMS)

Incidence/prevalence
The prevalence of multiple sclerosis varies by geographic location. The disease is commonest in the higher latitudes of the temperate zones, on both sides of the equator. In North America, the prevalence is about 100 per 100,000.

Economic impact
- As a disease primarily of young adults, MS has a significant economic impact.
- With appropriate medical care, MS now has little effect on lifespan.

Mount Sinai Expert Guides: Neurology, First Edition. Edited by Stuart C. Sealfon, Rajeev Motiwala, and Charles B. Stacy.
© 2016 John Wiley & Sons, Ltd. Published 2016 by John Wiley & Sons, Ltd.
Companion website: www.mountsinaiexpertguides.com

- It incurs significant long-term healthcare costs and disabilities affecting work productivity.
- The currently available disease-modifying therapies for MS are very expensive.

Etiology

- The cause of multiple sclerosis is unknown.
- Current evidence supports a dysimmune state. While many categorize MS as an autoimmune disease, the strict criteria for autoimmunity have not yet been fulfilled. This includes our lack of a full understanding of the immunopathogenesis of the illness and of the central nervous system (CNS) target in multiple sclerosis.
- Over the years, a number of microbes, mostly viruses, have been proposed as etiologic agents of multiple sclerosis. None has stood the test of time. Despite that, there is much in the character of the disorder that would fit a latent infection. This includes the fact that children emigrating from a high-risk region to a lower risk region pick up the lower risk of multiple sclerosis while adults keep the risk of the region in which they were raised.
- There is a genetic element to MS. Monozygotic twins have a concordance rate of approximately 30%. Dizygotic twins have a concordance rate of 3–5%, similar to that seen for non-twin siblings. Those with MS in the family have a 20 to 30-fold greater risk of developing the disease. The genetics are not mendelian. Modern genetic analyses suggest that there are over 100 MS susceptibility genes, none of which is required for development of the illness.

Pathology/pathogenesis

The pathology that underlies MS is primarily inflammatory demyelination. Axonal degeneration and cortical and deep gray matter neuronal loss also occur.

Predictive/risk factors

- There are no predictive factors for multiple sclerosis.
- The disease occurs most commonly in Whites and less often in other racial groups.
- Females are affected more commonly than males at a ratio of about 3 to 1.

Section 2: Prevention and screening

Not applicable for this topic.

Section 3: Diagnosis

BOTTOM LINE/CLINICAL PEARLS
- MRI lesions in the juxtacortical regions, periventricular, brainstem, cerebellum, or spinal cord are characteristic of multiple sclerosis.
- Dissemination in time can be confirmed on MRI scan by the finding of new T2 or gadolinium enhancing lesions on any scan subsequent to a baseline scan or if on an initial MRI scan, at the time of clinical presentation, there are both enhancing and non-enhancing T2 lesions.

Diagnosing multiple sclerosis depends on establishing that lesions in the central nervous system are *disseminated in time* (more than one episode) and *disseminated in space* (more than one location within the CNS). In practice, this can be accomplished by obtaining a history of two events and finding objective evidence on examination of involvement of more than one area of the central nervous system. Current diagnostic guidelines also allow for the presence of lesions on the MRI scan to serve as surrogates for clinical evidence of dissemination in time or space.

Differential diagnosis of CNS primary demyelinating diseases

- For differential diagnosis of optic neuritis refer to Chapter 11: Visual Loss and Double Vision.
- For differential diagnosis of spinal cord disorders, refer to Chapter 18: Suspected Spinal Cord Dysfunction.

Differential diagnosis	Features
Acute disseminated encephalomyelitis	A monophasic illness; more cortical signs such as encephalopathy and seizures; MRI scans can differ from MS and the lesions frequently all enhance with gadolinium
Neuromyelitis optica	Classically limited to severe involvement of the spinal cord and optic nerves, but can affect the brainstem and other areas in what are now referred to as neuromyelitis spectrum disorders. Attacks tend to be more severe than those seen in MS. Frequently associated with antibodies to the aquaporin 4 receptor, and more rarely to anti-myelin oligodendrocyte glycoprotein (MOG) antibodies
Other conditions to consider (see also Chapter 18)	Progressive myelitis can occur with B12 deficiency, HTLV myelopathy, spinal tumors, genetic disorders, and spinal vascular malformations. Also to be considered are systemic inflammatory conditions, such as sarcoid, Lyme disease, and rheumatologic conditions. Workup for any of these should be based on a careful medical history and physical examination

Typical presentation

- Multiple sclerosis can produce the signs and symptoms of involvement of any area of the CNS.
- Common presenting events include optic neuritis, partial myelitis, internuclear ophthalmoplegia, facial sensory loss, tremor, and cerebellar signs.

Clinical diagnosis

History

The mean age of onset of MS is age 32 and the disease tends to affect young adults. There can be pediatric onset and also late life onset. The typical history in MS is of an acute or subacute onset of CNS-mediated dysfunction. In addition to exploring the presenting complaint, thorough questioning about previous resolved neurologic symptoms, such as visual disturbances, dizziness, numbness, tingling, and weakness may help support the diagnosis of MS.

Physical examination

A careful examination of the entire neuraxis is necessary in suspected multiple sclerosis. Particular attention should be paid to the optic nerves, brainstem, and motor and sensory function. Typical findings include afferent pupillary defect, red desaturation, diplopia (particularly unilateral or bilateral failure of adduction from internuclear ophthalmoplegia), nystagmus, ataxia, sensory levels, and corticospinal tract signs.

Useful clinical decision rules: the clinical course of MS

MS is the most variable of the serious neurologic conditions. At one extreme, individuals may have a form of MS that never expresses itself clinically, whereas at the other they may have a type causing very severe impairment or disability. There are malignant forms of MS that produce serious disability evolving rapidly over a short period of time. Benign MS is a retrospective determination after 10–15 years of illness without significant disability. Caution is advised in diagnosing benign MS, as the risk for a serious exacerbation persists throughout life. MS overall has a minimal effect on longevity, reducing lifespan by about 6 years.

There are four clinical courses that MS may follow:

- *Relapsing-remitting* (RR) MS is the commonest form. In RR MS there are acute exacerbations (synonyms: relapse, flare, or attack) that are characterized by relatively sudden onset of CNS dysfunction (such as optic neuritis, partial myelitis, brainstem features). The symptoms last from days to weeks and are associated with varying degrees of recovery, from minimal to full. On average, 50% of exacerbations leave some residual deficit. A subsequent attack may occur any time after, but usually is separated by months to years (and even decades). Between attacks, there is clinical stability.
- *Secondary progressive* (SP) MS occurs in a subset of RR MS who at some point after onset develop a slow, progressive worsening of their function independent of any exacerbations (although there can be concurrent exacerbations).
- *Primary progressive* (PP) MS lacks acute exacerbations. Rather, there is a gradual onset of symptoms over months or longer. PP MS tends to have a later age of onset and affects men and women equally.
- *Progressive relapsing* (PR) MS results from the occurrence of acute exacerbations after the onset of PP MS. It is the least common form of MS.

The disease course can generally be separated into relapsing forms and progressive forms. As noted below, current therapies are most effective for relapsing forms of MS. In relapsing MS, the accrual of impairment occurs by incomplete recovery from exacerbations. Progressive MS tends to have a worse prognosis than relapsing-remitting MS.

Disease severity classification

MS is the most variable of the serious neurologic diseases. Individuals may go their entire lives and never manifest clinical features or, at the other extreme, MS can produce severe impairment and disability. The expanded disability status scale (EDSS, Kurtzke scale) is used for classifying disability from MS.

Laboratory diagnosis

List of diagnostic tests

- The most important paraclinical study for diagnosing and monitoring MS is the MRI scan. Both cranial and spinal MRI scanning are of value. The cranial MRI is exquisitely sensitive to the pathologic process underlying MS. There are 10–20 new MRI lesions seen for every clinical event. Cranial MRI abnormalities are present in over 90% of MS cases and, as discussed above, form an important adjunct to the diagnostic process. The commonest locations for MRI lesions are periventricular, juxtacortical, brainstem, cerebellar, and spinal cord. Gadolinium-enhancing lesions are common in MS, especially with relapsing forms. Their presence indicates a relatively acute lesion, as they resolve over 4–6 weeks. In addition, MRI lesion load and signs of cerebral atrophy correlate with greater degrees of disability.
- Spinal fluid (CSF) analysis can be useful in diagnosing MS, but has no prognostic value. CSF examination can also help to exclude alternative diagnoses. There can be a modest elevation of CSF protein in MS, but rarely above 100 mg/mL. Similarly, there can be mild pleocytosis, but usually less than 20 white cells/mm³. Greater elevations of either white cells or protein should raise suspicion of another diagnosis. Intrathecal synthesis of immunoglobulin is common in MS leading to an elevated IgG index and the presence of oligoclonal bands in the CSF that are not seen in the serum. CSF analysis is not required to establish the diagnosis of MS according to current guidelines (Tables 23.1 and 23.2).

Table 23.1 MS diagnostic criteria.

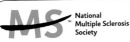 National Multiple Sclerosis Society   **2010 Revised McDonald MS Diagnostic Criteria[1]**   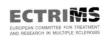 EUROPEAN COMMITTEE FOR TREATMENT AND RESEARCH IN MULTIPLE SCLEROSIS

Diagnosis of MS requires elimination of more likely diagnoses and demonstration of dissemination of lesions in space (DIS) and time (DIT)*

CLINICAL (ATTACKS)	LESIONS	ADDITIONAL CRITERIA TO MAKE DX
2 or more	Objective clinical evidence of ≥2 lesions or objective clinical evidence of 1 lesion with reasonable historical evidence of a prior attack	None. Clinical evidence alone will suffice; additional evidence desirable but must be consistent with MS
2 or more	Objective clinical evidence of 1 lesion	DIS; OR await further clinical attack implicating a different CNS site
1	Objective clinical evidence of ≥2 lesions	DIT; OR await a second clinical attack
1	Objective clinical evidence of 1 lesion	DIS OR await further clinical attack implicating a different CNS site AND DIT; OR await a second clinical attack
0 (progression from onset)		One year of disease progression (retrospective or prospective) AND at least two of: DIS in the brain based on ≥1 T2 lesions in periventricular, juxtacortical or infratentorial regions; DIS in the spinal cord based on ≥2 T2 lesions; or positive CSF

1. Polman et al. Diagnostic criteria for multiple sclerosis: 2010 revisions to the McDonald Criteria Ann Neurol 2011;69:292–302. *See reverse for DIS and DIT

Source: Data from Polman et al. Diagnostic Criteria for Multiple Sclerosis: 2010 Revisions to the McDonald Criteria. Annals of Neurology 2011;69:292–302.

Table 23.2 Evidence in MS diagnosis.

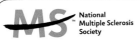 National Multiple Sclerosis Society   **Paraclinical Evidence in MS Diagnosis**   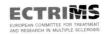 EUROPEAN COMMITTEE FOR TREATMENT AND RESEARCH IN MULTIPLE SCLEROSIS

Evidence for Dissemination of Lesions in Space (DIS)[2]	Evidence for Dissemination of Lesions in Time (DIT)[3]
≥ 1 T2 lesion in at least two out of four areas of the CNS: periventricular, juxtacortical, infratentorial, or spinal cord • Gadolinium enhancement of lesions is not required for DIS • If a subject has a brainstem or spinal cord syndrome, the symptomatic lesions are excluded and do not contribute to lesion count	• A new T2 and/or gadolinium-enhancing lesion(s) on follow-up MRI, with reference to a baseline scan, irrespective of the timing of the baseline MRI or • Simultaneous presence of asymptomatic gadolinium-enhancing and non-enhancing lesions at any time
Evidence for Positive CSF Oligoclonal IgG bands in CSF (and not serum) or elevated IgG index	[2] Swanton KL et al. Lancet Neurology 2007;6:677–686 /Swanton KL et al. J Neurol Neurosurg Psychiatry 2006;77:830–833 [3] Montalban X. et al. Neurology 2010;74:427–434

These diagnostic criteria were developed through the consensus of the International Panel on the Diagnosis of MS. See cited articles for details. Funding through National Multiple Sclerosis Society (USA) and European Committee for Treatment and Research in MS; additional support from the Multiple Sclerosis International Federation and MS Ireland

National Multiple Sclerosis Society (USA) Professional Resource Center. 733 Third Avenue, New York, NY 10017-3288
http://www.nationalMSsociety.org/PRC. MD_info@nmss.org
© 2011 National Multiple Sclerosis Society

BR0040

Source: Data from Polman et al. Diagnostic Criteria for Multiple Sclerosis: 2010 Revisions to the McDonald Criteria. Annals of Neurology 2011;69:292–302.

- Evoked potential (visual, somatosensory) testing can provide useful information for subclinical evidence of dissemination in space.

Diagnostic algorithm

Patients presenting with an initial acute or subacute event of optic neuritis, brainstem or cerebellar dysfunction, or partial myelitis (any of which is characterized as a "clinically isolated syndrome", CIS) should have a cranial MRI and if they have a myelitis, a cervical or thoracic MRI (depending on the clinical location of the myelitis). If there are asymptomatic lesions seen on the imaging, the chances of this becoming MS are quite high (80% over the next 15 years). If the MRI has no asymptomatic lesions, the risk is 20%. Further testing beyond this would depend on whether the clinical examination or imaging showed atypical features for MS or whether there were systemic comorbidities that might suggest an alternative diagnosis. For example, if the patient had pulmonary symptoms, rash, joint swelling, or bone lesions, a workup for systemic illness would be in order. There are no agreed standard ancillary tests that should be performed on all patients being worked up for MS. One is well advised to keep in mind that the diagnostic criteria for MS, as outlined above, recommend that there be "no better diagnosis."

Potential pitfalls/common errors made regarding diagnosis of disease

- A common error in diagnosing MS is to misinterpret non-specific or trivial white matter changes on MRI as indicative of MS. This is particularly troublesome in the circumstance referred to as the "radiologic isolated syndrome" or RIS. This occurs when an MRI of the brain is performed for an unrelated reason, most commonly a headache or head trauma, and is reported to show changes consistent with MS. Often the findings are non-specific and not of great consequence. However, in some instances, the MRI changes are characteristic of the findings used in the MS diagnostic criteria. In this case, there is a reasonably high risk that the MRI will change over time or that the individual will go on to develop a clinical event typical of MS. The important point here is that in the absence of a clinical event, one cannot diagnose MS. Individuals with RIS should be followed, with serial MRIs, to see if change occurs or if there are subsequent clinical findings.
- A second pitfall is to ignore indications of systemic illness and diagnose MS in the presence of other organ involvement.

Section 4: Treatment
Treatment rationale

Treatment of MS can be divided into three categories:
1. Treatment of acute exacerbations
2. Disease-modifying therapies
3. Symptomatic therapy.

Although there are no modern studies on treating acute exacerbations of MS, most clinicians will treat serious exacerbations with 3–5 days of intravenous methylprednisolone.

There are currently 10 disease-modifying agents available for treating relapsing forms of MS (see Table of treatment).

Table of treatment: MS disease-modifying agents

Name	Mechanism of action	Delivery method	Dose	Frequency	Side effects
β-Interferon-1a (Avonex)	Inhibits proliferation of lymphocytes; inhibits pro-inflammatory cytokines and increases anti-inflammatory cytokines; inhibits cellular trafficking across blood–brain barrier	Intramuscular injection	30 μg	Weekly	Fever, chills, HAs, mild flu-like symptoms, muscle aches, anemia, depression
β-Interferon-1a (Rebif)	Same as above	Subcutaneous injection	44 μg	Three times weekly	Injection-site reactions, mild flu-like symptoms, muscle aches, anemia, depression
β-Interferon-1b (Betaseron)	Same as above	Subcutaneous injection	250 μg	Every other day	Injection-site reactions, flu-like symptoms, menstrual disorders, headaches, mild neutropenia/anemia/thrombocytopenia, depression
Glatiramer acetate (Copaxone)	Inhibits anti-inflammatory cytokines; promotes a shift from Th1 to Th2 helper T cells; may affect antigen presentation	Subcutaneous injection	20 mg 40 mg	Daily 3 times weekly	Injection-site reactions, immediate post-injection reaction (IPIR), which includes chest pain, rarely lymphadenopathy
Natalizumab (Tysabri)	Monoclonal antibody directed against the cellular adhesion molecule α4-integrin, inhibiting lymphocyte trafficking from the bloodstream into the CNS	Intravenous infusion	300 mg	Every 28 days	Allergic reactions especially after second dose, infections, progressive multifocal leukoencephalopathy, liver abnormality, questionable relationship to melanoma
Mitoxantrone (Novantrone)	Inhibits DNA and RNA synthesis, intercalates DNA; cytotoxic agent; suppresses lymphocyte proliferation	Intravenous infusion	Based on body surface area: 12 mg/m²	Every 3 months with total lifetime maximum of 140 mg/m²	Myelosuppression, alopecia, secondary amenorrhea, cardiotoxicity, leukemia
Fingolimod (Gilenya)	Modulates the sphingosine 1-phosphate receptor; inhibits lymphocyte trafficking out of lymph nodes	Oral	0.25 mg	Daily	Bradycardia and other cardiac rhythm issues, macular edema, infections (especially herpetic), hypertension, pulmonary function changes, hepatotoxicity, leukopenia
Teriflunomide (Aubagio)	Pyrimidine synthesis inhibitor, reduces lymphocyte activation and proliferation	Oral	7 or 14 mg	Daily	Gastrointestinal symptoms, leukopenia, hair thinning, hepatotoxicity
Dimethyl fumarate (Tecfidera)	Inhibits immune cells, possibly antioxidant	Oral	240 mg	Twice daily	Gastrointestinal symptoms, flushing, leukopenia, elevated liver enzymes

- There are no established treatment algorithms for choosing a therapy.
- Efficacy, safety, and convenience are considerations that factor into the decision, in that order; comparative efficacy data are not extensive.
- High-dose high-frequency interferon is more effective than low-dose low-frequency interferon.
- Glatiramer acetate is superior to low-dose low-frequency interferon, but has similar efficacy to high-dose interferon.
- Fingolimod is superior to low-dose low-frequency interferon.
- Teriflunomide has similar efficacy to high-dose interferon.
- The other agents do not have good comparative efficacy data and one should never try to compare results from different clinical trials.
- Both glatiramer acetate and the interferons have excellent safety records.
- Oral agents offer better convenience than injectable agents.

Relapsing patients with very active disease, who have not been exposed to the JC virus (and thus at extremely low risk of PML), are good candidates for natalizumab.

When to hospitalize

With access to specialized MS outpatient services, hospitalization is rarely required in MS. If an exacerbation is severe or timely outpatient management is impractical, hospitalization may be needed. If there are potential complications from use of high-dose steroids, such as in diabetics, management may be safer in hospital. Inpatient rehabilitation therapy may be of benefit.

Management of symptoms

In addition to therapy directed at the disease, it is also important to address the associated symptoms and complications of MS.

- Patients with fatigue may benefit from modafinil.
- Spasticity can be improved with oral baclofen (intrathecal pump for severe cases), tizanidine, or botulinum toxin injection.
- Patients with pseudobulbar affect may benefit from oral dextromethorphan.
- Gait and mobility may respond to dalfampridine.
- Other common complaints that may benefit from targeted symptomatic therapy include:
  - paroxysmal symptoms
  - bladder dysfunction
  - pain
  - psychological or psychiatric issues (depression)
  - cognitive impairment
  - complications of therapy.

CLINICAL PEARLS
- Multiple sclerosis can affect any area of the central nervous system.
- Early treatment with disease-modifying agents is recommended.
- Remember to consider symptomatic therapies.

Section 5: Special populations
Pregnancy
- Pregnancy tends to be protective of MS. Relapse rates decrease with each trimester of pregnancy, but increase for the 3-month post-partum period. Breast feeding may offset the post-partum risk.
- None of the disease-modifying therapies is approved for use during pregnancy. The wash-out period is different for each agent. This should be kept in mind when starting therapy and a discussion about family planning should occur.

Children
- While there have been no randomized clinical trials demonstrating the efficacy and safety of the MS disease-modifying agents in children, there are many observational studies documenting safe use of most of these agents in the pediatric population.

Elderly
- MS is primarily a disease of young adults, but onset may occur in any age group. In the elderly, careful diagnosis is most important. Most MS agents have been tested in adults up to 60–65 years, and in the absence of specific contraindications are used in older patients.

Section 6: Prognosis

> **BOTTOM LINE/CLINICAL PEARLS**
> **Prognosis in MS is better in:**
> - Younger individuals
> - Women
> - Relapsing disease (as opposed to progressive)
> - Sensory attacks (as opposed to motor or cerebellar involvement)
> - Recovery without residual
> - Long inter-attack period

Prognosis for treated patients
The disease-modifying therapies have reduced relapse rates and lessened the accrual of disability of MS. It is difficult to quantify the prognosis for any given individual (as opposed to the group responses seen in clinical trials). Further complicating this is the fact that the relapse rate for MS has decreased in both treated and untreated patients in the past decade.

Follow-up tests and monitoring
There are no standards for monitoring MS patients. MRIs can provide useful information, but there is no established guideline for determining when the occurrence of new MRI lesions should lead to a treatment-altering decision. Each of the MS therapies has specific monitoring criteria.

Section 7: Reading list

Key reading sources for this chapter can be found online at www.mountsinaiexpertguides.com

Suggested websites

National Multiple Sclerosis Society: http://www.nationalmssociety.org/ms-clinical-care-network/clinical-resources-and-tools/core-curriculum/diagnosing-multiple-sclerosis/diagnostic-criteria/index.aspx

Additional material for this chapter can be found online at:
www.mountsinaiexpertguides.com

This includes advice for patients, a case study, multiple choice questions, a reading list.

CHAPTER 24

Infections of the Nervous System

Michael P. Mullen[1] and Geena Varghese[2]
[1]Icahn School of Medicine at Mount Sinai, New York, NY, USA
[2]Westmed Medical Group, West Harrison, NY, USA

OVERALL BOTTOM LINE
- Infections of the nervous system include meningitis (inflammation of the meninges), encephalitis (inflammation of the brain parenchyma), and abscess (a focal, encapsulated infection).
- Most cases of meningitis are viral.
- The cause of encephalitis is usually not determined.
- The purpose of this chapter is to provide a basic understanding of clinically relevant CNS infections.
- Etiologies, presentation, and diagnosis of meningitis and encephalitis will be explored.
- The various causes of brain abscesses, their presentation, and treatment will be discussed.
- If left untreated CNS infections can be fatal; therefore rapid diagnosis is crucial for patient outcome.

Section 1: Background
Definition of disease
- *Meningitis* is an inflammation of the meninges, which causes an elevation of white blood cells in the cerebrospinal fluid. Infectious etiologies include viruses (most common), bacteria, spirochetes, fungi, parasites, and amoebas. It is sometime non-infectious, for example in association with lupus or the chemical meningitis associated with subarachnoid hemorrhage.
- *Encephalitis* is an inflammation of the brain parenchyma usually caused by infectious organisms, the most common being viruses, then bacteria, prions, parasites, and fungi. Encephalitis can at times overlap with meningitis, and this is known as *meningoencephalitis*. Determining the etiology of encephalitis is difficult and diagnosis is confirmed in only about 16% of cases.
- *Brain abscess* is a focal area of infection that progresses to collection of pus with a capsule. It can occur through direct spread from a single adjacent site, hematogenous seeding from a distant site, or have an unknown etiology. A detailed history to determine the inciting event will help the physician predict the microbiology of the abscess. Classification and microbiology of brain abscesses are typically based on the origin.

Mount Sinai Expert Guides: Neurology, First Edition. Edited by Stuart C. Sealfon, Rajeev Motiwala, and Charles B. Stacy.
© 2016 John Wiley & Sons, Ltd. Published 2016 by John Wiley & Sons, Ltd.
Companion website: www.mountsinaiexpertguides.com

Incidence/prevalence

Aseptic meningitis, particularly viral meningitis, is the most common type of meningitis. According to the Centers for Disease Control and Prevention (CDC) the leading cause is enterovirus, affecting 30,000–70,000 individuals each year in the USA. As many cases go unreported, the actual incidence is likely higher.

Annually, 1.2 million cases of bacterial meningitis occur worldwide as reported by the CDC, causing significant morbidity and mortality. In the USA there are over 4000 cases of bacterial meningitis annually resulting in about 500 deaths.

Etiology

Meningitis

- *Aseptic meningitis* refers to meningeal inflammation in the absence of any infecting organism identified by Gram stain or bacterial culture. Virus infection is the most common cause, and lymphocytic pleocytosis (infectious or non-infectious) is usually present.
  - Enteroviruses appear to be the leading cause of aseptic meningitis and are prevalent during the summer and fall seasons. Enteroviruses, coxsackieviruses, and echoviruses are the most common organisms isolated from individuals with meningitis.
  - Herpesviruses include herpes simplex virus 1 and 2, varicella zoster virus, cytomegalovirus, Epstein–Barr viruses, and human herpes viruses 6, 7, and 8. Of these herpes simplex virus is the most significant. Herpes simplex virus type 2 is associated with meningitis, as opposed to type 1, which is seen more frequently in encephalitis. Cytomegalovirus and Epstein–Barr virus typically cause meningitis in immunocompromised individuals.
  - Human immunodeficiency virus (HIV) more commonly causes meningitis during the acute stages of infection, but HIV meningitis can also occur during later stages.
- Bacterial meningitis can cause significant morbidity and mortality if not immediately recognized. The more common etiologies worldwide include *Haemophilus influenzae*, *Neisseria meningitidis*, and *Streptococcus pneumoniae*.
  - *Haemophilus influenzae* remains one of the leading causes of meningitis throughout the world, but the rate has decreased significantly in the USA since the advent of *H. influenzae* type B vaccine.
  - *Neisseria meningitidis* typically causes meningitis in children and young adults. Those individuals who have terminal complement (C5–9) deficiencies develop more invasive disease.
  - *Streptococcus pneumoniae* is the leading cause of meningitis in the USA therefore leading to the greatest mortality. Serious infections are associated with predisposing conditions such as splenectomy, diabetes, alcoholism, chronic renal disease, chronic liver disease, and multiple myeloma.
  - *Listeria monocytogenes* has been found in poultry, decaying vegetables, soil, and groundwater. It occurs more frequently in infants less than 1 month of age, adults greater than 50 years, and immunocompromised individuals. *Listeria* is unusual among bacteria in that it typically causes a predominantly lymphocytic pleocytosis.
  - *Staphylococcus aureus* meningitis is typically seen in trauma or neurosurgical patients, as well as in those with renal failure requiring dialysis, or with malignancy, or with intravenous drug abuse.
  - Gram-negative bacilli – aerobic Gram-negative bacilli are an increasingly recognized cause of meningitis, more often seen in trauma or neurosurgical patients, and immunocompromised individuals.

- Spirochete meningitis
  - *Treponema pallidum* can invade the CNS early in the course of infection. It can manifest in four different stages – syphilitic meningitis, meningovascular syphilis, parenchymatous neurosyphilis, and gummatous neurosyphilis – all of which can overlap. Syphilitic meningitis typically occurs in the setting of secondary syphilis.
  - *Borrelia burgdorferi* – the CNS is involved in about 10–15% of Lyme infections, either in the initial stages or up to 6 months later.
- Amoeba – two types of amoeba have been shown to infect humans: *Naegleria* and *Acanthamoeba*.
  - *Naegleria fowleri* is more likely to cause meningoencephalitis. It has been isolated from soil and various bodies of water such as lakes, ponds, and springs, but excluding seawater and properly chlorinated water.
- Fungal meningitis can present as acute or chronic meningitis.
  - *Exserohilum* species was the primary fungus implicated in the 2012 outbreak of meningitis related to contaminated methylprednisolone injections produced at a New England center. Another fungal meningitis, aspergillosis, was also identified during the outbreak.
  - Cryptococcal meningoencephalitis – *Cryptococcus* typically causes a meningoencephalitis, with *C. neoformans* and *C. gattii* being the more common species. It is the most common fungal meningitis and is an opportunistic infection in immunocompromised individuals, though it can occur in immunocompetent persons.
- Chronic meningitis is defined as meningitis lasting longer than 4 weeks, and it can include both infectious and non-infectious etiologies.
  - Tuberculosis – tuberculous meningitis is the most common cause of chronic meningitis. It is difficult to diagnose. The patient's country of origin, contact with infected individuals, and immune status are all relevant in determining the likelihood of this disease.
  - *Histoplasma* meningitis is a type of fungal meningitis that typically occurs in immunocompromised individuals, such as AIDS patients, transplant recipients, or those receiving chronic steroids.

Encephalitis

- Herpesviruses are a common cause of encephalitis. These include: HSV-1, HSV-2, VZV, CMV, EBV, HHV6, HHV7, and HHV8.
  - Herpes simplex virus is a common cause of encephalitis: HSV-1 accounts for about 90% of all HSV encephalitides. Unlike other encephalitides, HSV encephalitis is not seasonal.
  - Varicella zoster encephalitis can occur either as primary infection or as reactivation of latent disease, the latter being more common. VZV as a primary infection typically occurs in children; it then becomes dormant in dorsal root ganglia, and reactivation occurs in the form of herpes zoster, also known as shingles.
  - CMV encephalitis typically occurs in immunocompromised individuals, AIDS and transplant patients specifically. It can occur as primary infection or reactivation of disease.
  - HHV6 is a viral infection of T lymphocytes that can reactivate and cause symptoms of encephalitis typically in individuals that are immunocompromised, especially bone marrow transplant patients.
- Arbovirus encephalitis – arthropod-borne viruses are transmitted by mosquitoes or ticks and can cause infection in humans. The most notable ones in the USA are West Nile, St Louis encephalitis, and La Crosse encephalitis viruses. The viruses replicate in the tissues or lymph nodes and then disseminate into the blood and occasionally cause encephalitis.
  - West Nile virus has become an increasing cause of viral encephalitis in the USA and is transmitted by infected mosquitoes. It causes clinically apparent CNS disease in less than 1% of people infected.

- St Louis encephalitis is an important cause of encephalitis found throughout South and North America. Similar to West Nile it is a flavivirus and is transmitted by infected mosquitoes.

Brain abscess

- When originating from paranasal sinus infections, the organisms typically encountered include streptococci, *Haemophilus*, *Bacteroides*, and *Fusobacterium* spp. species.
- Otogenic infections include streptococci, Enterobacteriaceae, *Bacteroides*, and *Pseudomonas aeruginosa*.
- Distant metastatic spread can come from endocarditis, urinary tract, abdominal abscess, or the lungs. Organisms involved in lung infections typically include *Streptococcus* species, fusiform, and *Actinomyces*. If it is secondary to endocarditis then the most common organisms are viridans streptococci or *S. aureus*. Urinary tract infections causing brain abscess would likely involve Enterobacteriaceae or *Pseudomonas*. Abdominal sources of infection would be streptococci, Enterobacteriaceae, and anaerobes.
- In penetrating head trauma the most common organism is *S. aureus*, though *Clostridium* species and *Enterobacter* species can also be seen.
- Post-neurosurgical procedure infections can include *S. aureus*, *Streptococcus* spp., *Pseudomonas*, and *Enterobacter*.
- Special populations such as immunocompromised patients, HIV patients, and immigrants have different microbiological flora to consider.
- In immunocompromised patients it is important to note that fungal infections such as aspergillosis and candidiasis can occur.
- Mucormycosis is another fungal infection seen in immunocompromised hosts as well as diabetics, chronic steroid users, and intravenous drug abusers.
- Tuberculosis is a rare cause of brain abscess and occurs in immunocompromised individuals, HIV patients, or those from endemic areas. It should especially be considered in those that have extracranial tuberculosis.
- *Nocardia* brain abscess is seen mostly in those that are receiving steroids or in transplant recipients. It is typically disseminated from the lungs, but can be a primary brain lesion.
- AIDS patients with brain abscess often have toxoplasmosis, which is typically reactivation of a previous infection. Note: An important differential in space-occupying lesions in AIDS patients is infectious abscess versus primary CNS lymphoma (PCNSL) related to Epstein–Barr virus (EBV).
- Parasitic infections such as cysticercosis and *Entamoeba histolytica* should be a consideration in immigrants with brain abscess.

Pathology/pathogenesis

- Meningitis – the most common forms of community-acquired bacterial meningitis cause disease by initial mucosal colonization and subsequent invasion of the CNS. Bacterial morphology as well as host immune defense are important factors for development of invasive disease. Nosocomial meningitis occurs either by hematogenous spread or by direct entry as seen in post-neurosurgical procedures. In either case once the organism crosses the blood–brain barrier it causes inflammation and edema leading to the typical symptoms of meningitis.
- Encephalitis can cause infection by direct invasion of the brain tissue as seen in meningitis, from colonization, previous infection, or viremia. It is important to distinguish infectious encephalitis

from ADEM (acute disseminated encephalomyelitis), which is an immunologic response to an antigen secondary to a previously infecting organism or immunization.
- Brain abscesses result from direct seeding of the brain from infections of the sinuses, teeth, or ear. Neurosurgery or penetrating brain trauma can also cause a direct seeding of infection leading to an abscess. Hematogenous spread can occur from an infection at any other site in the body, such as endocarditis, abdominal abscesses, and skin infections. About 20–30% of cases of brain abscess have no identifiable origin (cryptic).

Section 2: Prevention and screening

> **BOTTOM LINE/CLINICAL PEARLS**
> - *H. influenzae* type b (Hib) vaccine was introduced in 1990 and since then there has been a significant decrease in bacterial meningitis.
> - Meningococcal and pneumococcal vaccines given to high-risk individuals have been shown to have an impact on rates of bacterial meningitis.
> - Antibiotic prophylaxis is recommended for close contacts of those with invasive meningococcal infection. It is ideally administered within 24 hours after diagnosis of the index patient.

Section 3: Diagnosis

> **BOTTOM LINE/CLINICAL PEARLS**
> - Absence of fever does not exclude brain abscess – fever occurs in only ~50% of cases.
> - Unless contraindicated, lumbar puncture should be performed without delay to improve outcome in bacterial meningitis.
> - Antibiotics are to be administered immediately while awaiting diagnostic workup.
> - Suspected meningitis with petechial rash should be considered a medical emergency.

Typical presentation

Meningitis

Clinical manifestations vary between meningitis and encephalitis, and at times overlap in meningoencephalitis.
- Typically patients have fever, headache, meningismus, and altered mental status.
- Symptoms usually occur for hours to days prior to the patient seeking medical attention.
- Different etiologies of meningitis will have distinguishing presentations.
- Enteroviruses in general cause non-specific symptoms such as exanthemas, myopericarditis, rash, diarrhea, and upper respiratory symptoms.
- Amebic meningitis patients can complain of olfactory hallucinations. Tuberculous meningitis can present with fevers, weight loss, and malaise, but also can have no symptoms outside of CNS complaints.
- Lyme and meningococcal meningitis patients can complain of diffuse arthralgias.
- Symptoms of chronic meningitis can wax and wane for weeks to months.
- Cryptococcal meningoencephalitis can present as a subacute process with minimal symptoms.

Encephalitis

- In contrast to those with meningitis, patients with encephalitis tend to have mental status changes such as personality alterations, speech disturbances, seizures, visual changes, hallucinations, or cranial nerve palsies.
- They can also present with fever, headache, or meningismus, but these are usually less prominent than in meningitis.
- Symptoms may have been present for a longer duration before seeking medical attention than with meningitis.
- Notable features of HSV encephalitis include seizures, behavioral changes, personality changes, and disorientation along with olfactory hallucinations.
- Patients with HHV6 can present with limbic encephalitis, characterized by seizures, memory loss, and insomnia.
- West Nile virus encephalitis typically causes a flu-like illness that progresses to fevers, headache, myalgias, lymphadenopathy, and a maculopapular rash.
- *Listeria monocytogenes* can produce ataxia, tremors, nystagmus, and cranial nerve palsies, which indicate rhombencephalitis, an encephalitis of the brainstem or cerebellum.

Brain abscess

Symptoms of brain abscess vary considerably depending on the location, size, and number of abscesses.

- One common complaint noted among most patients is a headache, dull in quality.
- Surprisingly, fevers occur in less than half of patients.
- The symptoms for a brain abscess are non-specific, which would explain why patients do not seek medical attention until symptoms become more severe.

Clinical diagnosis

History

For any individual with a suspected CNS infection a detailed history will help determine the cause. Patients can be exposed to a certain organism at one point in their life and after becoming immunocompromised the infection can reactivate.

- Ask where the patient was born, where they have lived throughout their life, and when they have travelled outside their area. Certain infections are endemic to a particular location, such as histoplasmosis in the Midwestern states bordering the Ohio River valley.
- Sexual history, including sexual preferences, should also be obtained for every patient to determine those at high risk for HIV and syphilitic meningitis.
- Behavioral practices such as hiking or hunting should be asked about to raise the suspicion of tick-borne illnesses.
- Food consumption is another important question; those that drink unpasteurized milk might be at higher risk for certain bacterial infections such as *Listeria* meningitis.
- Animal exposure can be a clue to diagnosis; dog exposure can be related to *Coxiella* or cat to toxoplasmosis.
- A thorough immunization history is vital information especially in the immigrant population.

Physical examination

- Meningitis
  - Meningismus can be demonstrated through positive Kernig's and Brudzinski's signs. Kernig's sign is a maneuver done when the patient is lying supine and the thigh and knees are flexed.

The legs are then passively extended; when this elicits pain or resistance it indicates meningeal inflammation. Brudzinski's sign is positive when passive flexion of the neck causes flexion of the hips and knees. A negative test should not exclude meningitis.

- Papilledema is seen in less than 5% of those with meningitis.
- Other physical examination findings can be seen specific to a certain organism:
  - In meningococcus meningitis a rash that is described as erythematous macular becoming petechial involving the extremities can be observed.
  - For Lyme meningitis 40% of patients can have the characteristic rash of erythema migrans.
  - HSV-2 meningitis patients can have genital lesions/ulcers at the time of diagnosis, though not always seen.
  - If parotiditis is noticed then mumps meningitis should be suspected, especially in unvaccinated individuals.
- Encephalitis
  - The physical examination outside of the nervous system can be normal.
  - Patients can have a broad range of neurologic findings such as confusion, ataxia, nystagmus, cranial nerve palsies, and reduced consciousness.
  - VZV encephalitis is typically accompanied by a herpes zoster rash, which starts as erythematous papules, then evolves into vesicles, also known as shingles.
  - West Nile virus encephalitis and St Louis encephalitis can present with flaccid paralysis.
- Brain abscess
  - The systemic examination is quite variable and may provide a clue to the source of the infection.
  - Focal neurologic deficits depend on the location of the lesion.
  - Rupture of the brain abscess or those with a large abscess causing edema can present obtunded with seizures and critically ill.

Laboratory diagnosis
List of diagnostic tests
- Upon initial evaluation serum laboratory tests should be done including a complete blood count (CBC), basic metabolic panel (BMP), and two sets of blood cultures.
- Other non-invasive tests to perform depend on the particular organism under suspicion. If there are risk factors for *Cryptococcus* meningitis, a serum cryptococcus antigen test can be performed. If histoplasmosis is suspected then urine histoplasma antigen can be sent. Serum *Toxoplasma gondii* IgG should be ordered if considering reactivation of disease.
- Unless there is a contraindication (such as coagulopathy, local infection, concern for unstable intracranial hypertension), lumbar puncture for cerebrospinal fluid (CSF) analysis and opening pressure measurement should always be performed. Cervical puncture is an alternative when lumbar puncture is not feasible.
- The color of the CSF is normally clear. Cloudy CSF can indicate the presence of white blood cells. Xanthochromia may indicate lysed red blood cells or elevated protein.
- Standard tests to send in the CSF include: white blood cell count with differential, red blood cells, glucose, protein, Gram stain, and bacterial culture. Additional tests to be sent depend on clinical suspicion such as fungal culture, VDRL, cryptococcal antigen, and cytology. Also polymerase chain reactions for various viral etiologies such as HSV and VZV encephalitis can be performed if suspected. Specific CSF antibody tests, especially IgM, can be indicative of active CNS disease, as in West Nile encephalitis (Table 24.1).

Table 24.1 Cerebrospinal fluid findings in patients with meningitis.

Type of meningitis	White blood cell count (cells/mm³)	Glucose	Protein	Opening pressure
Bacterial	1000–5000 neutrophilic predominance	↓↓	↑	↑↑
Viral	50–1000 lymphocytic predominance	n/↓	n/↑	n
Fungal	<500 lymphocytic predominance	↓	↑	n/↑
Tuberculosis	50–300 lymphocytic predominance	↓	↑	↑

- A small percentage of patients with bacterial meningitis might have lymphocytic predominance of WBCs in the CSF. Early viral meningitis can have primarily neutrophils in the CSF.
- False elevation of WBCs and protein in the CSF can be seen after a traumatic lumbar puncture.
- CSF glucose must be compared to the serum glucose; a ratio <0.4 strongly favors bacterial meningitis.
- The most vital procedure when suspecting meningitis is lumbar puncture (LP) for CSF analysis. In general the lumbar puncture should be performed without delay to decrease the mortality and morbidity, especially in bacterial meningitis.
- CNS imaging is recommended prior to the LP to evaluate for potential space-occupying lesions, herniation, or bleed. If a patient has neurologic deficits, immunocompromise, seizure activity, or signs of increased intracranial pressure it is prudent to perform a CT head prior to the LP.
- For patients with suspected encephalitis MRI brain should be performed during the workup in addition to the CSF analysis.
- For confirmed or suspected brain abscess an MRI of the brain can better characterize the lesion. As a general rule, since there is typically a delay in performing procedure and imaging, antibiotics should be started immediately.

Potential pitfalls/common errors made regarding diagnosis of disease

- The CSF cell count is valuable to narrow the cause of the meningitis.
- There is often a limited amount of CSF obtained and therefore it is important to prioritize the CSF studies.
- Sending inappropriate CSF tests with little clinical significance or poor yield should be avoided, such as viral cultures which are of limited value.

Section 4: Treatment
Treatment rationale
Bacterial meningitis
- Suspected bacterial meningitis is a neurologic emergency, and parenteral antimicrobials should be initiated as soon as possible. Delaying antibiotics for the workup, including lumbar puncture, may worsen the outcome.
- Careful history-taking could provide clues to the etiology of the meningitis but usually it is unknown at initial encounter and empiric therapy is given. Guidelines for empiric therapy are based on our current knowledge of the more common pathogens.

- Initial antibiotic therapy for all adults should include intravenous vancomycin and ceftriaxone. Ceftriaxone would cover the most common etiology, which would be *Strep. pneumoniae*, as well as *Neisseria meningitidis* and other Gram-negative organisms. Vancomycin is part of the initial therapy based on the assumption that *Strep. pneumoniae* is resistant to penicillin. Additional empiric therapy is considered based on patient demographics and clinical history. For those patients that have head trauma, recent neurosurgery, immunocompromise, where *Pseudomonas* would be considered, cefepime or meropenem is recommended as initial therapy instead of ceftriaxone to cover for *Pseudomonas*. When *Listeria* meningitis is suspected or the patient is immunocompromised it is recommended to add ampicillin or penicillin to the empiric regimen. Duration of treatment depends on the specific organism.
- Studies show dexamethasone should be given for suspected pneumococcal meningitis. Improvement in outcome is seen for those who receive early dexamethasone, given before or in conjunction with antimicrobials.

Encephalitis
Most viral etiologies of encephalitis have no definitive treatment other than supportive care. It is recommended that empiric aciclovir should be administered to all those with suspected encephalitis until definitive diagnosis is established, because HSV is a common cause of treatable encephalitis. Other therapies for encephalitis (e.g. ganciclovir for CMV) should be specific for the organisms that are strongly suspected or confirmed. Routine steroids have no proven role in encephalitis, but may be lifesaving in acute cerebral swelling, especially in HSV encephalitis.

Brain abscess
- Neurosurgical consult is warranted as soon as the diagnosis is made.
- Empiric treatment for bacterial brain abscess depends on the suspected origin of the infection.
  - For paranasal sinus or otitis media sources, it is recommended to treat with metronidazole and ceftriaxone or cefotaxime.
  - With a dental source of infection, the initial antimicrobial therapy should be metronidazole and penicillin.
  - For metastatic spread of infection or for empiric therapy, metronidazole along with ceftriaxone or cefotaxime with vancomycin is suggested.
  - For abscesses following neurosurgical procedures or penetrating trauma, vancomycin with an agent that will cover *Pseudomonas*, such as cefepime or meropenem, is recommended.
  - In general, if *Pseudomonas* is suspected then antipseudomonal agents should be used.
  - If methicillin-resistant *Staphylococcus aureus* (MRSA) is suspected vancomycin should be used.
- Duration of treatment depends on whether there is any surgical intervention and on the patient's response. In general, most studies recommend 4–6 weeks for surgically treated abscesses and longer, 6–8 weeks, for larger abscesses and those that are not surgically treated.
- Follow-up imaging is recommended during treatment and after completing treatment.

When to hospitalize
Virtually all, except cases of mild viral meningitis, should be hospitalized.

Table of treatment (Algorithm 24.1)

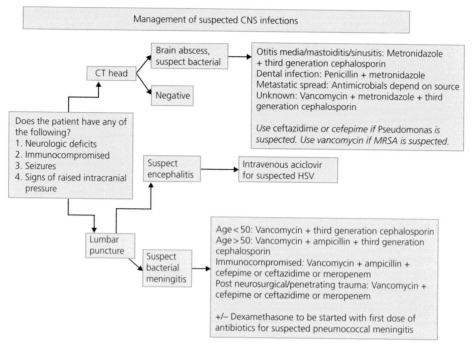

Algorithm 24.1 Managing suspected CNS infections.

Prevention/management of complications
- Hydrocephalus may present acutely or in the chronic phase as deteriorating consciousness, and typically is confirmed by imaging and usually requires shunting.
- Seizures require appropriate anticonvulsant treatment.
- Dexamethasone is used for pneumococcal meningitis to prevent hearing impairment.
- Signs of increased intracranial pressure must be treated aggressively and steroids are NOT contraindicated in HSV encephalitis when brain swelling develops, typically several days after presentation and antiviral therapy.

> **CLINICAL PEARLS**
> - Unless there is a strong contraindication, CSF analysis should be obtained for all suspected cases of meningitis or encephalitis.
> - Antimicrobial therapy should not be delayed under any circumstances.
> - When etiology or organisms are unknown, broad empiric treatment should be given initially until further information is available.

Section 5: Special populations
Pregnancy
Pregnant women are at increased risk of developing *L. monocytogenes* meningitis. Treatment is the same as for non-pregnant individuals in coordination with an obstetrician.

Children

In newborns and infants diagnosis is challenging since the classic symptoms can frequently be missed. Other clues such as irritability, decreased appetite, vomiting, and lethargy, or bulging fontanelles can be seen. The most common bacterial organisms for vaccinated children would be *S. pneumoniae* and *N. meningitidis*. In infants less than 3 months of age, *L. monocytogenes*, *E. coli*, and group B streptococci are important pathogens. Empiric treatment would include vancomycin and a third generation cephalosporin with weight-based dosing. Dexamethasone can be considered for patients with pneumococcal meningitis, according to the American Academy of Pediatrics. A pediatric specialist should be consulted when meningitis is suspected.

Elderly

Mortality is greater for the elderly with meningitis compared to younger individuals, as it is for most infections. The etiology is different than the typical adult population, with the more common organisms being *Strep. pneumoniae*, *L. monocytogenes*, Gram-negative bacilli, and *Streptococcus agalactiae*. Empiric treatment is similar to that for adults with the addition of ampicillin to cover for *L. monocytogenes*.

Others

- Immunocompromised. Patients that are immunocompromised with suspected bacterial meningitis can get standard empiric treatment. Antimicrobial coverage for *Pseudomonas*, MRSA, and *Listeria* should be considered in these patients depending on clinical presentation.
- Acquired immune deficiency syndrome (AIDS):
  - Patients with AIDS are at higher risk for CNS infections, with rates increasing with the degree of immunosuppression.
  - HIV itself can cause aseptic meningitis, usually seen at the onset of infection, which can be self-limiting. Symptoms can improve with initiation of antiretroviral therapy at diagnosis.
  - The most common opportunistic infection in AIDS patients is *Cryptococcus* meningoencephalitis, as mentioned previously. According to the Infectious Disease Society of America (IDSA) guidelines, treatment includes induction therapy with intravenous amphotericin B (or lipid formulations of amphotericin B, which have less renal complications) with or without flucytosine. Induction is recommended for 2 weeks followed by oral fluconazole. Opening pressure is typically elevated in *Cryptococcus* meningoencephalitis, and it is recommended to perform repeated lumbar puncture to reduce the opening pressure to less than 200 mm H_2O.
  - Bacterial meningitis treatment in AIDS patients is the same as it is for the immunocompetent patients.
  - CNS space-occupying lesions in AIDS patients are typically due to CNS toxoplasmosis or PCNSL, the former being more common. In non-life-threatening cases patients can be treated for CNS toxoplasmosis with a combination of pyrimethamine and sulfadiazine. After 10–14 days, if there are persistent symptoms or no change in imaging, a brain biopsy should be pursued.

Section 6: Prognosis

> **BOTTOM LINE/CLINICAL PEARLS**
> - CNS infections can cause severe neurologic compromise and be fatal if left untreated.
> - The case fatality rates for bacterial meningitis vary by region, pathogen, and age group. According to the CDC case fatality can be as high as 70% if left untreated, and one in five individuals who survive can be left with permanent neurologic effects. The fatality rate of meningococcemia can be up to 40% even with appropriate antibiotic therapy. According to the WHO the case fatality rate for *Haemophilus influenzae* meningitis is 5% and can cause deafness in 20% of survivors.
> - Viral meningoencephalitides also have high fatality rates; according to the CDC, West Nile virus carries a 3–15% case fatality rate.
> - With the high rates of morbidity and mortality with all types of meningitis prompt recognition and antimicrobial therapy is essential.

Section 7: Reading list

Key reading sources for this chapter can be found online at www.mountsinaiexpertguides.com

Section 8: Guidelines

Mount Sinai Hospital Infection Control guidelines

- Known or suspected *N. meningitidis* or *H. influenzae* meningitis patients should be placed on droplet precautions.
- Patients with *M. tuberculosis* meningitis with suspected pulmonary involvement or potential to aerosolize are to be placed on airborne isolation.
- When disseminated varicella zoster is suspected, including CNS disease, contact and airborne precautions are recommended. Hospital personnel in contact with the patient must be immune to varicella.

> **Additional material for this chapter can be found online at:**
> **www.mountsinaiexpertguides.com**
>
> **This includes a case study, multiple choice questions, and a reading list.**

CHAPTER 25

Parkinson's Disease and Related Disorders

Barbara Kelly Changizi
The Ohio State University Wexner Medical Center, Columbus, OH, USA

OVERALL BOTTOM LINE

- Parkinsonism is characterized by bradykinesia, rigidity, tremor, and postural instability.
- Parkinson's disease (PD) is the most common cause of parkinsonism.
- The cause of the dopaminergic cell loss underlying PD is unknown, but the genetic and environmental contributors continue to be better understood.
- Symptomatic benefit via dopaminergic pathways is the mainstay of pharmacotherapy. There is no cure for PD.
- Deep brain stimulation provides benefit for advanced PD with motor fluctuations or severe tremor when pharmacotherapy has reached its limits of efficacy.

Section 1: Background

Definition of disease

Parkinsonism is characterized by the cardinal features of bradykinesia, rigidity, 4–6 Hz resting tremor, and postural instability. Parkinsonism can be caused by a variety of disorders, the most common being PD.

The UK Parkinson's Disease Society Brain Bank Criteria constitute a commonly used set of criteria to accurately diagnose PD. Diagnostic criteria are bradykinesia and at least one of the following: muscular rigidity, 4–6 Hz resting tremor, and postural instability. Other causes of parkinsonism include the Parkinson-plus syndromes of multiple system atrophy, progressive supranuclear palsy, cortical basal ganglionic degeneration, and Lewy body dementia as well as toxin, drug, and vascular-induced parkinsonism.

Disease classification

PD and the Parkinson-plus syndromes are classified as movement disorders because they affect the ability to control movement, and involve dysfunction of the basal ganglia (BG). These disorders comprise the hypokinetic movement disorders, because they cause a poverty of movement.

Incidence/prevalence

- PD affects 5 million people worldwide.
- The prevalence of PD is 0.3% of the general population, and the prevalence increases with age, with reports of 1.6% of people older than 65 years, and 3.5% of those older than 85 years having PD.
- There is a 1.5:1 ratio of men to women with PD.

Mount Sinai Expert Guides: Neurology, First Edition. Edited by Stuart C. Sealfon, Rajeev Motiwala, and Charles B. Stacy.
© 2016 John Wiley & Sons, Ltd. Published 2016 by John Wiley & Sons, Ltd.
Companion website: www.mountsinaiexpertguides.com

Economic impact

- The financial burden of Parkinson's disease exceeds $14 billion annually in the USA, and is estimated to double by 2040.

Etiology

- The cause of PD is unknown.
- There is degeneration of the substantia nigra pars compacta (SNRpc), which leads to dopamine deficiency in the basal ganglia (BG) circuitry.
- Loss of dopamine leads to reduced activity in the direct pathway and overactivity in the indirect pathway of the BG, ultimately leading to inhibition of the thalamus and features of parkinsonism.
- Patients with PD may have an underlying genetic predisposition to develop the disease combined with exposure to environmental risk factors.
- The majority of PD patients have no known genetic cause; however, several identified mutations (alpha synuclein, PINK1, parkin, LRRK2, DJ-1, glucocerebrosidase enzyme, and PITX3) in a minority of cases may eventually provide clues to a comprehensive understanding of a common pathogenic mechanism.
- The causes of neurodegeneration may be multifactorial; proposed mechanisms include mitochondrial respiratory failure and oxidative stress, protein misfolding, impaired proteasomal degradation, iron dysregulation, lack of trophic factors, excitotoxicity, and inflammation.

Pathology/pathogenesis

PD is a neurodegenerative disease. Motor symptoms result from reduced dopamine in the BG circuitry. Dopamine deficiency is caused by degeneration of neurons in the substantia nigra pars compacta of the midbrain, which shows loss of pigmentation at autopsy. Neurodegeneration is also seen in the other pigmented brainstem nuclei and the pyramidal cells of the presupplementary cortex.

The BG contain two dopaminergic pathways, the direct and indirect pathways, which are thought to promote and inhibit motor functioning respectively. Dopamine deficiency leads to reduced excitatory activity in the direct pathway via D1 receptors, and increased inhibitory activity in the indirect pathway via D2 receptors. The imbalance between the pathways leads to pathologic firing patterns of the subthalamic nucleus and globus pallidus interna, ultimately leading to excessive inhibition of the thalamus and to the features of parkinsonism.

Lewy bodies, which are eosinophilic inclusions found in neurons, are the pathologic hallmark of PD. They contain alpha synuclein, ubiquitin, torsin A, and pentraxin II. While Lewy bodies are the traditional hallmark of PD, they are not pathognomonic; they are observed in other parkinsonian syndromes, and can be absent in some forms of PD. They are found in the substantia nigra pars compacta, fitting with the fact that PD is associated with dopamine deficiency. Some researchers have noted a sequence of Lewy body appearance as PD progresses, starting in the dorsal motor nucleus of the vagus nerve and olfactory bulbs, followed by the raphe nucleus and locus coeruleus, and later in the midbrain and nucleus basalis of Meynert, and finally the mesocortex and neocortex. This progression may explain the non-motor features of PD, including lack of olfaction, constipation, autonomic dysfunction, and eventual cognitive decline.

Predictive/risk factors

- Older age
- Family history of PD
- Male gender

- Farming, rural living
- Exposure to copper, manganese, lead
- Pesticide exposure
- High milk intake
- Significant traumatic brain injury

Section 2: Prevention and screening

BOTTOM LINE/CLINICAL PEARLS

As the cause of PD is unknown, prevention measures are unclear. The following has been gleaned from epidemiologic studies.
- Cigarette smoking, coffee and caffeine intake, and exercise may lower the risk of developing PD.
- Studies have shown lower risk of PD associated with higher plasma levels of vitamin D at baseline. Also, PD patients have been observed to have lower vitamin D levels than the normal population.
- PD patients have lower levels of serum uric acid than controls. Uric acid is an antioxidant and free radical scavenger. Lower plasma urate levels are linked to a higher risk of developing PD. Higher serum uric acid concentration has been associated with slower clinical progression of PD.

Section 3: Diagnosis

BOTTOM LINE/CLINICAL PEARLS
- The diagnosis of PD is established on clinical grounds.
- History may include soft speech, resting tremor, small handwriting, loss of olfaction, dragging of a leg, shuffling, constipation, slowness, or poor dexterity.
- Examination findings include bradykinesia, rigidity, tremor, and postural instability.

PD differential diagnosis

Differential diagnosis	Features
Dementia with Lewy bodies	Dementia and hallucinations early in the course, susceptibility to hallucinations with low doses of levodopa, fluctuating mental status
Multiple system atrophy (MSA): MSA-A (Shy–Drager syndrome) MSA-P (striatonigral degeneration) MSA-C (olivopontocerebellar atrophy)	Short-lived or poor response to dopaminergic therapy Early and prominent autonomic dysfunction including orthostasis, impotence, urinary incontinence Cerebellar dysfunction Pyramidal dysfunction Bulbar dysarthria Brain MRI may show pontine or cerebellar atrophy, or hot-cross-buns sign within pons, or putaminal slit sign [131]m-iodobenzylguanidine (MIBG) cardiac scintigraphy is normal in MSA, but abnormal in PD

(Continued)

Differential diagnosis	Features
Progressive supranuclear palsy (PSP)	Axial rigidity, supranuclear gaze palsy, early falls due to postural instability. Brain MRI may show midbrain atrophy
Corticobasal ganglionic degeneration	Apraxia, alien limb, dystonia in one limb, cortical sensory loss (agraphesthesia, astereognosia)
Essential tremor	Tremor is typically symmetric, and is a kinetic tremor worsened by actions requiring fine dexterity plus a postural tremor involving flexion and extension in the upper extremities. Distribution includes the hands, head, and voice
Normal pressure hydrocephalus (NPH)	Triad of magnetic gait, urinary incontinence, and dementia Brain imaging shows disproportionate ventriculomegaly Lumbar drain or lumbar puncture with large-volume CSF removal relieves symptoms temporarily, especially gait difficulty
Drug-induced parkinsonism	Exposure to neuroleptics or other dopamine-receptor blocking agents, lithium, dopamine depletors Presence of other drug-induced movement disorders such as tardive dyskinesia or akathisia Functional imaging of striatal dopamine transporter uptake (fluorodopa PET, beta-CIT SPECT, [123I]FP-CIT SPECT or DaTscan) is normal (abnormal in PD)
Wilson's disease	Presence of Kayser–Fleischer rings, liver disease, and other neurologic signs such as dystonia, wing-beating tremor, or ataxia. Ceruloplasmin is low and 24-hour urine copper is elevated
Vascular parkinsonism	Mild parkinsonism, particularly shuffling gait and lower extremity bradykinesia, stepwise progression of symptoms, tremor usually absent MRI shows extensive small vessel disease or lacunae in the BG
Toxins	History of exposure to 1-methyl-4-phenyl-1,2,3,6-tetrahydropyridine (MPTP), carbon disulfide, carbon monoxide, manganese Brain MRI may show changes in the BG (e.g. T2 hyperintensity in globus pallidus)

Typical presentation

Parkinson's disease typically presents with cardinal features of bradykinesia, rigidity, tremor, and postural instability. Bradykinesia is an abnormal slowness of movement. Rigidity is an increased resistance to passive movement. Postural instability reflects loss of the postural reflexes that allow the patient to maintain balance. Tremor is typically resting, 4–6 Hz, with a pill-rolling quality in the hand that typically starts asymmetrically in the upper or lower extremities.

Clinical diagnosis

History

Patients may report a history of constipation and poor sense of smell. They may report that speech is soft or raspy, and handwriting is smaller. Patients may report shuffling or dragging of a leg, or tremor in an arm or leg that dampens with activity. The patient will report changes in dexterity or slowness described as difficulty fastening buttons and zippers, or tying shoelaces.

Physical examination

Bradykinesia is apparent when testing rapid alternating movements; there is reduced amplitude, fatiguing, or arrests during such tasks as repeated finger tapping, hand opening, and foot or toe tapping. When ambulating, the patient will show decreased arm swing or a shuffling gait. The classic parkinsonian tremor is a 4–6 Hz tremor observed at rest that dampens with activity. Rigidity presents as resistance to passive movement of the limb around the joints. When there is superimposed resting tremor, rigidity may demonstrate a cogwheeling quality.

Postural instability causes retropulsion, which is assessed using the pull test, in which the patient is tugged backwards while standing. If the patient takes more than two steps or falls backwards, the test is abnormal. Masked facies, micrographia, and stooped posture may also be observed. Freezing of gait (FOG) is episodic halting gait, or inability to generate effective stepping.

Disease severity classification

The Unified Parkinson Disease Rating Scale (UPDRS), and the recently modified Movement Disorder Society UPDRS (MDS-UPDRS) are routinely used to assess the severity of parkinsonism (see Guidelines). A higher score indicates greater severity of disease.

Laboratory diagnosis

List of diagnostic tests

- Brain MRI is performed to exclude other causes of parkinsonism (toxin exposure, tumor, vascular parkinsonism, NPH). The MRI is not affected by PD.
- Serum ceruloplasmin and 24-hour urine copper are tested to exclude Wilson's disease, especially in any patient presenting with parkinsonism younger than age 50. Ceruloplasmin is low and urine copper is elevated in Wilson's disease.
- Olfactory testing may show hyposmia or anosmia, which can be one of the earliest signs of PD.
- Functional neuroimaging may be helpful to differentiate essential tremor or drug-induced parkinsonism from PD. FP-CIT SPECT, beta-CIT SPECT, or fluorodopa PET will show decreased BG presynaptic dopamine uptake in PD.

Potential pitfalls/common errors made regarding diagnosis of disease

- Patients with postural or action tremor may be misdiagnosed with essential tremor.
- Patients with Wilson's disease, which is a treatable condition and potentially lethal, may be misdiagnosed as PD.
- Patients with normal pressure hydrocephalus may have mild parkinsonism and a magnetic gait that mimics the shuffling gait of parkinsonism. Patients should be screened for ventriculomegaly by brain imaging.

Section 4: Treatment (Algorithm 25.1)

Treatment rationale

There is no cure for PD; treatment focuses on symptoms, and potential neuroprotection. Most pharmacotherapy focuses on replacement of dopamine to improve motor functioning. Levodopa is converted to dopamine in the brain, and is the most effective treatment for PD. Pulsatile high-dose levodopa is associated with increased risk of motor fluctuations over time, and so some experts prefer alternative agents for milder disease in younger patients. These include monoamine oxidase-B inhibitors (MAOI-Bs), dopamine agonists, and amantadine. Anticholinergic drugs

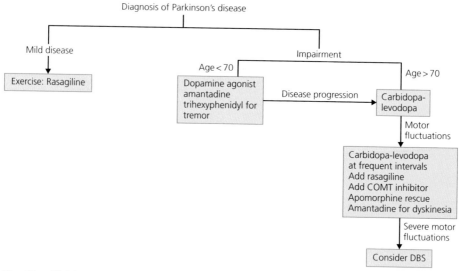

Algorithm 25.1 Management of Parkinson's disease.

may provide relief of tremor but are not particularly effective for bradykinesia and rigidity, and are poorly tolerated in the elderly.

As the disease progresses, symptoms worsen and require a cocktail of medications at higher doses, including levodopa. Motor fluctuations and dyskinesia develop. Motor fluctuations consist of wearing off of drug benefit several hours after medication dose. Patients alternate between being "on" with relief of parkinsonism, and being "off," when the symptoms of parkinsonism return. Dyskinesias are involuntary movements that are typically choreiform or dystonic, and may occur in the "on" state. At this stage of disease, levodopa must be taken at regular intervals. MAOI-Bs and catechol-O-methyl transferase (COMT) inhibitors may be added to extend levodopa effect. Dopamine agonists have a longer half-life, and are helpful as adjunct therapy. Amantadine reduces dyskinesia. Apomorphine, an injectable dopamine agonist, may provide rapid rescue from freezing. Eventually, the best medical management may provide poor relief from motor fluctuations, and surgical options are considered. Deep brain stimulation (DBS) of the globus pallidus or subthalamic nucleus (STN) has been shown to be superior to optimal medical management in PD patients with severe motor fluctuations.

When to hospitalize
- Parkinsonism-hyperpyrexia syndrome (PHS) is a rare but potentially life-threatening condition caused by abrupt cessation of dopaminergic therapy in the PD patient. This consists of rigidity, confusion, hyperpyrexia, dysautonomia, and elevated creatine kinase. Treatment includes rapid replacement of dopaminergic therapy.
- PD patients may develop confusion with severe hallucinations or paranoia that poses a safety risk to the patient or family. Psychosis in PD patients may be due to pharmacotherapy as well as progression of disease.
- Medical complications such as pneumonia, other infections, and falls often precipitate hospitalization.

Managing the hospitalized patient
- Patients with PD frequently have prolonged hospital stays due to motor complications, inappropriate use of neuroleptics, falls, and aspiration pneumonia.

- Staff must be educated about the necessity of specific dosage schedules to avoid reduced mobility.
- Avoid dopamine receptor blocking agents, including antiemetics and neuroleptics. Quetiapine is the preferred antipsychotic in the PD patient.

Table of treatment

Medical	
• Levodopa (combined with carbidopa in standard-release, controlled-release, dissolvable-in-mouth formulations, also as an enteral suspension)	• Most efficacious drug for PD • Always combined with carbidopa, a peripheral decarboxylase inhibitor, to block conversion to dopamine in the systemic circulation and allow more levodopa to cross the blood–brain barrier • Dosing varies according to patient's tolerance and stage of PD – use the lowest dose that is effective for symptoms • Side effects include nausea, orthostasis, hallucinations, fatigue
• Dopamine agonists (pramipexole, ropinirole, rotigotine, apomorphine)	• Stimulate dopamine receptors • Long duration of action (except apomorphine) • Not as potent as levodopa and more prone to side effects of nausea, hallucinations, orthostasis, sedation (driving precautions) • Used as monotherapy or adjunct therapy • Screen for impulse control disorders (see below)
• MAO-B inhibitors (selegiline, rasagiline)	• Decrease degradation of dopamine in brain by inhibiting monoamine oxidase • Used as monotherapy or adjunct therapy • Rasagiline may be neuroprotective
• COMT inhibitors: Entacapone (200 mg with carbidopa/levodopa); Tolcapone (up to 100 mg t.i.d.)	• Decrease degradation of dopamine by inhibiting catechol-O-methyl transferase (COMT) • Must be taken with levodopa to be effective • Used to treat motor fluctuations by extending the life of levodopa • A few patients develop diarrhea • Turn urine orange • Tolcapone avoided as first-line therapy due to rare risk of fulminant hepatitis
• Anticholinergic agents (trihexyphenidyl)	• Effective for tremor, little benefit for bradykinesia or rigidity • Side effects of confusion, urinary retention, constipation, dry mouth, especially in elderly • Used as monotherapy or adjunct therapy, typically in tremor-predominant younger patients
• Amantadine (recommended 100 mg b.i.d. typically; t.i.d. for severe dyskinesia)	• Antiviral agent with dopaminergic activity (increases dopamine release and inhibits dopamine reuptake) • Effective for dyskinesia through NMDA receptor antagonist effect
Surgical • Deep brain stimulation (DBS)	• Provides high-frequency stimulation to the GPi or STN to regulate pathologic firing • Effective for dopamine-responsive symptoms of rigidity, tremor, and bradykinesia • Used for patients with medication-refractory tremor, severe motor fluctuations, or troublesome dyskinesia • Contraindicated in dementia, uncontrolled hypertension

(Continued)

• Lesioning of the posteroventral portion of the GPi, thalamotomy	• Lesioning has been essentially replaced by high-frequency stimulation (see above). Thalamotomy provides relief of contralateral tremor only, and pallidotomy provides relief of dyskinesia and bradykinesia. Subthalamotomy leads to improvement in tremor, rigidity, bradykinesia, and reduction of levodopa dose • Bilateral pallidotomy has a high risk of bulbar dysfunction, and subthalamotomy carries a significant risk of hemiballism • Lesioning is irreversible and does not allow the flexibility in programming that DBS provides
Management of associated symptoms • Sialorrhea • Rhinorrhea • Constipation • Depression	Atropine 1% ophthalmic solution drops sublingually, glycopyrrolate 1 mg t.i.d., and botulinum toxin injections to salivary glands every 3 months may improve sialorrhea Ipratropium nasal spray may improve rhinorrhea Polyethylene glycol and lubiprostone provide relief of constipation Selective serotonin reuptake inhibitors (SSRIs) improve depression, and are less likely to cause side effects than the tricyclic amines. SSRIs may aggravate parkinsonism, particularly fluoxetine and paroxetine. Sertraline is least likely to worsen parkinsonism

Prevention/management of complications

- Dopaminergic medication should be taken with food to avoid nausea. However, high protein intake can limit absorption of levodopa. The antiemetics ondansetron and trimethobenzamide do not worsen parkinsonism. Antiemetics that act by blocking dopamine receptors should be avoided.
- Orthostasis is caused by PD and/or by dopaminergic medication. Fludrocortisone, midodrine, and droxidopa are effective treatments.
- Hallucinations and paranoia may present in later stages of the disease, and are aggravated by amantadine, dopamine agonists, and high doses of levodopa. Quetiapine and clozapine are the preferred antipsychotics to avoid worsening parkinsonism; however, clozapine carries a low but potentially fatal risk of agranulocytosis and requires close blood count monitoring.
- Impulse control disorders (ICDs) occur in a minority of patients prescribed dopamine agonists. These include pathologic gambling, shopping, hypersexuality, and hyperphagia. Treatment involves lowering or discontinuing the dopamine agonists. Amantadine may be an effective therapy.

CLINICAL PEARLS
- There is no cure for PD; treatment at this time is mainly symptomatic.
- Levodopa is the most effective therapy for PD, but is associated with higher risk of motor fluctuations and dyskinesia after long-term use.
- Dopamine agonists, MAOI-Bs are alternatives to levodopa.
- Amantadine may be used as monotherapy for mild disease, or to treat dyskinesia in advanced patients.
- Anticholinergics are effective for tremor.
- DBS is considered for patients with refractory tremor, or motor fluctuations that are not well controlled with pharmacotherapy.

Section 5: Special populations

Elderly

The elderly are more susceptible to side effects. Avoid anticholinergics in the elderly, as these can lead to confusion, constipation, and urinary retention. The elderly are more prone to hallucinations, confusion, and orthostasis from dopamine agonists.

Others

For the younger PD patient, consider potential neuroprotective strategies and levodopa-sparing treatments. Neuroprotective strategies include selegiline or rasagiline. Dopamine agonists are the next most efficacious therapy after levodopa, and are less likely to induce dyskinesia. Anticholinergics may be an option for the tremor-predominant patient.

Section 6: Prognosis

BOTTOM LINE/CLINICAL PEARLS

- There is no cure for PD.
- There is progressive decline in both motor and non-motor features over decades.
- Non-motor features include cognitive impairment, hallucinations, depression, and autonomic symptoms including orthostasis and urinary dysfunction.
- Symptomatic therapy and DBS improve tremor, bradykinesia, and rigidity, but postural instability and gait freezing may not respond.
- The majority of patients develop motor fluctuations after approximately 5 years of levodopa therapy.
- At least one-third of PD patients go on to develop dementia.

Section 7: Reading list

Key reading sources for this chapter can be found online at www.mountsinaiexpertguides.com

Suggested websites

CurePSP Foundation for PSP, CBD, and related brain diseases: www.psp.org
Parkinson Disease foundation: www.pdf.org
The Michael J. Fox Foundation: www.michaeljfox.org

Section 8: Guidelines

Title	Source	Weblink
Treatment of nonmotor symptoms of Parkinson disease	American Academy of Neurology (AAN), March 2010	https://www.aan.com/pressroom/home/getdigitalasset/8475
Neuroprotective strategies and alternative therapies for Parkinson disease	AAN, April 2006, reaffirmed October 2009	http://www.neurology.org/content/66/7/976.full.pdf
Treatment of Parkinson disease with motor fluctuations and dyskinesias	AAN, April 2006	http://www.neurology.org/content/66/7/983.full.pdf
Diagnosis and prognosis of new onset Parkinson disease	AAN, April 2006, reaffirmed October 2009	http://www.neurology.org/content/66/7/968.full
Evaluation and treatment of depression, psychosis, and dementia in Parkinson disease	AAN, 2006	http://tools.aan.com/professionals/practice/guidelines/Eval_Treatment_PD_Sum.pdf

Section 9: Evidence for therapies

Type of evidence	Title and comment	Weblink
RCT	Parkinson Study Group. Effects of tocopherol and deprenyl on the progression of disability in early Parkinson's disease. N Engl J Med 1993;328(3):176–83 **Comment**: Selegiline reduced the risk of developing disability requiring levodopa therapy by 50%, but many believe due to symptomatic effect	http://www.ncbi.nlm.nih.gov/pubmed/8417384
RCT	Olanow CW et al. A double-blind, delayed start trial of rasagiline in Parkinson's disease. N Engl J Med 2009;361:1268–78 **Comment**: Early treatment with rasagiline at a dose of 1 mg daily may have disease-modifying benefit	http://www.nejm.org/doi/full/10.1056/NEJMoa0809335
RCT	Parkinson Study Group. Pramipexole vs levodopa as initial treatment for Parkinson disease. JAMA 2000;284(15):1931–8 **Comment**: Pramipexole monotherapy is effective. Initial pramipexole treatment resulted in significant reduction in risk of motor fluctuations compared to levodopa	http://jama.jamanetwork.com/article.aspx?articleid=193185
RCT	Lieberman A, Olanow CW, Sethi K, et al. A multicenter trial of ropinirole as adjunct treatment for Parkinson's disease. Ropinirole Study Group . Neurology 1998;51:1057–62 **Comment**: Ropinirole is effective in patients with motor fluctuations and reduces levodopa requirement	http://www.ncbi.nlm.nih.gov/pubmed/9781529
RCT	Parkinson Study Group. A randomized placebo-controlled trial of rasagiline in levodopa-treated patients with Parkinson disease and motor fluctuations: the PRESTO study. Arch Neurol 2005;62:241–8 **Comment**: Rasagiline reduces off time by 1.85 hours in patients with motor fluctuations	http://www.ncbi.nlm.nih.gov/pubmed/15710852
RCT	Stocchi F et al. Initiating levodopa/carbidopa therapy with and without entacapone in early Parkinson disease: the STRIDE-PD study. Ann Neurol 2010;68(1):18-27. **Comment**: Entacapone was associated with shorter time to onset and frequency of dyskinesia compared to levodopa alone.	http://www.ncbi.nlm.nih.gov/pubmed/20582993
RCT	Weaver FM, et al., CSP 468 Study Group. Bilateral deep brain stimulation vs best medical therapy for patients with advanced Parkinson disease: a randomized controlled trial. JAMA 2009;301(1):63–73 **Comment**: DBS is superior to best medical therapy for patients with motor fluctuations	http://www.ncbi.nlm.nih.gov/pubmed/19126811

Additional material for this chapter can be found online at:
www.mountsinaiexpertguides.com

This includes advice for patients, a case study, multiple choice questions and a reading list.

CHAPTER 26

Hyperkinetic Movement Disorders

Ritesh A. Ramdhani and Steven J. Frucht

Icahn School of Medicine at Mount Sinai, New York, NY, USA

OVERALL BOTTOM LINE

- Hyperkinetic movement disorders, which include dystonia, tremor, chorea, myoclonus, and tics, are often a diagnostic challenge.
- Understanding and deciphering the phenomenology of these involuntary movements is critical to formulating an accurate differential diagnosis and pursuing a management strategy.

Section 1: Background
Definition of disease

- *Essential tremor* is a rhythmic oscillatory movement most commonly seen in the hands when doing tasks such as writing, pouring, or eating.
- *Dystonia* is a syndrome of involuntary, sustained muscle contractions, frequently causing twisting and repetitive movements or abnormal postures.
- *Myoclonus* is a sudden, shock-like muscle jerk, usually lasting less than a tenth of a second.
- *Chorea* is an involuntary, random, flitting movement that may involve the face, neck, trunk, or limbs.
- *Tics* are quick, stereotyped motor movements or vocalizations that briefly interrupt normal activity, are temporarily suppressible, and usually accompanied by a premonitory sensation.

Incidence/prevalence

- Tic disorders are more common in children, at a prevalence of 3% with a predilection to affect boys more than girls.
- Essential tremor prevalence is reported to range from 0.3 to 4% in persons over 40 years of age.
- Prevalence of primary dystonia is approximately 16 per 100,000.
- Chorea and myoclonus are symptoms of underlying conditions and prevalence and incidence data are not applicable.
- Huntington's disease is one of the common causes of adult-onset chorea, with a prevalence of 5–6 per 100,000 in North American, European, and Australian populations. Asian populations have a prevalence of about 0.4 per 100,000.

Mount Sinai Expert Guides: Neurology, First Edition. Edited by Stuart C. Sealfon, Rajeev Motiwala, and Charles B. Stacy.
© 2016 John Wiley & Sons, Ltd. Published 2016 by John Wiley & Sons, Ltd.
Companion website: www.mountsinaiexpertguides.com

Etiology

Essential tremor (ET)

- Genetic studies have suggested an autosomal dominant inheritance with linkage to chromosomes 3q13 and 2p22.
- The *LINGO1* gene on chromosome 15 has recently been found to be associated with ET.

Dystonia

Monogenic forms of dystonia (i.e. primary torsion with or without tremor, dystonia-plus syndromes, primary paroxysmal dystonias) are associated with numerous mutated loci designated DYT loci, which are predominantly autosomal dominant in inheritance. Genetic studies have led to the identification of the genes located at many of these loci (i.e. DYT 1, 4, 5, 6, 8, 10, 11, 12, 18, 23, 24, 25).

- Primary torsion with or without tremor. Early onset dystonia is commonly caused by the *TOR1A* gene (torsin 1A, DYT1) or *THAP1* (thanatos associated protein domain containing, apoptosis associated protein 1; DYT6). Mutations in *CIZI/DYT23* (Cip-interacting zinc finger), *ANO3/DYT24* (anoctamin 3), and *GNAL/DYT25* (guanine-nucleotide binding) genes have been implicated in adult-onset focal/segmental dystonia.
- Dystonia-plus syndrome (dystonia associated with another movement disorder). The three most common are dopa-responsive dystonia (DRD; DYT5), myoclonus-dystonia (M-D; DYT11) and rapid onset dystonia-parkinsonism (RDP; DYT12). Genetic mutations in the tetrahydrobiopterin synthetic pathway, specifically the *GCH1* gene in the autosomal dominant variant, and the *TH* gene in the autosomal recessive form, are responsible for DRD. In addition, M-D results from a mutation in the epsilon-sarcoglycan (*SGCE*) gene, while RDP is caused by mutation of the *ATP1A3* gene, which encodes a Na^+/K^+-ATPase pump.
- Primary paroxysmal dystonia (dystonia with or without dyskinesias occurring in brief episodes with normalcy in between). Most syndromes of paroxysmal dystonia have a known gene mutation. DYT8 results from mutations in the myofibrillogenesis regulator (MR-1) gene, whereas the *PRRT2* gene, encoding a synaptic membrane protein, is responsible for DYT10, and *SLC2A1*, a gene encoding a glucose transporter type 1 protein, causes DYT18.
- Heredodegenerative dystonia. This is a feature of other neurologic diseases, such as Huntington's disease, neurodegeneration with brain iron accumulation (NBIA), Wilson's disease, McLeod's syndrome, Lesch–Nyhan syndrome, and Leigh's disease.
- Secondary dystonia may result from an identified neurologic precipitant, such as a brain injury, cerebrovascular disease, or neuroleptic inducer.

Myoclonus

- Physiologic (e.g. hypnic jerks, hiccups).
  Essential (e.g. alcohol-sensitive myoclonus dystonia).
- Epileptic (e.g. progressive myoclonic encephalopathies).
  Secondary (e.g. metabolic derangements, medications, anoxia, neurodegenerative diseases).

Chorea

- Metabolic:
  - Non-ketotic hyperglycemia (hemichorea).
  - Elevated or decreased calcium, magnesium, or sodium.
  - Thyroid disease, B12 deficiency.
  - Pregnancy (chorea gravidarum).

- Infectious:
  - Sydenham's chorea (streptoccoccus), Creuztfeldt–Jakob disease (prion).
  - Striatal necrosis from encephalitis, measles, mycoplasma, or herpes.
- Medications:
  - Neuroleptics, oral contraceptives, stimulants.
- Inflammatory:
  - Lupus.
  - Anti-phospholipid syndrome.
- Hematologic:
  - Polycythemia vera.
  - Paraneoplastic syndromes (antibody-mediated):
  - Anti-CRMP, anti-Hu, anti-Yo, anti-LGI1, anti-NMDA.
- Genetic:
  - Autosomal dominant: Huntington's, neuroferritinopathy, benign hereditary chorea, SCA 1,2,3,17, Fahr's disease.
  - Autosomal recessive: Wilson's disease, chorea-acanthocytosis, NBIA.
  - X-linked: McLeod's syndrome, Lesch–Nyhan syndrome, Lubag or X-linked dystonia-parkinsonism (DYT3), mitochondrial diseases (Leigh's disease).

Tics
- Tics can evolve in an acute setting with encephalopathy or in other disorders such as encephalitis, prion disease, Sydenham's chorea, Huntington's disease, chorea-acanthocytosis, or NBIA.
- Simple or complex motor tics usually are seen in otherwise healthy young people with a family history of tics, obsessive compulsive disorder (OCD), or attention deficit hyperactivity disorder (ADHD).

Pathology/pathogenesis
- Essential tremor – neuroimaging and pathologic analyses have revealed cerebellar dysfunction as an important facet.
- Dystonia – striatal abnormalities, cortical inhibition, sensorimotor plasticity changes, as well as cerebellar outflow dysfunction are underpinnings of the pathogenesis.
- Myoclonus – the origin of myoclonic discharges can either be cortical, subcortical, or spinal with the aforementioned etiologies impacting numerous of these anatomic sites at various times.
- Chorea – striatal, subthalamic nucleus, and thalamocortical/brainstem dysfunction have been implicated in the pathogenesis of these involuntary movements but no unifying physiological model has been deciphered.
- Tics – believed to involve the basal ganglia-thalamocortical circuits with changes in limbic and sensorimotor interactions.

Section 2: Prevention and screening
The ethical considerations of genetic screening for Huntington's disease in asymptomatic family members are complex and need careful consideration.

Section 3: Diagnosis
See Chapter 9, Abnormal Movements and Incoordination, for the differential diagnosis of these conditions.

BOTTOM LINE/CLINICAL PEARLS
- Genetic testing for monogenic dystonia should be prompted by phenomenological categorization.
- Early-onset dystonia that generalizes without cranio-cervical involvement is suggestive of *DYT1/TOR1A* mutation, whereas those with cranio-cervical onset call into consideration *DYT6/THAP1*.
- Adult cranio-segmental onset without generalization may be related to *GNAL*, *CIZ1*, or *ANO3* mutations but these are not routinely checked due to low penetrance.
- Young-onset dystonia responsive to a levodopa trial is the hallmark for DRD, and mutations in the *GCH1* or *TH* genes should be checked to confirm the diagnosis.
- *DYT11/SGCE* and *DYT12/RDP* should be considered when myoclonus or parkinsonism with rapid rostrocaudal spread of symptoms accompanies dystonia, respectively.
- Among the paroxysmal dystonias, knowing the precipitating trigger(s) – sudden movement (*PRRT2*), exercise induced (*SLC2A1*), or caffeine/stress (MR-1) – is most helpful in guiding genetic testing.

Typical presentation

Essential tremor (ET)

ET is a kinetic tremor of the arms that can have a postural component at frequencies anywhere from 4 to12 Hz, although a 6 Hz tremor is most common. Older patients tend to have lower frequencies than younger patients. The kinetic component occurs during voluntary movements and can interfere with tasks such as writing, eating, and pouring. The tremor can also involve the head, legs, and vocal cords as well as causing mild ataxia and incoordination.

Dystonia

Dystonia can present as focal, segmental, or generalized. Focal dystonias can be divided into task-specific (i.e. writer's cramp, spasmodic dysphonia, musician's hand) or non-task-specific such as cervical dystonia and blepharospasm. Segmental dystonia affects contiguous body regions. Generalized dystonia involves at least one leg, the trunk, and another body part, while multifocal involvement, though rare, affects non-contiguous body parts. Hemidystonia refers to dystonia affecting an ipsilateral arm and leg.

Myoclonus

Clinically, myoclonus can present as spontaneous, action, reflex, rhythmic, or negative. No one type is pathognomonic of a specific etiology but often they occur in conglomeration. Deciphering the type(s) of myoclonus as well as its distribution (generalized, focal, segmental, multifocal) creates a compass for the examiner to use with the historical information to conceptualize the neuroanatomic and pathophysiologic origin.

Chorea

In chorea or chorea-athetosis, movements can flow from one body region to another, are irregular, non-suppressible, and non-stereotyped. Both proximal and distal parts of limbs can be affected, with variation in the amplitude of the movements. Patients usually present with movements that adversely impact their daily functioning. It is not uncommon for chorea to be accompanied by other neurologic disorders such as dystonia or ballism. Neurobehavioral changes may also occur.

Tic disorder

Tics can present as motor or phonic phenotypes. Motor tics can either be simple, such as unimodal stereotyped limb, neck, or facial movements, or a complex variant that consists of non-rhythmic patterns of movements. Phonic tics have a similar breakdown, with simple phonic tics being non-lexical vocalizations such as beeps, clicks, or barks, and coprolalia highlighting the complex variant.

Tourette's syndrome (TS) can be diagnosed in patients younger than age 18 with both vocal and motor tics for more than 1 year. Patients with TS not only have behavioral problems but also can manifest echolalia, echopraxia, pallalia, coprolalia, and copropraxia. Aggression and rage attacks are also on the spectrum of the condition.

Clinical diagnosis

History

- *Essential tremor:* Age of onset, location, characteristics of the tremor and conditions in which it occurs, impact on daily activities (i.e. writing, typing, holding items), and family history should be elicited. A comprehensive review of medications should focus on drugs that can exacerbate tremor, such as valproate, lithium, corticosteroids, selective serotonin reuptake inhibitors, antiemetics, and neuroleptics. Essential tremor is often suppressed by alcohol, and patients should be specifically queried about this.
- *Dystonia:* It is important to understand the timeline of progression as well as spread of dystonia to other limbs and/or cranial-facial regions. Family history, exposure to dopamine receptor blocking agents, cerebral trauma, cognitive changes, and other neurologic symptoms should be obtained.
- *Myoclonus:* See Typical presentation (above).
- *Chorea:* The movements are often first noted by family members. Central pontine myelinolysis can be associated with chorea, and in hospitalized patients the history of rapid sodium correction should be explored. Recent infections, autoimmune disorders such as lupus, and thyroid disease should be queried. Family history for abnormal movements and Huntington's disease is important.
- *Tic disorder:* It is important to ask patients who are being evaluated for tics whether a premonitory feeling is present prior to executing the tic. Daily occurrence patterns, degree of suppressibility, as well as persistence during sleep should be ascertained. Comorbid OCD or ADHD symptoms should also be queried along with a family history for psychiatric behaviors or tics, as they commonly run in families.

Physical examination

- *Essential tremor:* When evaluating tremor, the patient should first be observed with their hands at rest. Postural and kinetic components of hand tremors are investigated with enhancing maneuvers including juxtaposing arms in a wing-beat position with fingers spread apart and finger to nose repetition. Tone and rapid movements (i.e. finger and toe tapping, hand closure, and pronation-supination of each arm) are important to rule out bradykinesia. Head and vocal tremors should be specifically assessed. Vocal tremor can be assessed by having the patient say and hold the sounds "Ahh" and "Eee" while listening carefully. Tasks such as writing, holding a cup, pouring water from one cup into another, and drawing an Archimedes spiral with each hand should be performed.
- *Dystonia:* When examining a patient with dystonia, it is important that the speed, amplitude, and rhythm of the dystonia as well as its distribution be described while the patient is at rest and during the execution of certain postures (i.e. outstretched arms, writing, pouring, walking,

jogging). The use of sensory tricks, also referred to as *geste antagonistes*, as well as the presence of task specificity are pathognomonic features of dystonia. Additional features supportive of this clinical diagnosis include overflow and mirror movements.

- *Myoclonus:* Examination calls for careful observation of the patient at rest and during voluntary movements. Spontaneous myoclonus occurs at rest and can be sporadic or continuous with a wide distribution from focal to generalized. Action myoclonus appears during activation of muscle groups, with multifocal and generalized myoclonus being the commonest distribution sites. External sensory stimuli should be applied at a somesthetic, visual, or auditory level to determine whether reflex or stimulus-sensitive myoclonus is present. Rhythmic or spinal myoclonus is focal or segmental with a continuous jerking of 1–4 Hz that usually comes from spinal cord pathology. Asterixis or negative myoclonus can be elicited by having patients keep their arms outstretched with wrists hyperextended.
- *Chorea:* Amplitude of the movements, superimposed ballistic or athetotic movements, and consistency or lack thereof should be characterized. Signs of motor impersistence or inability to maintain voluntary muscle contraction are evident in a darting tongue during protrusion or milk-maid's grip. Deep tendon reflexes tend to be hung-up while a dance-like, prancing gait is also characteristic.
- *Tic disorder:* Careful observation should be employed during the visit when the patient is distracted. A patient's ability to suppress tics may mask the true phenotype. Assessing for other neurologic signs, including cognitive dysfunction, parkinsonism, chorea, or dystonia, is also important.

Disease severity classification

- *Essential tremor:* A number of assessment tools are available to determine disease severity. The commonest are the Fahn–Tolosa–Marin Tremor Rating Scale and the Rating of Spirals and Handwriting, specifically axis tilt, oscillations of the spirals, and level of tremulousness of the written letters. Physiologic measurements can be performed using accelerometry or electromyography.
- *Dystonia:* The Burke–Fahn–Marsden Scale is commonly used for generalized dystonia while the Toronto Western Spasmodic Torticollis Rating Scale (TWSTRS) is a valid rating tool for cervical dystonia.
- *Myoclonus:* The Unified Myoclonus Rating Scale can be used to quantify the severity of myoclonus.
- *Tic disorder:* The Yale Global Tic Severity Scale is used to evaluate tics.

Laboratory diagnosis: Diagnostic tests

Essential tremor

It is advisable that patients younger than 50 years be screened for Wilson's disease by checking serum ceruloplasmin, undergo evaluation for Kayser–Fleischer rings by an experienced ophthalmologist, and have their 24-hour urine copper measured.

Dystonia

Primary dystonia cannot be confirmed with laboratory results, but is based on history and examination. A workup for secondary causes should include CBC, electrolytes, renal and liver function, ESR, ANA, RPR, and serum ceruloplasmin. Brain MRI is the most valuable tool in establishing etiology. Further investigations for genetic disorders should be based on clinical findings, imaging and laboratory results, and family history.

Myoclonus

An acute or subacute generalized myoclonus should prompt an evaluation for metabolic and toxic insults such as renal and liver dysfunction, thyroid and electrolyte abnormalities, severe glycemic fluctuations, and hypoxemia. Presence of unexplained encephalopathy with signs of systemic illness warrants excluding infectious encephalitides (i.e. HSV, SSPE) and autoimmune/paraneoplastic syndromes. HIV, Whipple's disease, celiac disease, and CJD should also be considered in the setting of an acute dementing myoclonic condition.

Childhood onset or progressive young onset dementia with myoclonus requires an EEG, cerebral MRI imaging, and possibly genetic testing to evaluate for childhood epilepsy syndromes (i.e. Lennox–Gastaut syndrome, juvenile myoclonic epilepsy), mitochondrial cytopathies (i.e. MERRF), progressive myoclonic encephalopathies (i.e. Lafora disease, Unverricht–Lundborg disease, neuronal ceroid lipofuscinosis), or lysosomal storage diseases (i.e. Gaucher's disease, Tay–Sachs disease).

When additional neurologic deficits such as dystonia, bradykinesia, and rigidity are present with myoclonus, Wilson's disease, NBIA, and Huntington's disease (Westphal variant) should be under diagnostic consideration. Myoclonus in the elderly with slowly progressive dementia is primarily due to Alzheimer's disease, CBD, or olivopontocerebellar atrophy (OPCA), and manifested as polyminimyoclonus of the hands.

Neuroimaging is required when the etiology is not evident and to rule out structural and cerebrovascular causes. Spinal MRI is indicated in patients with rhythmical segmental myoclonus.

Chorea

Based on the history and clinical examination a systematic approach to the workup should be undertaken. Screening for metabolic derangements such as hyperglycemia, thyroid and parathyroid dysfunction, B12 deficiency, and electrolyte abnormalities should be done. In cases of acute onset, a toxicology screen to exclude cocaine and stimulants is also necessary.

Sydenham's chorea is the commonest infectious cause of chorea in children. Anti-streptolysin O (ASO) titers and an echocardiogram are necessary if there is a clinical suspicion. Measles, parvovirus, mycoplasma, and herpes simplex are other common causes in children, while HIV and syphilis can trigger chorea in adults.

Systemic lupus erythematosus, antiphospholipid syndrome, and Sjögren's can cause an autoimmune chorea and require evaluating for antinuclear antibody, lupus anticoagulant, anticardiolipin antibody, anti-DNA antibody, sedimentation rate, and SS-A/B. Paraneoplastic antibodies associated with chorea include antibodies against CRMP-5/CV2, Yo, Hu, NMDA, and LG1.

Suspicion for hereditary choreas requires genetic tests based on the probable inheritance pattern. The differential and supplementary tests include:
- autosomal dominant Huntington's disease;
- autosomal recessive diseases such as Wilson's disease (check 24-h urine copper and serum ceruloplasmin), chorea-acanthocytosis (check peripheral smear for acanthocytes, serum CPK), ataxia-telangiectasia (check cholesterol and alpha-fetoprotein), and brain iron accumulation disorders (i.e. pantothenate kinase-associated neurodegeneration (PKAN), aceruloplasminemia);
- X-linked disorders (e.g. McLeod's disease);
- mitochondrial diseases (e.g. Leigh's disease).

Most of these conditions manifest multiple movement disorders, cognitive changes, and multisystem dysfunction.

A brain MRI should be done in all patients to exclude structural etiologies such as subdural hematomas, striatal infarcts, and AVMs and tumors. A complete blood count may detect polycythemia vera.

Tic disorder

Tics evolving in an acute setting with encephalopathy and/or other movement disorders require an infectious workup for encephalitis, prion disease, and Sydenham's chorea. Toxicology, heavy metal screen, spinal fluid, antistreptococcal titers, and brain MRI should be obtained. Tics on the backdrop of a static encephalopathy or autism require brain imaging. Progressive neurologic deterioration with signs of chorea, parkinsonism, or dystonia should prompt genetic testing for neurodegenerative conditions such as Huntington's disease, chorea-acanthocytosis, or NBIA. The occurrence of simple or complex motor tics in an otherwise healthy young person with a family history of OCD, ADHD, or tics does not require further workup unless other neurologic signs are present.

Potential pitfalls/common errors made regarding diagnosis of disease

Essential tremor
- Distinguishing ET from Parkinson's disease, dystonia, and enhanced physiologic tremor can be challenging.
- ET patients may have mild cogwheeling but no other neurologic signs consistent with Parkinson's disease such as asymmetric bradykinesia, overt increase in tone, masked facies, and reduced arm swing when walking.
- A dystonic tremor tends to be irregular and more jerky, usually with a specific position (null point) in which the tremor is absent. Dystonia patients may use a sensory geste.
- Enhanced physiologic tremor has a low amplitude and high frequency (10–13 Hz) compared to the high-amplitude lower-frequency kinetic tremor of ET.
- Weight-bearing of the tremulous hands will dampen ET tremor, while it enhances physiologic tremor.

Myoclonus
- The phenotypic presentation of myoclonus can be mistaken for chorea, tics, or dystonic spasms.
- Tics can be as quick as myoclonus but have distinguishing features in that they are (1) suppressible, (2) have a premonitory sensation prior to being executed, and (3) always disappear in sleep.
- Chorea's flitting movements are irregular, multifocal and unpredictable compared to myoclonic jerks, while dystonic spasms are longer lasting and associated with twisting and abnormal postures.
- Cortical myoclonus sometimes causes a rare postural and action tremor on the order of 9–18 Hz. Electrophysiologic testing is often needed to clarify this diagnosis.

Chorea
- Close attention should be paid to all movements as compensatory semi-purposeful movements may camouflage chorea.

Tic disorder
- It is important that the clinician can distinguish tics and Tourette's syndrome (TS) from other conditions such as stereotypies, myoclonic jerks, automatisms of epilepsy, or psychiatric behaviors.
- Stereotypies are repetitive movement patterns that are distractible.
- Psychiatric illness such as schizophrenia and OCD can cause delusional-triggered repetitive behaviors.
- Automatisms can occur in complex partial or absence seizures.

Section 4: Treatment (Algorithms 26.1–26.3)
Treatment rationale
Essential tremor
First-line treatment is propranolol or primidone. Propranolol is discouraged in patients with comorbid asthma, depression, or aortic stenosis. Patients who are alcohol responsive do very well on primidone but anecdotal evidence suggests that those who have a modest response to 100 mg daily of primidone will not benefit from further increases. Combination treatment with primidone and propranolol with further additions of gabapentin, topiramate, or clonazepam can be considered if sufficient tremor reduction is not achieved. Thalamic deep brain stimulation (DBS) and intramuscular botulinum toxin injections are considered in medication-resistant tremor.

Dystonia
Prior to treating any dystonia, secondary causes should be ruled out. If a secondary etiology is found, treatment should be tailored towards it. Treatment of dystonia itself is symptomatic and requires a multifaceted approach. This includes assessing the patient's underlying psychiatric comorbidities (i.e. anxiety, depression), pain, and orthopedic complications. Physical therapy and use of orthotics can help prevent contractures and reduce pain. Pharmacologic therapies include levodopa, anticholinergics (i.e. trihexyphenidyl), baclofen, benzodiazepines, tetrabenazine, and muscle relaxants. Botulinum toxin injections can be used to treat focal dystonias or to alleviate disabling symptoms in segmental or generalized dystonia. Implantation of deep brain stimulators is reserved for refractory cases, particularly severe generalized dystonia in children.

Myoclonus
Treatment of myoclonus is primarily pharmacologic, with the goal of suppressing the movements in order to improve quality of life and overall functioning. Clonazepam, valproate, levetiracetam, piracetam, zonisamide, topiramate, acetazolamide, and tetrabenazine are effective for cortical and subcortical myoclonus. Spinal myoclonus is amenable to clonazepam, valproate, 5-HT, and tetrabenazine (in cases of diaphragmatic involvement). Alcohol-sensitive myoclonus and essential myoclonus have demonstrated responsiveness to clonazepam and to gamma-hydroxybutyrate. Botulinum toxin injections may be considered in treating focal myoclonus.

Chorea
Chorea treatment is predicated on the severity and clinical setting of the condition. Treating the underlying condition is the most efficacious approach. For symptomatic improvement, usually postsynaptic dopamine receptor blocking agents such as atypical or typical neuroleptics are effective, but consideration of extrapyramidal adverse effects must be weighed. The NMDA antagonist amantadine, anticonvulsants such as valproate and levetiracetam, and dopamine-depleting agents such as tetrabenazine are viable alternatives. The Parkinson's patient with dyskinesias may benefit from a reduction in levodopa dosages or addition of amantadine.

Tic disorders
Treatment of tics must take into account the age of the patient as well as potential side effects of the numerous medications available. Clonidine, guanfacine, and clonazepam are usually first-line treatments for tics. Tetrabenazine can be used in cases of refractory or breakthrough tics. Neuroleptic agents such as risperidone, haloperidol or pimozide are last resorts given their propensity to induce extrapyramidal syndromes. Tourette patients with

rage attacks or agitation often benefit from mood stabilizers such as lamotrigine or valproate. Comorbid OCD responds to SSRIs while alpha-2 agonists and occasionally stimulants are used to treat underlying ADHD.

DBS is a viable alternative when medication has failed in TS patients. Botulinum toxin injections into the vocal folds have demonstrated efficacy for coprolalia and malignant phonic tics.

Table of treatment

Essential tremor	
Oral medications (therapeutic range mg/day): • Primidone (50–1000) • Propranolol (160–320) • Topiramate (100–400) • Gabapentin (1800–3600) • Alprazolam (0.75–2.75) • Clonazepam (0.25–3.0) • Nimodipine (120)	
Deep brain stimulation	Target: nucleus ventralis intermedius (VIM)
Botulinum toxin intramuscular injections	Site: wrist flexors, supinators/pronators, wrist extensors Dose: 50–100 U
Dystonia	
Oral medications: • Trihexyphenidyl (up to 80–140 mg/day in children) • Levodopa • Baclofen, oral or intrathecal • Benzodiazepines • Tetrabenazine	
Botulinum toxin injections	Focal dystonias, symptomatic regions in segmental/generalized dystonia
Deep brain stimulation	Indications: primary generalized dystonia, cervical, myoclonus-dystonia Targets: bilateral globus pallidus interna (GPi)
Myoclonus	
Oral medications (therapeutic doses): • Clonazepam (1.5–15 mg/d) • Valproate (10–15 mg/kg/d) • Piracetam (4.8–24 g/d) • Levetiracetam (1000–3000 mg/d) • Zonisamide (300–400 mg/d) • Topiramate (250–300 mg/d) • Tetrabenazine (50–150 mg/d) • Gamma-hydroxybutyrate (4.5–9 mg/d)	
Botulinum toxin injection	Focal
Deep brain stimulation	Investigational for myoclonus-dystonia (DYT-11, essential myoclonus) Target: GPI, VIM thalamus

(Continued)

Essential tremor	
Chorea	
Oral medications: • Tetrabenazine • Amantadine • Levetiracetam • Valproate • Neuroleptics (typical or atypical)	
Tic disorders	
Oral medications (therapeutic range mg/day): • Clonidine (0.1–0.3) • Guanfacine (1–6) • Clonazepam (0.5–3) • Tetrabenazine (12.5–300) • Risperidone (0.5–6) • Pimozide (1–6) • Haloperidol (0.5–10)	
Deep brain stimulation	Investigational targets: Globus pallidus interna, centromedian nucleus-parafascicular (CM-PF) thalamic nuclei, and the anterior limb of the internal capsule
Botulinum toxin	Phonic tics – vocal cords; focal limb tics

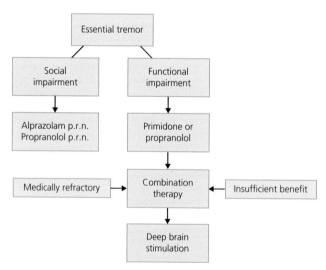

Algorithm 26.1 Treatment approaches for essential tremor.

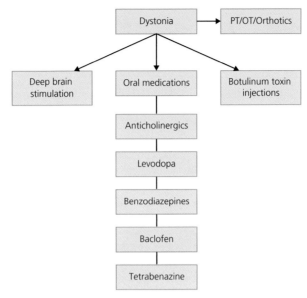

Algorithm 26.2 Treatment options for dystonia.

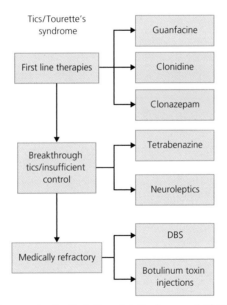

Algorithm 26.3 Treatment approaches for tics in Tourette's Syndrome and other tic disorders.

CLINICAL PEARLS

- Positive family history, response to alcohol, and absence of other neurologic features such as bradykinesia or dystonia suggest essential tremor.
- Involuntary muscle contractions causing twisting and abnormal postures and that have a sensory geste, task specificity, and null point are seen in dystonia. Always query for secondary causes of dystonia especially exposure to neuroleptics or trauma to brain or limb.
- Diagnostic evaluation of myoclonus should include a complete electrolyte panel, glucose level, liver function, and thyroid studies. Infectious and paraneoplastic investigations are predicated on clinical suspicion.
- In patients with chorea, essential historical information includes medication (especially dopamine receptor blockers) and recreational drug use, and family history, as well as neurobehavioral changes.
- Tics are rapid stereotyped motor movements or vocalizations that can be volitionally suppressed and accompanied by a premonitory sensation. Tics in the presence of encephalopathy warrant a brain MRI and CSF examination in addition to electrolyte panel, thyroid studies, and inflammatory markers to investigate potential infectious, structural (stroke, tumors), genetic, and toxic etiologies.

Section 5: Special populations
Not applicable for this chapter.

Section 6: Prognosis

BOTTOM LINE/CLINICAL PEARLS

- The prognosis for nearly all of these conditions is related to the underlying etiology as well as their level of severity.
- Screening for reversible causes in the appropriate clinical setting is important.
- Confirmation of a neurodegenerative process requires close monitoring and comprehensive symptomatic treatment.

Additional material for this chapter can be found online at:
www.mountsinaiexpertguides.com

This includes a case study with two accompanying video clips, multiple choice questions, and a reading list.

CHAPTER 27

Alzheimer's Disease and Frontotemporal Dementia

Sam Gandy

Icahn School of Medicine at Mount Sinai; and James J. Peters VA Medical Center, New York, NY, USA

OVERALL BOTTOM LINE

- The most common differential diagnosis of dementia involves the distinction among Alzheimer's disease (AD), frontotemporal dementia (FTD, also known as Pick's disease), and vascular dementia (VaD).
- AD and VaD may frequently coexist.
- The clinical phenotype of FTD may be caused by either frontotemporal lobar degeneration (FTLD) or AD pathology, and the age at onset usually provides a major clue, with AD most frequently presenting in patients over age 75 and FTLD most frequently presenting around age 60.

Section 1: Background
Definition of disease

- AD, VaD, and FTLD are defined by their neuropathologic findings. Individual patients with these disorders can have disturbances of short-term memory, behavior, and executive function. In general, each is characterized by differences in the prominence of these features.
- AD affects about half of the over-85 population and is characterized by a typical short-term amnestic syndrome and the accumulation of amyloid plaques and neurofibrillary tangles.
- FTLD is a rare cause of dementia, presenting around age 60, and involving disorders of language and behavior out of proportion to any amnestic disorder. FTLD is a pure tauopathy with no amyloid plaques. The intraneuronal inclusions also include aggregates of TDP43, ubiquitin, and other proteins.
- VaD may present alone or as part of a mixed dementia in which AD and VaD coexist. There is a prominent dysexecutive syndrome out of proportion to the amnestic syndrome.

Disease classification
AD: Clinical, pathologic, and genetic classification

- Alzheimer's is generally classified clinically as early-onset AD (before age 65 years) or late-onset AD (after age 65 years).
- AD can be divided into three groups according to genetic etiology. All forms of AD have identical neuropathology:
  - *Deterministic genes* are responsible for typical familial AD and include the genes encoding amyloid precursor protein (*APP*) and presenilins 1 and 2 (*PSEN1*, *PSEN2*). When mutations are present in these genes, their actions are completely penetrant. Onset tends to be in the 40s and 50s but onset as young as 18 years is known.

Mount Sinai Expert Guides: Neurology, First Edition. Edited by Stuart C. Sealfon, Rajeev Motiwala, and Charles B. Stacy.
© 2016 John Wiley & Sons, Ltd. Published 2016 by John Wiley & Sons, Ltd.
Companion website: www.mountsinaiexpertguides.com

- A single *major risk factor gene* has been identified: the epsilon 4 polymorphism in the apolipoprotein E gene (*APOE*). *APOE* epsilon 4 is present in about half of all patients with late-onset AD. Each copy of *APOE* epsilon 4 triples the risk for AD. Some *APOE* epsilon 4 heterozygotes escape AD, but most *APOE* epsilon 4 homozygotes develop AD. The only exception is a family in Iceland with a protection mutation in APP that reduces amyloid beta accumulation by 50%.
- In a recent genome-wide association study of about 75,000 AD patients, about two dozen *linked genes* were identified with statistically significant impact on risk. However, the impact of each is small compared to that of *APOE* epsilon 4.

FTLD: Clinical classification
- Behavioral variant FTD (bvFTD) can resemble mania, depression, or schizophrenia and may progress without any measurable cognitive change. There may be hypersexuality; life expectancy is normal.
- Primary progressive aphasia (PPA) has several subtypes:
  - Semantic dementia (SD) patients have fluent speech, progressive impairment of single-word comprehension, preserved articulatory abilities, and a multimodal breakdown of semantic memory. They may show behavioral changes in the course of the disease similar to bvFTD and may become egocentric and develop fixed daily routines.
  - Progressive non-fluent aphasia (PNFA) patients present with apraxia of speech or expressive agrammatism. Single-word comprehension and object knowledge are relatively preserved, and behavioral symptoms are less common.
  - Logopenic or phonological variant (LPA) is a more recently defined subtype of PPA characterized by a slow rate of speech output, word-finding difficulties, deficits in sentence repetition, and occasional phonemic errors in spontaneous speech and naming, whereas motor speech, expressive grammar, and single-word comprehension are relatively spared.

FTLD: Clinico-genetic and clinico-pathologic classification
There are ongoing efforts to link clinical phenotypes, pathologic phenotypes, and genotypes. FTLD is a neuropathologically heterogeneous disorder, which can be divided into two major subtypes: *FTLD with tau-positive inclusions* (*FTLD-tau*), and *FTLD with ubiquitin-positive and TDP-43-positive, but tau-negative inclusions* (*FTLD-TDP*). FTLD is increasingly recognized to represent a spectrum of overlapping clinical and neuropathologic disorders that include:
- ALS: amyotrophic lateral sclerosis
- FTD-MND: FTD-motor neuron multiplex disease
- SD: semantic dementia FTD
- bvFTD: behavioral variant FTD
- PNFA: primary non-fluent aphasia FTD
- CBD: corticobasal degeneration
- PSP: progressive supranuclear palsy
  The genetic mutations associated with these clinical syndromes include:
- *MAPT* (microtubule-associated protein tau) – see Figure 27.1.
- *TDP-43* (TAR DNA-binding protein 43) – see Figure 27.1.
- *GRN* (progranulin) – see Figure 27.1.
- *VCP* (valosin-containing protein) – mutations associated with frontotemporal dementia.
- *FUS* (fused in sarcoma) – see Figure 27.1.
- *CHMP2B* (charged multivesicular body protein 2B) – mutations associated with FTLD.

The relationship among these clinical, genetic, and pathologic phenotypes is complex and evolving. A diagrammatic summary illustrating some of the proposed relationships among these spectrum disorders is shown in Figure 27.1.

VaD classification

The role of vascular disease in dementia is especially challenging since no molecular markers are available as affirmative evidence of the diagnosis and since VaD increases the risk for AD. Criteria have recently been proposed for diagnosing a predominantly vascular etiology of dementia (VaD), and these are shown in Box 27.1.

BOX 27.1 CRITERIA FOR DIAGNOSING A PREDOMINANTLY VASCULAR ETIOLOGY OF DEMENTIA (VAD)

A. One of the following clinical features:

   1. The onset of the cognitive deficits is temporally related to cerebrovascular events (CVEs). (Onset is often abrupt with a stepwise or fluctuating course owing to multiple such events, with cognitive deficits persisting beyond 3 months after the event. However, subcortical ischemic pathology may produce a picture of gradual onset and slowly progressive course, in which case A2 applies.) The evidence of CVEs is one of the following:

     (a) Documented history of a stroke, with cognitive decline temporally associated with the event.

     (b) Physical signs consistent with stroke (e.g. hemiparesis, lower facial weakness, Babinski sign, sensory deficit including visual field defect, pseudobulbar syndrome – supranuclear weakness of muscles of face, tongue, and pharynx, spastic dysarthria, swallowing difficulties, and emotional incontinence).

   2. Evidence for decline is prominent in speed of information processing, complex attention, and/or frontal-executive functioning in the absence of history of a stroke or transient ischemic attack. One of the following features is additionally present:

     (a) Early presence of a gait disturbance (small-step gait or *marche petits pas*, or magnetic, apraxic-ataxic, or parkinsonian gait); this may also manifest as unsteadiness and frequent, unprovoked falls.

     (b) Early urinary frequency, urgency, and other urinary symptoms not explained by urologic disease.

     (c) Personality and mood changes: abulia, depression, or emotional incontinence.

B. Presence of significant neuroimaging (MRI or CT) evidence of cerebrovascular disease (one of the following):

   1. One large vessel infarct is sufficient for mild VCD, and 2+ large vessel infarcts are generally necessary for VaD (or major VCD).

   2. An extensive or strategically placed single infarct, typically in the thalamus or basal ganglia, may be sufficient for VaD.

   3. Multiple lacunar infarcts (>2) outside the brainstem; 1–2 lacunes may be sufficient if strategically placed or in combination with extensive white matter lesions.

   4. Extensive and confluent white matter lesions.

   5. Strategically placed intracerebral hemorrhage, or >2 intracerebral hemorrhages.

   6. Combination of the above.

Exclusion criteria (for VaD)

1. History

     (a) Early onset of memory deficit and progressive worsening of memory and other cognitive functions such as language (transcortical sensory aphasia), motor skills (apraxia), and perception (agnosia) in the absence of corresponding focal lesions on brain imaging or history of vascular events.

     (a) Early and prominent parkinsonian features suggestive of Lewy body disease.

     (b) History strongly suggestive of another primary neurologic disorder, such as multiple sclerosis, encephalitis, or toxic or metabolic disorder, sufficient to explain the cognitive impairment.

2. Neuroimaging

     (a) Absent or minimal cerebrovascular lesions on CT or MRI.

3. Other medical disorders severe enough to account for memory and related symptoms:
   (a) Other disease of sufficient severity to cause cognitive impairment, e.g. brain tumor, multiple sclerosis, encephalitis.
   (b) Major depression, with a temporal association between cognitive impairment and the likely onset of depression.
   (c) Toxic and metabolic abnormalities, all of which may require specific investigations.
4. Other medical disorders severe enough to account for memory and related symptoms:
   (a) Other disease of sufficient severity to cause cognitive impairment, e.g. brain tumor, multiple sclerosis, encephalitis
   (b) Major depression, with a temporal association between cognitive impairment and the likely onset of depression
   (c) Toxic and metabolic abnormalities, all of which may require specific investigations
5. The presence of biomarkers for Alzheimer's disease (cerebrospinal Abeta and pTau levels or amyloid imaging at accepted thresholds) exclude diagnosis of probable VaD, and indicate AD with CVD.

Source: Sachdev P, Kalaria R, O'Brien J, Skoog I, Alladi S, Black SE, et al. Diagnostic criteria for vascular cognitive disorders: a VASCOG statement. Alzheimer Dis Assoc Disord 2014 Jul–Sep;28(3):206–18. Reproduced with permission from Wolters Kluwer Health.

Incidence
- Age 45–64:
  - All causes of dementia: 350 per 100,000 adults
  - AD: 250 per 100,000 adults
  - VaD: 60 per 100,000 adults
  - FTD: 20 per 100,000 adults
- Over age 65:
  - All cause dementia: 3500 per 100,000 adults
  - AD: 2500 per 100,000 adults
  - VaD: 600 per 100,000 adults

Economic impact
In 2010, the worldwide cost of all cause dementia was over $600 billion.

Etiology
- Alzheimer's disease risk factors:
  - 3% of AD cases due to mutations in *APP*, *PS1*, *PS2*
  - 50% of AD cases associated with *APOE4* polymorphisms
  - 20 other high-risk genes, but all less potent than *APOE4*
  - Hypercholesterolemia
  - Hypertension
  - Obesity
  - Diabetes
  - Sedentary lifestyle
  - Social isolation
  - Mentally inactive, low educational level

- Frontotemporal dementia:
  - Associated with mutations in *GRN, MAPT, FUS, TDP43, CHMP2B, VCP*.
- Vascular dementia major risk factors:
  - Hypertension
  - Atrial fibrillation
  - Diabetes
  - Hypercholesterolemia
  - Cigarette smoking
  - Prior stroke or myocardial infarction

Pathology/pathogenesis

VaD is caused by the accumulated effects of multiple small or large cerebral infarctions or diffuse white matter ischemic damage. The mechanisms by which genetic and idiopathic AD and FTLD develop are subjects of intense study and debate, with more known about AD.

The pathology of AD includes amyloid plaques that are derived from abnormal beta amyloid deposition and neurofibrillary tangles that are composed of abnormal tau protein aggregates. Elements proposed to contribute to the pathophysiology of AD include:

- Changes in beta amyloid (Aβ) metabolism:
  - Increase in total Aβ.
  - Increase in the ratio of specific beta amyloid fragments (Aβ42/Aβ40) ratio.
  - Reduced degradation.
- Oligomerization of Aβ42 and diffuse plaque deposits.
- Effects of soluble oligomers on neuronal function.
- Aberrant tau protein phosphorylation and dephosphorylation.
- Propagation of abnormal oligomers, neuronal dysfunction, neuronal loss, and neurofibrillary tangle formation.

Predictive/risk factors

Disease: risk factor(s)	Comment
AD: *APOE4*	Each *APOE4* allele triples risk
AD: *APP, PS1, PS2*, Down's syndrome	Complete penetrance early onset AD
FTLD: *MAPT, GRN, FUS, TDP43*	Complete penetrance FTLD

Section 2: Prevention and screening

BOTTOM LINE/CLINICAL PEARLS
- Improved cardiovascular health and maintaining social and mental activity reduce the risk and severity of both AD and VaD.
- Physical activity prescription: three sessions per week, 30 min per session, e.g. brisk walking or weight training, slows progression of AD or VaD.
- No evidence that early diagnosis or early initiation of cholinesterase inhibitors changes course.
- Vitamin E (2000 IU/day) slows loss of self-care, activities of daily living.
- Vitamin E does not reduce the incidence of mild cognitive impairment; its benefit is confined to patients with mild stage dementia or later.
- No effective screening or prevention for FTD.

Section 3: Diagnosis

BOTTOM LINE/CLINICAL PEARLS
- Alzheimer's disease (AD) may initially present with isolated memory disturbance.
- Frontotemporal dementia (Pick's disease, FTD) typically presents with personality change and language disturbance.
- Sometimes dementia presents as aphasia.
- Amnestic mild cognitive impairment (MCI), when restricted to memory, is a frequent harbinger of dementia. The transition from MCI to mild dementia is usually considered to be the progression of the amnestic disorder to a point that interferes with daily function.
- Most common differential will be Alzheimer's versus vascular. Remember that both may coexist, and that vascular dementia increases the risk for Alzheimer's.
- Patients presenting in their 60s with aphasia in addition to impulse control often have FTD.

Differential diagnosis of AD, FTD, and VaD

For complete differential diagnosis see Chapter 7.

Typical presentation

Dementia patients often lose insight into their illnesses and are brought in by caregivers, who are the main sources of the complaints.
- If language or behavioral changes are preponderant, or if the patient is relatively young (i.e. around age 60 years), frontotemporal dementia should be considered.
- Alzheimer's is much more common, typically involves prominent amnesia, and typically affects people over age 70 years.
- VaD may present with stepwise progression of cognitive deficits and have other associated focal symptoms and signs. Often coexists with AD.
- Please refer to Chapter 7 for an overview of the history, physical evaluation, and diagnostic testing of dementia patients.

Clinical diagnosis

History

Disease	Symptoms	Duration/tempo	Other key features
Alzheimer's disease	Amnesia for recent events	Subacute-chronic	Often lack of insight, noted typically by a family member, may have a positive family history
Frontotemporal dementia	Behavioral or language changes out of proportion to dementia	Subacute-chronic	Often lack insight, age at onset around 60 years, genotyping of *MAPT*, *PRGRN*, *C9ORF*, *TDP43*
VaD	Varied cognitive deficits, executive function affected more than memory, other focal neurologic symptoms	Evolution over years, classically stepwise onset, associated with strokes, but may be progressive	Vascular risk factors, history of previous stroke or strokes

Physical examination
- Alzheimer's disease: Mini mental status examination (MMSE) abnormal, remainder of examination normal.
- Vascular dementia: MMSE abnormal, may be focal motor signs.
- Frontotemporal dementia: MMSE abnormal, disinhibition or aphasia.

Laboratory diagnosis (Figures 27.2 and 27.3)

Alzheimer's disease	Atrophy on MRI; amyloid biomarker in CSF or on amyloid imaging, genetic testing for *APP*, *PSEN1*, *PSEN2* may be definitive if mutation detected
Vascular dementia	Evidence of multiple strokes or white matter changes as well as atrophy on MRI; no biomarker evidence for amyloidosis
Frontotemporal dementia	MRI evidence for frontal or temporal atrophy, PET shows hypometabolism (Figure 27.2); genetic testing; amyloid studies negative

Potential pitfalls/common errors made regarding diagnosis of disease
- Missing a reversible dementia is an important "must avoid" in dementia evaluation and care.

Section 4: Treatment
Treatment rationale
The response to cholinesterase inhibitors is evaluated in most AD and VaD patients. Patients are titrated onto a cholinesterase inhibitor over 1 month. Memantine is typically added as well. Evidence suggests that benefit from these wears off over 18 months, but many patients are maintained indefinitely on both drugs.

Antidepressants and antipsychotics are used for symptom control. Regularization of sleep is often a high priority for the patient and caregivers. However, many patients have paradoxical responses or increased sensitivity and cognitive side effects with sedative and hypnotic medications.

When to hospitalize
- Avoid if possible due to a high propensity toward delirium and agitation when the patient is taken out of her or his accustomed environment. May be necessary due to acute decompensation or intercurrent medical illness.
- Hospitalization often precipitates placement for chronic care at moderate-stage disease as a result of safety, care regimen, and monitoring concerns, as well as disruptive behavior.

Prevention/management of complications
Complications of dementia include depression, agitation, anxiety, and psychosis. No medications are specifically approved for use in these conditions in the geriatric population. SSRIs, benzodiazepines, and atypical antipsychotics are used to manage symptoms in the same fashion that they are used to manage these symptoms in other settings.

The main point of caution is that atypical antipsychotics (quetiapine, risperidone) have a Black Box warning since they have increased risks for side effects of stroke and extrapyramidal disorders in the elderly. As such, these drugs are usually used as last resorts and only with the expressed consent of the next of kin.

Nuedexta is a new drug combination that is promising for behavioral management in Alzheimer's disease. Nuedexta does NOT have a black box warning and is already approved for pseudobulbar palsy.

See also Section 9: Guidelines.

Table of treatment: Cholinesterase inhibitors and NMDA receptor blockade for treatment of AD

Agent	Suggested dose	Side effects	Comments and cautions
Cholinesterase inhibitors			
Donepezil hydrochloride (Aricept) • Oral; FDA-approved for mild, moderate, and severe Alzheimer's disease	Start: 5 mg daily Escalation: 10 mg daily after 4–6 weeks if tolerated	Nausea, vomiting, and diarrhea (sometimes can be reduced when taken with food, reducing dose, slower titration, or dividing the dose to twice daily) Muscle cramps Urinary incontinence Syncope Bradycardia (doses >10 mg/day) Fatigue Sleep disturbance Vivid dreams	5 mg dose is effective. Caution when using in people with cardiac conduction conditions such as symptomatic bradycardia, or with a history of falls or syncope (may want to avoid, or seek cardiac consult)
Galantamine (Razadyne, Razadyne ER) • Oral; FDA-approved for mild and moderate Alzheimer's disease only	• Immediate release: Start: 4 mg twice daily. Escalation: 8 mg twice daily after 4 weeks. May increase to 16 mg twice daily after an additional 4 weeks. Max.: 24 mg/day • Extended release: Note: Razadyne ER is once daily. Start: 8 mg daily or 4 mg twice daily. Escalation: 16 mg daily after 4 weeks or 8 mg twice daily after 4 weeks May increase to 24 mg per day (32 mg per day not more effective in Alzheimer's disease)	Same as for donepezil Sleep disturbances may be less compared to donepezil	Starting dose is not therapeutic. Maximum dose 16 mg/day if renal impairment is present Other cautions same as donepezil

	Dosing	Side effects	Comments
Rivastigmine tartrate (Exelon) • Oral; FDA-approved for mild and moderate Alzheimer's disease only	Start: 1.5 mg twice daily. Escalation: 3 mg twice daily after 4 weeks. May increase to 4.5 mg twice daily after an additional 4 weeks. May increase to 6 mg twice daily after an additional 4 weeks	Nausea, vomiting, and diarrhea (must be taken with food) More nausea and vomiting than with other ChEIs Anorexia May be less muscle cramping than with other ChEIs Bradycardia (rare at therapeutic doses) Other side effects the same as other ChEIs	Starting dose is not therapeutic. Cautions same as for donepezil and galantamine
Rivastigmine (Exelon) • Transdermal; FDA-approved for mild and moderate Alzheimer's disease only	Start: 4.6 mg/24 hour patch daily. Escalation: 9.5 mg/24 hour patch daily after 1 month. When switching from oral to the patch: for a total daily dose of less than 6 mg oral rivastigmine switch to 4.6 mg/24 hour patch (first check medication adherence); for a total daily dose of 6–12 mg of oral rivastigmine switch to 9.5 mg/24 hour patch Apply the first patch on the day following the last oral dose	Nausea, vomiting, at 4.6 mg/24 hour patch same as with placebo Other side effects the same as donepezil and galantamine	Starting dose is not therapeutic. Cautions same as for donepezil and galantamine
NMDA receptor blocker			
Memantine hydrochloride (Namenda) • Oral solution; FDA-approved for moderate and severe Alzheimer's disease only	Start: 5 mg once daily Escalation: The recommended target dose is 20 mg/day. The dose should be increased in 5 mg increments to 10 mg/day (5 mg twice daily), 15 mg/day (5 mg and 10 mg as separate doses), and 20 mg/day (10 mg twice daily). The minimum recommended interval between dose increases is 1 week	Confusion, insomnia, headache, constipation (one or more of these is significant – all occur in practice)	Starting dose is not therapeutic The dosage of memantine hydrochloride shown to be effective in controlled clinical trials is 20 mg/day

Source: Data from FDA-approved package inserts. Modified from the California Workgroup on Guidelines for Alzheimer's Disease Management. Guideline for Alzheimer's Disease Management. State of California, Department of Public Health. 2008. http://www.alz.org/socal/images/professional_GuidelineFullReport.pdf. Accessed January 06, 2016.

Section 5: Special populations
Not applicable for this topic.

Section 6: Prognosis

> **BOTTOM LINE/CLINICAL PEARLS**
> - Average time from diagnosis to death in AD or FTD is 10 years.
> - Institutionalization is usually prompted by uncontrollable behavior or nursing needs.
> - There is a relentless downward course and ultimately, vegetative state and death.

Section 7: Reading list
Key reading sources for this chapter can be found online at www.mountsinaiexpertguides.com

Suggested websites
Alzheimer's Association: https://www.alz.org/
The Association for Frontotemporal Degeneration: http://www.theaftd.org/

Section 8: Guidelines

Title	Source	Weblink
Guideline for Alzheimer's Disease Management	California Workgroup, Final report 2008	http://www.alz.org/socal/images/professional_GuidelineFullReport.pdf
Toward defining the preclinical stages of Alzheimer's disease: recommendations from the National Institute on Aging-Alzheimer's Association workgroups on diagnostic guidelines for Alzheimer's disease.	Sperling RA, Aisen PS, Beckett LA, et al., 2011	http://www.ncbi.nlm.nih.gov/pubmed/10921745
Advancing research diagnostic criteria for Alzheimer's disease: the IWG-2 criteria	DuboisB, Feldman HH, Jacova C, et al., 2014	http://www.ncbi.nlm.nih.gov/pubmed/24849862

International society guidelines for dementia
The main differences between the international working group (IWG) criteria and the NIA-Alzheimer's Association (NIA-AA) criteria involve the incorporation of biomarkers into the latter criteria. Guidelines for diagnosis and treatment are well summarized in http://www.alz.org/socal/images/professional_GuidelineFullReport.pdf, accessed January 01, 2016.

Section 9: Evidence for effectiveness of therapies

Type of evidence	Title and comment	Weblink
Double-blind, placebo-controlled trial	A 24-week, double-blind, placebo-controlled trial of donepezil in patients with Alzheimer's disease. Donepezil Study Group. **Comment**: Key evidence for effectiveness of donepezil in AD	http://www.ncbi.nlm.nih.gov/pubmed/9443470
Double-blind, placebo-controlled, parallel-group, randomized clinical trial	Effect of vitamin E and memantine on functional decline in Alzheimer disease: the TEAM-AD VA cooperative randomized trial **Comment**: Findings suggest benefit of alpha-tocopherol in mild to moderate AD by slowing functional decline and decreasing caregiver burden	http://www.ncbi.nlm.nih.gov/pubmed/24381967

Section 10: Images

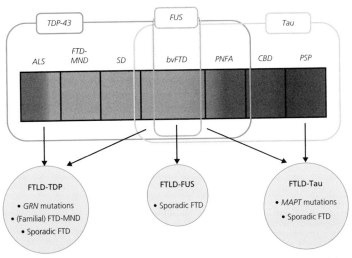

Figure 27.1 Relationship of genetic, neuropathologic, and clinical forms of frontotemporal dementia (FTD). ALS, amyotrophic lateral sclerosis; FTD-MND, FTD-motor neuron multiplex disease; SD, semantic dementia FTD; bvFTD, behavioral variant FTD; PNFA, primary non-fluent aphasia FTD; CBD, corticobasal degeneration; PSP, progressive supranuclear palsy. Note: The overlap with CBD and PSP is largely genetic but without an obvious clinical relationship between FTD and either CBD or PSP. A color version of this figure is available on the companion website. *Source*: Seelaar H, et al. 2011. Reproduced with permission of the BMJ Publishing Group Ltd.

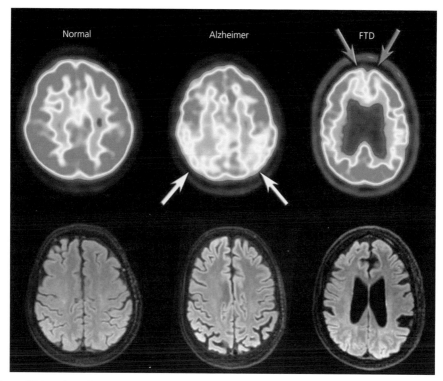

Figure 27.2 FDG-PET imaging in a normal subject, and in patients with either Alzheimer's disease or frontotemporal lobar degeneration (FTD). Arrows indicate marked parieto-occipital hypometabolism in AD and frontal hypometabolism in FTD compared to normal. A color version of this figure is available on the companion website. *Source*: http://www.radiologyassistant.nl/en/p43dbf6d16f98d/dementia-role-of-mri. html. Reproduced with permission of *Radiology Assistant*.

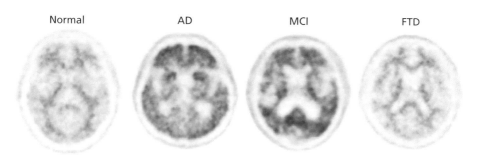

Figure 27.3 Florbetapir imaging in a normal subject, and in patients with Alzheimer's disease, with mild cognitive impairment (MCI) due to Alzheimer's disease, or frontotemporal lobar degeneration (FTD). Abnormally increased signal is seen in AD and in this case of MCI, which supports the diagnosis of early AD. *Source*: Kim et al. 2009. Molecular Imaging in Neurodegenerative Diseases. © 2009 Korean Medical Association.

Additional material for this chapter can be found online at: www.mountsinaiexpertguides.com

This includes advice for patients, a case study, multiple choice questions, and a reading list. Also included are color versions of Figures 27.1 and 27.2.

CHAPTER 28

Cerebellar and Brainstem Disorders

Florence Ching-Fen Chang[1] and Catherine Cho[2]
[1]Icahn School of Medicine at Mount Sinai, New York, NY, USA
[2]NYU Langone Medical Center, New York, NY, USA

OVERALL BOTTOM LINE

- A large number of diseases can affect posterior fossa (cerebellar and brainstem) function.
- The first steps in the diagnosis of disease in the posterior fossa are based on localization, disease tempo, and associated findings.
- Acute cerebellar and brainstem syndromes, particularly when associated with an altered level of consciousness, require urgent neuroimaging to exclude acute hydrocephalus or impending herniation and may require immediate neurosurgical intervention.
- Bilateral internuclear ophthalmoplegia (INO; i.e. unilateral failure of adduction, contralateral nystagmus) is most commonly seen in multiple sclerosis.
- In patients with vertigo, it is crucial to distinguish peripheral inner ear problems from vestibular nerve and brainstem causes. A positive head impulse test denotes a peripheral cause, whereas skew deviation usually indicates a brainstem localization.
- Alcoholic cerebellar degeneration causes gait ataxia out of proportion to appendicular dysmetria.
- A subacute cerebellar syndrome in a woman should prompt a careful search for ovarian or breast cancer. Early detection of carcinoma and its treatment in paraneoplastic cerebellar degeneration can prevent irreversible cerebellar function.
- CT scan is relatively insensitive for visualization of posterior fossa pathology and MRI is the preferred modality when clinically feasible.
- Acute cerebellar or brainstem symptoms and signs need urgent CT brain and vertebrobasilar imaging to exclude vascular pathology and vertebrobasilar artery dissection or thrombosis.
- To prevent Korsakoff's syndrome, administer intravenous thiamine before intravenous glucose in patients with alcohol abuse presenting to the hospital with acute medical illness.

Section 1: Background
Definition of disease

A diverse group of diseases can affect the cerebellum or brainstem. These include: vascular disease, infection, toxin or drug toxicity, autoimmune disorders, metabolic abnormalities, neoplasia, and degenerative conditions.

Mount Sinai Expert Guides: Neurology, First Edition. Edited by Stuart C. Sealfon, Rajeev Motiwala, and Charles B. Stacy.
© 2016 John Wiley & Sons, Ltd. Published 2016 by John Wiley & Sons, Ltd.
Companion website: www.mountsinaiexpertguides.com

Disease classification

Cerebellar and brainstem diseases can be classified by general etiologic categories. A classification of representative diseases affecting these structures follows:

- Cerebrovascular disease
  - Hemorrhage
  - Ischemic stroke
  - Vascular malformations
- Toxin exposure
  - Alcohol
  - Anticonvulsants
  - Benzodiazepines
  - Mercury
  - Lead
- Autoimmune disorders
  - Multiple sclerosis and neuromyelitis optica (NMO)
  - Behçet's disease
  - Sjögren's syndrome
  - CLIPPERS (chronic lymphocytic inflammation with pontine perivascular enhancement responsive to steroids)
  - Anti-GAD antibody associated cerebellar syndrome
  - Celiac disease
- Metabolic disorders
  - Hypothyroidism
  - Central pontine myelinolysis
- Inherited disease
  - Spinocerebellar ataxia
  - Friedreich's ataxia
  - Fragile X associated tremor-ataxia (FXTAS)
- Neoplasia
  - Primary central nervous system neoplasia
  - Secondary metastasis
  - Paraneoplastic syndrome
- Degenerative disease
  - Multiple system atrophy.

Section 2: Prevention and screening

Not applicable for this topic.

Section 3: Diagnosis, etiology, and treatment (Algorithms 28.1 and 28.2)

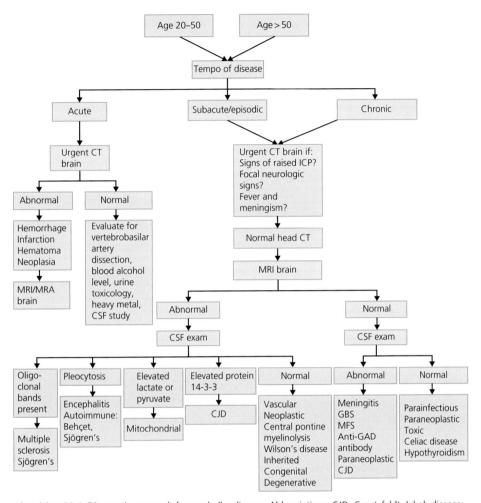

Algorithm 28.1 Diagnostic approach for cerebellar disease. Abbreviations: CJD, Creutzfeldt–Jakob disease; GBS, Guillain–Barré syndrome; ICP, intracranial pressure; MFS, Miller Fisher syndrome.

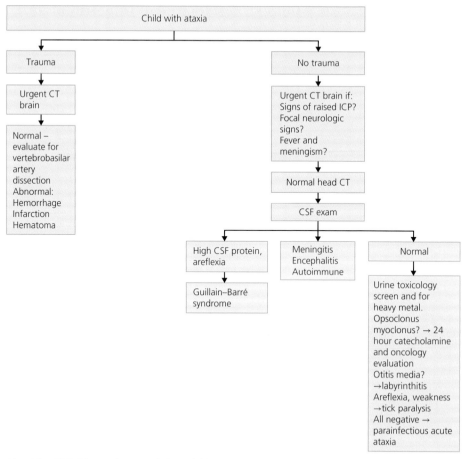

Algorithm 28.2 Diagnostic approach for a child with ataxia

BOTTOM LINE/CLINICAL PEARLS
- The tempo of the disease and age of onset are important clues for etiology.
- An acute presentation of cerebellar or brainstem features is most likely due to vascular or toxic etiologies.
- A subacute presentation (days to weeks) is usually secondary to infectious, autoimmune, neoplastic, paraneoplastic, metabolic, or toxic etiologies.
- In chronic presentation of cerebellar or brainstem disorder, consider inherited, toxic, neoplastic, or neurodegenerative causes.
- Childhood onset is most likely congenital, metabolic, infectious, or posterior fossa tumors.
- Young adult onset is most likely demyelination, alcohol toxicity, or hereditary ataxias.
- Over age 50 is most commonly ischemic or hemorrhagic stroke and more frequently is due to neoplasia or neurodegenerative or autoimmune disease.
- These disorders present with common constellations of signs and symptoms:
- Cerebellar symptoms include: slurred speech, vertigo, imbalance, falls, incoordination of upper extremities, action tremor.

- Cerebellar signs include:
  - dysarthria
  - dysdiadochokinesis
  - ataxia of gait or trunk
  - dysmetria
  - action tremor
  - hypotonia
  - nystagmus that changes direction with different direction of gaze.
- Brainstem symptoms include:
  - diplopia
  - dysphagia
  - unilateral or bilateral weakness
  - disturbance of consciousness
  - unilateral facial numbness and contralateral body numbness.
- Brainstem signs include:
  - altered level of consciousness;
  - cranial neuropathies;
  - ipsilateral cranial nerve findings with contralateral hemiparesis;
  - Horner's syndrome;
  - ipsilateral facial sensory loss and contralateral body pain and temperature loss;
  - unilateral or bilateral weakness;
  - ataxia.

Vascular disease

CLINICAL PEARLS
- Consider vascular disease with acute onset, risk factors, and deficits that follow a vascular territory.
- Classical brainstem vascular syndromes have been described, e.g. lateral medullary syndrome (ipsilateral facial sensory loss, Horner's, contralateral sensory loss, skew deviation, dysphagia, ataxia).
- Large vessel disease can progress from mild symptoms to catastrophic infarction.
- Both cerebellar hemorrhage and cerebellar infarction with edema can lead to sudden decompensation and death, which may be preventable by immediate neurosurgical intervention.

Disease classification
- Ischemic stroke
- Hemorrhage
- Cerebral venous thrombosis
- Vascular malformations.

Pathogenesis
- The mechanisms for cerebellar or brainstem infarction are: cardiogenic embolism – 30%; artery to artery embolism – 20%; large artery atherothrombosis – 23%; with the remainder idiopathic or other causes.

- Hemorrhagic stroke secondary to hypertension accounts for half of hemorrhagic strokes, and vascular malformations cause one-fifth of cases.
- Venous thrombosis may occur due to hypercoagulable states or adjacent inflammation.
- Vascular malformations most commonly present with hemorrhage.

Diagnostic tests

- Urgent cerebral CT or MRI as well as CT or MR angiography or conventional angiography when needed to establish diagnosis or guide therapy.
- CBC to exclude thrombocytosis, thrombocytopenia, or polycythemia.
- EKG for atrial fibrillation.
- Erythrocyte sedimentation rate is elevated in vasculitis, but is non-specific.
  For a full discussion of vascular diseases, see Chapter 20.

Infections

> **CLINICAL PEARLS**
> - Brainstem or cerebellar infection causes subacute cerebellar or brainstem dysfunction.
> - Identify HIV risk factors, history of opportunistic infection.
> - Post-viral acute cerebellar ataxia is more common in young children. In adults this can be caused by Epstein–Barr virus (EBV) and in children most commonly by varicella infection. Other causes include roseola, enterovirus, rubeola (measles), parvovirus, and mycoplasma.
> - Progressive ataxia, fever, diarrhea, and arthritis may be due to Whipple's disease (*Tropheryma whippleii* infection), which can be excluded by stool PCR assay.
> - Lyme borreliosis may rarely involve the cerebellum and cause chronic ataxia.
> - A brainstem or cerebellar abscess can present with localized brainstem or cerebellar features or hydrocephalus.

Etiology

Causes of infection of the brainstem and cerebellum include:
- HIV
- Prion
- Varicella zoster
- Epstein–Barr virus (EBV)
- HHV-6
- Measles
- Mumps
- Herpes simplex – although having a preference for the frontal and temporal lobes, brainstem infection can occur
- Coxsackievirus
- Enterovirus
- Enteric fever
- Echovirus
- Poliovirus
- Typhoid fever (isn't this the same as enteric fever-typhoid and paratyphoid?)
- Parvovirus B19
- Rotavirus
- Mycoplasma

- Legionella
- Borreliosis
- *Listeria*
- *Schistosoma*, especially *S. japonicum.*

Pathogenesis
- Varicella zoster is the most common cause of acute cerebellitis and comprises one-quarter of cases. Other viruses, including HIV, EBV, measles, mumps, herpes simplex, coxsackievirus, enterovirus, enteric fever, echovirus, poliovirus, typhoid fever, parvovirus B19, and rotavirus have been reported. Mycoplasmas, *Legionella*, borreliosis, and prion diseases like Creutzfeldt–Jakob disease (CJD) have also been implicated. HIV causes Purkinje cell loss in the cerebellum.
- A pyogenic brainstem abscess presents with brainstem or cerebellar localized symptoms or signs of hydrocephalus, and can develop by direct spread from otitis media, dental sources, neurosurgical procedures, trauma, or hematogenous seeding. The risk of abscess formation is increased in immunocompromised patients.
- *Listeria monocytogenes*, EBV and brucellosis can cause rhombencephalitis.
- Post-infectious cerebellar ataxia is autoimmune and in some cases antineuronal antibodies can be identified.

Presentation
- Creutzfeldt–Jakob disease presents with cognitive deficits and involuntary myoclonic jerks. In addition, upper motor neuron, extrapyramidal, and cerebellar signs are variably present.
- In pediatric patients with subacute cerebellar or brainstem signs look for: altered mental status, signs of head trauma, focal neurologic findings, fever with meningismus, weakness or areflexia, opsoclonus myoclonus, acute otitis media.

Diagnostic tests
Testing of suspected brainstem or cerebellar infection should be tailored to the presentation and may include CBC, electrolytes, MRI imaging, cerebrospinal fluid analysis, and specific serum or CSF PCR assays and serologies.
- Post-infectious ataxia:
  - If the child has altered mental status, head trauma, symptoms of raised intracranial pressure, focal neurologic findings, or fever with meningism, brain CT or MRI is necessary to look for a space-occupying lesion, ischemic infarction, or hemorrhage. If accompanied by weakness or areflexia, workup for Guillain–Barré syndrome or tick paralysis is warranted. If all of the above conditions are unlikely, a CSF study may be required to exclude viral encephalitis.
- CJD:
  - Brain MRI can show cortical changes on diffusion-weighted images.
  - EEG may show synchronous bi- or triphasic periodic sharp waves.
  - CSF protein 14-3-3 has moderate to high sensitivity and high specificity for CJD.

Prognosis
- 10% of children with acute cerebellar ataxia secondary to viral illness do not recover completely and have mild learning difficulties.
- Those having an older age at onset of ataxia have a worse prognosis.
For a full discussion of infections of the nervous system, see Chapter 24.

Toxins

> **CLINICAL PEARLS**
> - Many CNS active medications affect cerebellar function at therapeutic doses, and cause serious toxicity at higher levels.
> - Recreational drugs and heavy alcohol use are frequently denied by the affected patient, making toxicological screening very important.
> - Certain environmental toxins typically present with brainstem and cerebellar features that provide clues to their identity (e.g. botulism with ophthalmoplegia, fixed dilated pupils, and dysarthria).

Etiology

The following toxins may cause acute dysfunction or chronic damage to the brainstem and cerebellum; ancillary features help to distinguish the cause in a particular case:

- Medications:
  - Antiepileptics – gaze-evoked nystagmus is especially prominent.
  - Benzodiazepines.
  - Barbiturates.
  - Lithium – fine tremor accompanies ataxia.
  - Neuroleptics.
  - Tricyclic antidepressants.
  - Nitrous oxide – repeated use causes syndrome equivalent to B12 deficiency.
  - Calcineurin inhibitors.
  - Cytosine arabinoside (high dose).
- Recreational drugs:
  - Alcohol – acutely, the subject smells of alcohol and affect is disinhibited. Wernicke's encephalopathy may be present. Chronic exposure cerebellar syndrome has truncal ataxia with wide-based gait but fairly normal control in arms.
  - Phencyclidine – exceptionally disinhibited behavior and dissociation.
  - Ketamine.
  - Paint thinner.
  - Opioids – miosis, marked respiratory depression.
  - Nicotine.
  - Stimulants – cocaine may present with hypertension, tachycardia, hyperthermia, agitation, and seizures.
- Environmental toxins:
  - Heavy metals (lead, mercury, manganese) – associated sensory or motor neuropathies, anemia, look for gum "lead line."
  - Carbon monoxide – cherry red carboxyhemoglobin.
  - Benzene derivative solvents (toluene, xylene).
  - Organophosphates – fasciculations, salivation, lacrimation.
- Biological toxins:
  - Botulinum – fixed dilated pupils, ophthalmoplegia, dysarthria.
  - Tetanus – trismus, opisthotonus.
  - Diphtheria.
  - Ciguatera – inversion of temperature perception.
  - Eucalyptus oil.

Pathogenesis/pathology

Mechanisms of toxicity vary with the agent. For many neurotoxins, acute exposure can cause neuronal death, and the risk increases with chronic or repeated exposure. The cerebellar Purkinje cells are particularly vulnerable to many such agents.

Diagnostic tests

- A complete metabolic profile and CBC are essential; blood gases may assist management.
- In cases of suspected acute intoxication, blood and urine toxicology screens should be performed.
- When a CNS-active medication is known to be prescribed, drug levels should be drawn as early as possible.
- Many environmental toxins can be confirmed by specific tests, such as heavy metal assays, hippuric acid for benzene derivatives, methemoglobin for carbon monoxide.
- MRI may reveal particular patterns of abnormal brainstem or cerebellar signal in acute toxicity, or atrophy in chronic cases.

Treatment

In all cases, prompt cessation of toxin exposure and supportive care should be followed by attempted removal or neutralization of the toxin in the body.

- For acute ingestions, this may involve emptying the stomach contents and forcing diuresis.
- Eliminating body stores of heavy metals involves chelation. There are several recommendations for the treatment of lead intoxication.
- In cases of mercury toxicity affecting the nervous system, chelation is less effective, but still utilized.
- Blocking the effect of the toxin may be possible, for example with tetanus antitoxin.
- Supportive measures are always appropriate to ensure airway protection, adequate ventilation, maintenance of blood pressure, and so forth.
- Treatment of associated disorders must be considered, such as administering thiamine prior to glucose solutions in acute alcoholic toxicity to prevent Wernicke's encephalopathy.

Autoimmune disorders

CLINICAL PEARLS
- Multiple sclerosis classically presents with neurologic symptoms and signs separated in time and space (see Chapter 23).
- Acute or subacute presentation of a cerebellar or a brainstem syndrome in a patient with a history of recurrent oral or genital ulcers, fever, and skin lesions should raise a suspicion of Behçet's disease.
- Sjögren's syndrome can mimic multiple sclerosis in its clinical and radiologic findings.
- Enteropathic symptoms in association with cerebellar features can be seen in patients with celiac disease and other malabsorptive states. Vitamin E deficiency can contribute to the neurologic syndrome.

Disease classification

Some of the categories of autoimmune disease with brainstem and cerebellar features include:

- multiple sclerosis or neuromyelitis optica (NMO);
- Behçet's disease;

- Sjögren's syndrome;
- CLIPPERS (chronic lymphocytic inflammation with pontine perivascular enhancement responsive to steroids)
- anti-GAD antibody associated cerebellar syndrome;
- celiac disease.

Presentation

- Multiple sclerosis:
  - Patients present with neurologic symptoms and signs separated in time and space.
  - Trigeminal neuralgia at a young age, bilateral INO, tremor, and ataxia are common manifestations.
- Behçet's disease:
  - Subacute or acute presentation may include fever, neck stiffness, headache, weakness, numbness, altered level of consciousness, and diplopia.
- Sjögren's syndrome:
  - Patients may or may not have the classic complaints of dry eyes, dry mouth, and Raynaud's phenomenon.
  - In addition to brainstem and cerebellar involvement, features of mononeuritis multiplex causing dysesthesia, sensory loss, and focal weakness may be present. There may be associated sensory symptoms secondary to small fiber peripheral neuropathy.
  - Patients may also have optic neuritis, trigeminal sensory neuropathy, seizures, and cognitive dysfunction.
- CLIPPERS:
  - Facial paresthesia and episodic diplopia are often the presenting symptoms.
  - Subsequent development of other brainstem features is typical. Cerebellar involvement and myelopathy are also known to occur.
- Anti-GAD antibody associated progressive cerebellar syndrome:
  - The condition is more common in women, who may have a personal or family history of autoimmune conditions. Chronic progressive moderately severe gait ataxia with mild upper extremity ataxia is a typical presentation. Patients may or may not have associated features of "stiff person syndrome."
- Celiac disease:
  - Gradual-onset cerebellar ataxia with or without enteropathic symptoms of abdominal discomfort, weight loss, and diarrhea has been described in "gluten ataxia."
  - There is gait ataxia on examination, and patients may have stimulus-sensitive myoclonus and action tremor of the extremities.

Pathology/pathogenesis

- Multiple sclerosis:
  - The pathologic findings involve demyelination as well as neurodegeneration.
  - Plaques are areas of well-defined myelin loss, inflammatory cells, gliosis, and relative preservation of neurons and axons.
  - Plaques are found in both gray and white matter.
  - Plaques disrupt brainstem internuclear connections, cranial nerve nuclei, autonomic, sensory, and motor long tracts, cerebellar nuclei, and their outflow tracts.
- Sjögren's syndrome:
  - Aquaporin-4 antibody may play a role and mimic neuromyelitis optica with involvement of the brainstem and optic nerves.

- There may be subacute involvement of cerebellum and brainstem secondary to inflammation leading to necrotic and demyelinating lesions.
- Pathogenesis is unknown, but the current theory involves B cell hyperreactivity secondary to environmental triggers, which activate glandular and epithelial cells in genetically predisposed individuals.
- Behçet's disease:
  - Only 20% of patients with Behçet's disease have CNS involvement. Perivenular lymphocytic cuffing, inflammatory cell infiltration, gliosis, and neuronal loss are common in brainstem, corticospinal tracts, and cerebellum.
  - Rhombencephalitis or dural venous thrombosis can play a role.
  - Subacute or acute presentation of brainstem or cerebellar symptoms may be due to arterial or venous inflammation.
- CLIPPERS:
  - Chronic lymphocytic perivascular infiltrates are seen in the pons and less often in the medulla, the brainstem, the cerebellum, and the spinal cord.
- Celiac disease:
  - There may be cerebellar cortical atrophy with Purkinje cell loss, possibly from lymphocytic infiltration.
- Anti-glutamic acid decarboxylase (GAD) antibody associated cerebellar syndrome
  - A current hypothesis proposes that anti-GAD antibody in cerebrospinal fluid selectively suppresses inhibitory post-synaptic current in cerebellar Purkinje cells.

Diagnostic tests

- Multiple sclerosis:
  - Brain and spine MRI with gadolinium contrast showing lesions separated in time, CSF studies for oligoclonal bands and cell count, visual evoked potentials. HTLV-1 serology, lupus antibodies to exclude mimicking differential diagnoses (see Chapter 23).
  - MRI findings are distinct in patients with NMO (see Chapter 23).
  - Aquaporin antibody (gamma immunoglobulin [IgG] antibody) in serum and CSF can be useful for the diagnosis of NMO.
- Behçet's disease:
  - No pathognomonic test is available. Clinical features and a positive pathergy test can help establish the diagnosis. Brain MRI usually shows brainstem T2 hyperintensities. Brainstem auditory evoked potentials may provide supportive evidence of brainstem involvement when MRI is unremarkable. CSF shows elevated protein level, high IgG levels, and a pleocytosis with an increased number of polymorphonuclear cells and lymphocytes.
- Sjögren's syndrome:
  - Schirmer's test or rose Bengal test shows reduced tear production. Extractable nuclear antigen antibodies may be present. The labial salivary gland biopsy shows lymphocytic infiltration with glandular atrophy.
  - Investigations to screen for other organ involvement include renal function tests, electrolytes, and urinalysis.
  - Tests to screen for differential diagnoses include hepatitis C serology, HIV and HTLV-1 serology, serum QuantiFERON-TB Gold (QFT®) test (if anergic on Mantoux test or in those who have received previous bacille Calmette–Guérin vaccination).
- CLIPPERS:
  - Brain MRI shows symmetric curvilinear gadolinium enhancement peppering the pons and to a variable extent involving the medulla, brachium pontis, cerebellar hemispheres, mid-brain, and occasionally the spinal cord.

- Anti-GAD antibody associated progressive cerebellar syndrome:
  - Elevated serum and CSF GAD antibody levels are typically seen. Brain MRI may show cerebellar atrophy.
- Celiac disease:
  - Anti-gliadin antibodies, anti-endomysial antibodies, and anti-tissue transglutaminase (TTG) antibodies may be detected. Anti-endomysial antibodies have the highest specificity.
  - Small bowel biopsy can confirm the diagnosis.

Treatment
- Multiple sclerosis: see Chapter 23.
- Behçet's disease: when there is CNS involvement, intravenous methylprednisolone 1 g daily for 3–5 days is initiated and followed by maintenance azathioprine. Mycophenolate mofetil or cyclophosphamide are alternatives if azathioprine cannot be tolerated.
- Sjögren's syndrome: intravenous glucocorticoids and cyclophosphamide in acute illness followed by maintenance immunosuppression is a common approach, although clinical trial support is lacking.
- CLIPPERS: high-dose steroids are used, and if symptoms recur when steroids are being tapered, addition of other immunosuppressive agents is considered.
- Celiac disease:
  - Gluten-free diet improves cerebellar ataxia.
  - Screening and treatment of vitamin E deficiency with daily vitamin E supplementation at 100–400 units a day is useful.
- Anti-GAD antibody associated cerebellar syndrome:
  - Role of IVIG or plasma exchange is uncertain in those with cerebellar syndrome. Benzodiazepines and intravenous immunoglobulin improve stiffness related to stiff person syndrome but have no effect on gait ataxia. Downbeat nystagmus and appendicular ataxia have been reported to improve following IVIG at 0.4 g/kg daily for 5 days.

Metabolic disorders

> **CLINICAL PEARLS**
> - The presentation of acquired hypothyroidism in adults often includes gait ataxia.
> - Central pontine myelinolysis (CPM) may occur 2 to 6 days after rapid correction of hyponatremia.
> - Wilson's disease presents with a cerebellar syndrome of gait ataxia and tremor in 30% of cases. Slit-lamp examination may reveal Kayser–Fleischer rings.
> - Thiamine deficiency typically presents with acute onset of ataxia, nystagmus, ophthalmoplegia, and confusion (Wernicke's encephalopathy).
> - Vitamin E deficiency presents as a cerebellar syndrome in patients with longstanding fat malabsorption from bowel resection or dysfunction.

Etiology
The following disorders of metabolism or nutrition may include features of brainstem or cerebellar dysfunction at their presentation or during their course:
- Hyponatremia and hypernatremia
- Hypocalcemia and hypercalcemia
- Hypoglycemia and hyperglycemia

- Hypomagnesemia and hypermagnesemia
- Hypophosphatemia
- Uremia
- Hepatic failure
- Hypothyroidism and hyperthyroidism
- Hypoparathyroidism and hyperparathyroidism
- Vitamin E deficiency
- Vitamin B12 deficiency
- Thiamine deficiency
- Wilson's disease
- Trace element deficiencies.

Pathogenesis

The mechanisms by which metabolic and nutritional disorders can cause CNS dysfunction are as varied as the causes themselves. The reasons for specific involvement of the brainstem or cerebellum are largely speculative, but may include:
- Proximity to regions lacking a fully functioning blood–brain barrier.
- Special metabolic requirements for certain nerve populations.
- Close contact with the CSF.
- Structural consequences of closely packed nuclei and tracts.
- Relatively less sympathetic vascular regulation.
   Characteristic pathogenic and pathologic features in a few representative instances are:
- CPM – confluent areas of demyelination in the central pons, sometimes extending into the diencephalon.
- Hypothyroidism – degenerative changes in the anterosuperior vermis, atrophy of the central pons, transverse pontine fibers, and superior peduncles.
- Wilson's disease – impairment of cellular copper transport due to *ATP7B* mutation causes reduction of copper excretion into the bile, and consequent accumulation of copper in the brain and liver with resulting cellular toxicity and necrosis.
- Wernicke's encephalopathy – neuronal loss, gliosis, and vascular damage in the regions surrounding the third and fourth ventricles and the aqueduct.

Diagnostic tests
- In all cases a comprehensive metabolic panel is the essential starting point for diagnosis. Further laboratory testing should be tailored to the situation: thyroid profile, vitamin B12 levels, vitamin E levels, vitamin B1 level, erythrocyte transketolase activity, ceruloplasmin, urinary copper excretion, other trace metals, ammonia, magnesium, or glycohemoglobin, depending on the setting.
- Imaging usually requires MRI, as CT scans lack sensitivity especially in the posterior fossa. Characteristic patterns exist for some metabolic disorders.
- CSF studies have little role in the evaluation of metabolic disorders of the brainstem and cerebellum.

Treatment

The general principle in metabolic disorders is of course the restitution of normal levels of the metabolic substance in question, whether by addition or removal (e.g. electrolytes) or by correcting regulatory factors (e.g. insulin), with a few provisos:
- Too rapid correction of hyponatremia can lead to central pontine myelinolysis.
- Correction of severe hypothyroidism must be done gradually to avoid cardiac complications. Sometimes T3 must be added to the T4 to achieve full metabolic restitution.

- Initial hemodialysis for uremia should be accomplished in stages to avoid a dysequilibrium syndrome.
- Wilson's disease is treated by chelation therapy with D-penicillamine titrated to 1000–1500 mg daily in 2–4 divided doses, over 4–6 weeks. Trientine can be used at 20 mg/kg (maximum 1500 mg/day) if the patient cannot tolerate penicillamine.
- Oral zinc is added to chelation therapy at 150 mg daily in three divided doses, to reduce copper absorption in the gastrointestinal tract.

  For a full discussion of metabolic disorders causing encephalopathy, see Chapter 36.

Inherited disease

CLINICAL PEARLS
- While the family history may be negative in patients who have genetic causes of ataxia or brainstem disease, a thorough history is nonetheless critical. Some disorders show incomplete penetrance or can skip generations.
- Toxic, inflammatory, metabolic, and other treatable causes of cerebellar ataxia should be excluded.
- Genetic testing should be pursued in collaboration with a genetic counselor.

Background

Many hereditary diseases cause degeneration affecting cerebellar or brainstem function. Diseases can affect primarily either specific brainstem functions such as eye movements or facial strength, or cerebellar function, or combinations of cerebellar, brainstem, and other nervous system and systemic organ functions. Here we will focus on representative hereditary disorders affecting the cerebellum.

Disease classification

Hereditary cerebellar disease can be classified by either the pattern of inheritance or by the pathogenesis.

Classification by inheritance
- Autosomal recessive including:
  - Friedreich's ataxia
  - Ataxia telangiectasia
  - Progressive ataxia due to vitamin E deficiency
  - Wilson's disease
  - Abetalipoproteinemia
  - Ataxia with oculomotor apraxia
- Autosomal dominant including:
  - Spinocerebellar ataxias
  - Episodic ataxias
- X-linked recessive including:
  - Fragile X tremor ataxia syndrome (FXTAS)
- Mitochondrial disorders with mutations of mitochondrial genes or nuclear-encoded mitochondrial proteins, including:
  - Kearns–Sayre syndrome (KSS).
  - Myoclonus epilepsy with ragged-red fibers (MERRF).
  - Mitochondrial encephalopathy, lactic acidosis, and stroke-like episodes (MELAS).

- Neurogenic weakness, ataxia, and retinitis pigmentosa (NARP).
- Mitochondrial DNA-dependent DNA polymerase gamma (POLG).

Classification by pathogenesis
- Mitochondrial
- Metabolic
- Defective DNA repair
- Abnormal protein folding and degradation
- Channelopathies.

Incidence/prevalence
- Friedreich's ataxia is the commonest autosomal recessive ataxia in Whites and has a prevalence in the USA of about 1 in 50,000.
- The overall prevalence of autosomal dominant ataxia has been estimated at about 1 in 30,000.

Etiology
- Friedreich's ataxia: Homozygous GAA expansion that leads to frataxin deficiency. Frataxin deficiency causes iron dysmetabolism in the cerebellum and heart.
- Spinocerebellar ataxias (SCAs): More than 30 loci causing autosomal dominant SCAs have been identified. The most common gene defect is the presence of unstable trinucleotide repeats, usually CAG encoding polyglutamine segments. The presence of these abnormal polyglutamine protein conformations in different genes causing similar SCA syndromes suggests a shared neurotoxic mechanism.
- Episodic ataxias can result from mutations affecting potassium or calcium channels.
- FXTAS: Expansion of the CGG repeats normally found in the *FMR1* gene (but reaching a repeat number less than that causing fragile X mental retardation) causes symptomatology usually later in life.
- Mitochondrial diseases: Deletions or mutations interfere with oxidative phosphorylation or calcium homeostasis. The cerebellar Purkinje cell, being highly metabolically active, is more susceptible to this type of defect.

Pathology
- Friedreich's ataxia shows loss of large glutamatergic neurons of the dentate nucleus of cerebellum and large motor cortex neurons as well as degeneration of the dorsal root ganglia.
- SCAs have widespread degeneration of gray matter of the basal ganglia and thalamus, loss of white and gray matter of the brainstem and cerebellum, and neuronal loss in the primary motor cortex.

Presentation
- Friedreich's ataxia: Usually presents in childhood with ataxia involving the upper and lower extremities, difficulty acquiring motor milestones, and severe truncal ataxia and scoliosis. On examination, patients have pyramidal weakness, lower extremity wasting, areflexia, Babinski responses, and loss of vibration and proprioception in the lower extremities.
- Spinocerebellar ataxias: Patients generally present in childhood or young adulthood and have chronic progressive cerebellar ataxia, nystagmus, dysmetria, and dementia. There is variable association with peripheral neuropathy, optic nerve atrophy, brainstem involvement with facial weakness, parkinsonism, choreoathetosis, seizures, and hyperreflexia.
- Mitochondrial disorders: Presentation varies with the specific disorder. These disorders can present at any age with exercise intolerance, episodic seizures, encephalopathy, stroke-like episodes, or organ failure. On examination look for proximal weakness suggesting myopathy, retinal pigmentary changes, ophthalmoplegia, and ptosis.

Diagnostic tests

The definitive diagnosis for hereditary disorders with a known locus is via genetic testing, which should be pursued in conjunction with genetic counseling. Other laboratory abnormalities are also found in specific diseases.

- Friedreich's ataxia:
  - Axonal sensory neuropathy is found on nerve conduction testing. Neuroimaging excludes other disorders and may show a characteristic pattern of atrophy. Vitamin E is normal. EKG and echocardiogram are important to detect arrhythmia or hypertrophic cardiomyopathy, which are common causes of mortality.
- Spinocerebellar ataxias:
  - Brain MRI shows cerebellar atrophy.
- Mitochondrial disorders:
  - In MELAS, MRI may show T2 hyperintensity not respecting vascular territories. Serum or CSF lactate and pyruvate are elevated. Muscle biopsy may show ragged red fibers with mitochondrial proliferation, increased succinate dehydrogenase, and muscle fibers deficient in cytochrome C oxidase.

Treatment

Treatment that alters the course of the disease is not yet available for any hereditary ataxia. Symptomatic and supportive treatment is tailored to the specific disorder.

- Spinocerebellar ataxia:
  - Acetazolamide (250–500 mg/day) is useful for suppression of episodic ataxia in spinocerebellar ataxia type 6 but has no effect on the progression of ataxia.
  - 4-Aminopyridine (5 mg p.o. t.i.d.) is useful for reduction in the frequency of ataxia in episodic ataxia type 2.
- Friedreich's ataxia:
  - Idebenone reduces cardiac hypertrophy but does not stop the progression of ataxia.
- Mitochondrial disorders:
  - Coenzyme Q10 replacement (200–900 mg/day) can be useful in those with cerebellar ataxia secondary to coenzyme Q10 deficiency. L-Arginine intravenous infusion within 48 hours after stroke-like episode onset can improve outcome. Hearing loss can be treated with cochlear implant.
  - Avoid sodium valproate and mitochondrial toxins such as tetracycline, gentamicin, and ciprofloxacin.

Neoplasia

CLINICAL PEARLS
- Posterior fossa tumors can often cause an early increase in intracranial pressure with headache, vomiting, and altered level of consciousness.
- Surgical removal of a symptomatic cerebellar metastasis may provide significant benefit.
- Several heredofamilial conditions are associated with posterior fossa neoplasms – for example bilateral acoustic neuromas in neurofibromatosis 2, cerebellar hemangioblastoma in von Hippel–Lindau disease (see Chapter 29).
- Unilateral tinnitus and hearing loss may be the presenting complaint in patients with acoustic neuroma.

Disease classification

- Primary central nervous system neoplasia of the cerebellum and brainstem.
- Secondary metastasis to the posterior fossa.
- Brainstem and cerebellar paraneoplastic syndromes.

Pathogenesis/pathology

- Primary central nervous system neoplasia of the cerebellum and brainstem:
  - A wide range of tumors originate from different cell types of the central nervous system, for example astrocytomas, oligodendromas, ependymomas, choroid plexus papilloma, lymphomas, meningiomas, and other neuroepithelial tumors. Juvenile pilocytic astrocytoma and brainstem gliomas are unique to children.
- Secondary metastasis to the posterior fossa:
  - Lung, breast, melanoma, ovarian, and renal cell carcinomas hematogenously metastasize to the brain, mostly at the gray/white matter junction.
  - Meningeal carcinomatosis may present with multiple cranial neuropathies and ataxia.
- Paraneoplastic syndromes: The pathogenesis of paraneoplastic syndromes is incompletely understood, but is thought to arise from immune-mediated attack of shared antigens between tumor and cells of the nervous system. Both cell- and antibody-mediated responses have been implicated. Some of the autoantibodies associated with specific posterior fossa syndromes include:
  - Anti-Yo antibodies associated with cerebellar degeneration in women with ovarian or breast cancer.
  - Anti-Hu antibodies with lung cancer.
  - Anti-Tr antibodies with Hodgkin's lymphoma.
  - Anti-Ma/Ta antibodies in brainstem encephalitis associated with testicular cancer.

Presentation

- Primary central nervous system neoplasia, secondary metastasis:
  - Patient may have a history of primary malignancy
  - Symptoms may be related to raised intracranial pressure: headache, vomiting, diplopia, or altered mental status.
  - Specific brainstem and cerebellar signs such as cranial neuropathy, upper motor neuron signs, and cerebellar ataxia depend on the exact location, extent, and laterality of the tumor.
- Paraneoplastic syndromes:
  - Subacute ataxia or incoordination is seen in cerebellar degeneration.
  - Oscillopsia, tremors, falls, and ataxia are noted in opsoclonus myoclonus syndrome (typically seen with neuroblastoma).
  - Cranial neuropathies may be accompanied by weakness, numbness, autonomic disturbance, or altered consciousness in brainstem encephalitis.
  - In most cases, diagnosis of an underlying malignancy is made within 5 years of onset of the presentation of the paraneoplastic syndrome.

Diagnostic tests

- MRI of brain with and without contrast, or CT scan with and without contrast (if MRI cannot be obtained).

- If a mass lesion has been excluded, CSF studies to look for cytology and paraneoplastic auto-antibodies may be indicated.
- Malignancy workup in suspected paraneoplastic syndrome should include CT scans of chest, abdomen, and pelvis, mammography, and appropriate gastroenterologic endoscopic evaluation. PET scan is desirable, although insurance authorization can be difficult to obtain in the absence of known malignancy.

Treatment

- The approach to primary central nervous system neoplasia and secondary metastasis is discussed in Chapter 22.
- Paraneoplastic syndromes:
  - Treatment of the underlying cancer is the most important step, although the presenting syndrome may persist.
  - If malignancy workup is unrevealing, CT chest, abdomen, and pelvis and PET scan are repeated at regular intervals.
  - Autoimmune-induced paraneoplastic syndrome may be treated with intravenous immuno-globulins, pulse steroids, rituximab, cyclophosphamide, or plasmapheresis with variable success. These modalities prevent further progression of the condition and sometimes provide symptomatic improvement.

Degenerative disease

CLINICAL PEARLS
- Multiple system atrophy (MSA) is the prototype of degenerative disorders affecting the cerebellum.
- Patients presenting with autonomic symptoms, cerebellar and extrapyramidal signs should be evaluated for MSA.

Disease classification

- MSA-P: parkinsonism is more prominent.
- MSA-C: cerebellar dysfunction is more prominent.

In some cases autonomic findings are the prominent and presenting features. The term Shy–Drager syndrome was used in the past to describe such patients.

Pathology/pathogenesis

- There are glial cell cytoplasmic inclusions, myelin degeneration, and intermediolateral column cell loss. The exact cause of these changes is unknown.
- Degeneration of Purkinje cells, inferior olivary nuclei, middle cerebellar peduncles, and basis pontis underlies the cerebellar dysfunction in this condition.
- Accumulation of alpha-synuclein in various cells is noted and MSA is considered one of the synucleinopathies.

Presentation

- Patients present with falls, ataxia, slurred speech, and dysphagia. There may be some degree of stiffness, slowness without tremor, unexplained erectile dysfunction, fecal or urinary incontinence, and inappropriate laughter or crying.

- Examination shows bilateral cerebellar signs, quavery voice, pseudobulbar features, bradykinesia, postural instability, and orthostatic hypotension to a variable degree.

Diagnostic tests
- Diagnosis of probable MSA is based on clinical features; no laboratory or imaging studies are diagnostic.
- Autonomic testing may show prominent orthostatic hypotension and absence of compensatory tachycardia.
- Brain MRI may show atrophy of the pons, putamen, or middle cerebellar peduncles.
- FDG-PET showing hypometabolism in putamen may provide supportive evidence.

Treatment
There is currently no disease-altering treatment. The cerebellar features in this condition do not respond to any pharmacologic intervention. A trial of levodopa can be useful in early stages of the illness if there are significant extrapyramidal features. Supportive therapy and multidisciplinary care are useful for management of orthostatic hypotension, urinary and fecal incontinence, and prevention of falls.

Section 4: Treatment
See Section 3.

Section 5: Special populations
Not applicable for this topic.

Section 6: Prognosis

BOTTOM LINE/CLINICAL PEARLS
- Paraneoplastic syndrome, neoplasm, central pontine myelinolysis, anti-GAD antibody associated cerebellar syndrome, multiple system atrophy, and inherited cerebellar conditions have a poor functional outcome despite treatment, with the exception of episodic ataxia and the slowly progressive spinocerebellar type 6.
- Multiple sclerosis and Sjögren's syndrome have a reasonably good prognosis when treated.

Section 7: Reading list
Key reading sources for this chapter can be found online at www.mountsinaiexpertguides.com
Not applicable for this topic.

Additional material for this chapter can be found online at:
www.mountsinaiexpertguides.com

This includes a multiple choice question and a reading list.

CHAPTER 29

Inborn Errors of Metabolism

Shannon E. Babineau
Goryeb Children's Hospital, Morristown, NJ, USA

OVERALL BOTTOM LINE
- This chapter deals with three related topics: inborn errors of metabolism, neurocutaneous syndromes, and structural lesions (CNS malformations).
- Inborn errors of metabolism (IEM):
  - Small molecule inborn errors of metabolism typically present as acute encephalopathies while large molecule disorders become symptomatic over time.
- Neurocutaneous syndromes:
  - Because of their similar embryologic origins, neurocutaneous syndromes have distinct skin markings associated with underlying neurologic dysfunction and abnormalities.
- Structural lesions (CNS malformations):
  - CNS malformations are the second most common congenital malformations after cardiac disease; prognosis varies depending on the specific lesion.

Section 1: Background
Definition of disease

Inborn errors of metabolism (IEM) occur when a gene product (usually an enzyme) in one of the metabolic pathways is totally or partially absent leading to an excess of the substrate of the missing enzyme or to the deficiency of the product. The build-up of substrate can occur in one or multiple organ systems, including the nervous system, leading to dysfunction. Similarly, the deficiency of the product may be particularly consequential for the nervous system.

Neurocutaneous syndromes include disorders that have manifestations in organs that are derived from the embryologic ectoderm (central and peripheral nervous system, skin and eye). The most common syndromes include tuberous sclerosis (TS), which involves multiple hamartomatous abnormalities affecting the brain, kidney, heart, retina, and skin along with neoplasms of the central nervous system and kidneys. Neurofibromatosis type 1 (NF1) involves cutaneous pigmented lesions and tumors along peripheral nerves. Sturge–Weber (SW) syndrome involves the vasculature of the skin, eyes, meninges, and brain and does not have any tumors associated with it.

Structural malformations of the central nervous system occur during the development of the fetus and can be primary or secondary. Disruption of the closure of the caudal neural tube can lead to meningomyelocele, which is a vertebral cleft where the meninges and spinal cord are exposed causing spinal cord dysfunction at the level of the lesion. Holoprosencephaly occurs when the cerebral hemispheres and paired diencephalic structures do not fully separate. Other

---

Mount Sinai Expert Guides: Neurology, First Edition. Edited by Stuart C. Sealfon, Rajeev Motiwala, and Charles B. Stacy.
© 2016 John Wiley & Sons, Ltd. Published 2016 by John Wiley & Sons, Ltd.
Companion website: www.mountsinaiexpertguides.com

defects affecting cerebellar formation include Dandy–Walker malformation, where there is dysgenesis of the cerebellar vermis and an enlarged posterior fossa cyst.

Disease classification
IEM are typically classified by the affected metabolic pathway. Commonly included are disorders of amino acid, carbohydrate, lysosomal, and peroxisomal metabolism and urea cycle defects.

Incidence/prevalence
- Overall incidence of IEM: 1:800–2500
- Incidence of various IEM:
  - amino acidopathies (not phenylketonuria(PKU)): 7.6–18.7/100,000
  - PKU: 7.5–8.1/100,000
  - lysosomal storage disease: 7.6–19.3/100,000
  - peroxisomal storage disease: 3.5–7.4/100,000
  - urea cycle defects: 1.9–4.5/100,000
- Neurocutaneous syndromes:
  - tuberous sclerosis incidence: 1/6000
  - neurofibromatosis type 1: 1/2500–1/4000
  - Sturge–Weber 1/50,000
- Structural lesions:
  - meningomyelocele incidence is 17.8/100,000 births
  - holoprosencephaly incidence 1.26:10,000 births
  - Dandy–Walker has an incidence of 1:30,000 births.

Etiology
- IEM are caused by alterations of the genes encoding various metabolic enzymes, leading to absent or reduced enzyme levels or decreased function. The gene defects responsible for the most common IEM are listed in Table 29.1.

Table 29.1 Gene defects responsible for the most common inborn errors of metabolism (IEM).

Disease name	Gene locus	Gene name
Citrullinemia	9q34.11	Argininosuccinate synthetase (*ASS1*)
Fabry disease	Xq22.1	Alpha-galactosidase A (*GLA*)
Galactosemia	9p13.3	Galactose-1-phosphate uridylyltransferase (*GALT*)
Hurler disease	4p16.3	Alpha-L-iduronidase (*IDUA*)
Krabbe disease	14q31.3	Galactosylceramidase (*GALC*)
Ornithine transcarbamylase deficiency	Xp11.4	Ornithine carbamoyltransferase (*OTC*)
Phenylketonuria (PKU)	12q23.2	Phenylalanine hydroxylase (*PAH*)
Propionic acidemia	3q22.3 13q32.3	Propionyl-CoA carboxylase B (*PCCB*) Propionyl-CoA carboxylase A (*PCCA*)
Tay–Sachs disease	15q23	Hexosaminidase A (*HEXA*)
Zellweger syndrome	7q21.2	Peroxisome biogenesis factor 1 (*PEX1*)

- NF1 is due to an autosomal dominant genetic mutation in the neurofibromin gene on 17q11.
- Tuberous sclerosis is caused by an autosomal dominant or spontaneous mutation of the *TSC1* gene for hamartin on chromosome 9q34 or mutation in the *TSC2* gene for tuberin on chromosome 16p13.
- Sturge–Weber syndrome is the result of spontaneous mutation in the *GNAQ* gene for guanine nucleotide binding protein q polypeptide on chromosome 9q21.2.
- Meningomyelocele is often multifactorial and can occur secondary to chromosomal disorders, environmental exposure, folic acid deficiency, or the use of certain medications during pregnancy (sulfasalazine, valproate, carbamazepine, phenobarbital, phenytoin).
- Holoprosencephaly can be related to genetic mutations, maternal diabetes, retinoic acid, or alcohol or drug abuse during pregnancy.
- Dandy–Walker can be associated with genetic mutations including trisomy 13, intrauterine exposure to rubella, isoretinoid, or alcohol. It is seen in some IEM (congenital disorders of glycosylation) and in Aicardi syndrome.

Pathology/pathogenesis

In IEM, typically a genetic mutation leads to the absence or reduced function of a single enzyme. This leads to an accumulation of metabolites upstream in the pathway and an inability to make the end-products of a specific pathway.

In NF1 and TS, the altered or missing gene product causes uncontrolled cell growth leading to tumor formation. In SW, the altered gene product is thought to disrupt downstream signaling pathways responsible for blood vessel growth and regulation.

Meningomyelocele occurs when the caudal neural tube does not close, allowing exposure of the spinal cord outside of the body. This causes incomplete formation of the spinal cord below the lesion along with adhesions that can further disrupt the neural connections. Continuous CSF leakage from the lower defect does not allow the posterior fossa to form properly and the cerebellum is malformed and downwardly displaced (Chiari 2 malformation).

In holoprosencephaly often the same defect that causes failure of separation can lead to midline facial defects as well, which will be clinically obvious at birth. Patients may have a poorly formed pituitary gland and hypothalami leading to endocrinologic symptoms.

Dandy–Walker is thought to be related to developmental arrest in the opening of the foramen of Magendie leading to dilation of the fourth ventricle and absence of the cerebellar vermis.

Section 2: Prevention and screening

BOTTOM LINE/CLINICAL PEARLS
- The only prevention possible is through prenatal testing. Progression can be reduced with alterations in diet, supplements, and in some cases gene replacement therapy.
- Folic acid supplementation in women of childbearing age and during pregnancy reduces neural tube defects. 400 µg/day is recommended for all women of childbearing age, and up to 4 mg/day in patients at high risk such as those taking antiepileptic medications.

Screening

Developed countries screen every newborn for IEM. However, which diseases are screened vary from country to country and state to state.

All pregnant women are screened at 15–20 weeks gestation for an elevated serum alphafeto-protein (AFP).

During pregnancy prenatal ultrasound can identify malformations such as holoprosencephaly and Dandy–Walker malformations.

Primary prevention

• Folic acid is thought to be useful for preventing possible neural tube defects even in low-risk women. Neural tube defects usually occur before a woman knows she is pregnant, so it is recommended that all women who might become pregnant take a folic acid supplement.

Secondary prevention

• Folate supplementation reduces the risk of recurrent neural tube defects in future pregnancies by 70%.

Section 3: Diagnosis

BOTTOM LINE/CLINICAL PEARLS
• IEM can be categorized into large molecule and small molecule disorders.
• Small molecule disorders include amino and organic acidopathies, urea cycle and fatty oxidation defects, and mitochondrial disorders.
• Small molecule disorders typically present as acute decompensation in a newborn or in a child during a hypercatabolic state (fever, fasting) with features such as hyperammonemia, metabolic acidosis, or hypoglycemia.
• Large molecule disorders include lysosomal and peroxisomal storage disorders as well as glycogen storage disorders.
• Large molecule disorders typically present with slow progression of symptoms or neurodegeneration. Systemic involvement of the liver, heart, and spleen is often seen.
• A diagnosis of TS is typically suspected either prenatally when cardiac rhabdomyoma is found on ultrasound or in the first year of life when a child presents with seizures. By childhood, the patient will have at least one characteristic skin finding. The diagnosis can be made clinically and confirmed with genetic testing.
• NF1 is inherited in an autosomal dominant fashion so a patient may be diagnosed very early if there is a parent with the condition. Otherwise multiple café-au-lait spots or axillary freckling will lead to a diagnosis. Diagnosis is based on clinical criteria.
• SW should be suspected in any child with a port-wine stain, typically in the V1, V2 distribution, who presents with seizures, glaucoma, or hemiparesis. The diagnosis is confirmed when an MRI with contrast shows the typical leptomeningeal angioma ipsilateral to the port-wine stain. Testing for the recently described activating mutation of *GNAQ* that causes SW can be performed at specialized centers.
• Women who have had a prior pregnancy with a neural tube defect or who are taking certain anticonvulsants such as carbamazepine or valproic acid have an increased risk for having a child with meningomyelocele. Neural tube defects may cause an elevated serum AFP at the 15-week checkup, which should prompt confirmatory ultrasound or fetal MRI.
• Holoprosencephaly can be detected on prenatal ultrasound and should be looked for if there is evidence of facial defects including cleft palate. After birth, midline facial defects or hypothalamic/pituitary dysfunction may lead to diagnosis with characteristic MRI findings.

Dandy–Walker malformation may be detected by routine ultrasound prenatally as a large posterior fossa cyst, or hydrocephalus may be present. In a child with symptoms of increased intracranial pressure, MRI will demonstrate the typical findings.

- Dandy–Walker syndrome should be distinguished from Joubert syndrome, in which there is vermian hypoplasia, but not hydrocephalus or a posterior fossa cyst. This condition is associated with an abnormal breathing pattern and a characteristic "molar tooth sign" on MRI. Dandy–Walker should also be distinguished from the Walker–Warburg syndrome. These patients have a posterior fossa arachnoid cyst, but a normal vermis. Walker–Warburg is associated with lissencephaly and is a form of congenital muscular dystrophy.

Differential diagnosis

While many IEM lead to hyperammonemia or hypoglycemia, many other diseases may present with metabolic disturbances.

Differential diagnosis	Features
Hyperammonemia:	
• Severe dehydration	Mild elevations of ammonia (<150 µmol/L) in dehydration
• Liver failure	Elevated LFTs in liver failure
• HSV infection	HSV titers
• Valproate toxicity	High valproate levels
Hypoglycemia:	
• Endogenous insulin production – insulinoma	Insulin and c-peptide evaluation identify
• Ingestion of oral hypoglycemic agent	ingestion of exogenous hypoglycemic agent.
• Hormone deficiencies	Glucagon challenge: if responds well likely
• Accidental poisoning (ethanol, salicylates, beta-blockers)	hyperinsulinism. If only mild/moderate ketosis likely hyperinsulinism. If significant ketosis,
• Hepatic failure	hormone deficiencies likely

Typical presentation

Inborn errors of metabolism

- Amino acidopathies and organic acidurias typically present in the newborn period with poor feeding or lethargy after protein meals and can progress to coma. In older children, they can present with acute confusion or severe vomiting in catabolic states as well as developmental delay or regression.
- Urea cycle defects present in infants after a brief period of wellness with the development of hyperammonemic encephalopathy. Those with partial enzyme deficiencies can exhibit encephalopathy or psychosis after protein meals, stress, or catabolic state.
- Fatty acid oxidation disorders present with lethargy and encephalopathy during fasting and can exhibit hyperammonemia and hypoglycemia. In addition, there may be chronic weakness, myopathy of heart and skeletal muscles, and liver failure.
- Peroxisomal disorders typically present in infants with dysmorphic features and microcephaly. As the child grows there will be developmental delay, seizures, and hypotonia. Eventually there can be developmental or intellectual regression, visual deterioration, and peripheral neuropathy as well as liver failure.
- Lysosomal disorders present initially with developmental delay, progressive hepatomegaly and splenomegaly, and a cherry-red spot in the macula. There can be cognitive deterioration, coarsening of facial features, restriction of joint movement, and peripheral neuropathy.

Neurocutaneous syndromes

NF1 criteria for diagnosis include two of the following:

- Six or more café-au-lait spots (CAL) >5 mm in prepuberty and >15 mm in post puberty.
- Two or more neurofibromas or one plexiform neurofibroma.
- Freckling in the axilla or inguinal region.
- Optic glioma.
- Two or more Lisch nodules, sphenoid dysplasia, or thinning of the long bone cortex.
- First degree relative with NF1.

CAL appear first followed by axillary freckling, Lisch nodules, and then the neurofibromas. Optic gliomas present by age 3 with decreased color vision or acuity.

Tuberous sclerosis diagnosis requires two of the following major criteria:

- Facial angiofibroma or forehead plaque.
- Non-traumatic ungual or periungual fibroma.
- Three hypomelanotic macules.
- Shagreen patch.
- Multiple retinal hamartomas.
- Glioneuronal hamartoma.
- Subependymal nodule.
- Subependymal giant cell astrocytoma (SEGA).
- Cardiac rhabdomyoma.
- Lymphangioleiomyomatosis.
- Renal angiomyolipoma.

There are also minor criteria that can be used when there is only one major criterion met.

Sturge–Weber typically presents when a child has a seizure or develops glaucoma and is also noted to have a port-wine stain. It should be distinguished from:

- Isolated facial port-wine stain (no evidence of seizures, glaucoma, or hemiparesis).
- Klippel–Trenaunay sydrome (hypertrophic limb with more extensive capillary malformation).

Structural lesions

- Meningomyelocele is typically diagnosed prenatally. At birth a raw fleshy plaque over the back with a protruding membranous sac is observed. Infants may not have any movement of lower limbs with contractures. There will be bowel and bladder dysfunction. Hydrocephalus may be present at birth or may develop shortly thereafter.
- Holoprosencephaly may be diagnosed prenatally or may be suspected in an infant with midline facial defects including single eye, single central incisor, hypotelorism or cleft lip or palate. In more mildly affected patients it may be suspected if there are endocrinopathies, or it may be diagnosed on imaging during evaluation for developmental delay.
- Dandy–Walker is typically diagnosed prenatally, but can also be revealed during MRI evaluation in childhood for macrocephaly or when hydrocephalus causes symptoms of increased intracranial pressure.

Clinical diagnosis

History

- Most children with small molecule IEM will present within the first few days of life or be detected on newborn screening.
- In older children that may have partial enzyme defects clinical history should focus on identifying episodes of periodic decompensation – typically of recurrent vomiting, altered mental status, or hypoglycemia – out of proportion to the inciting illness, possibly requiring hospitalization. One should identify whether the decompensations are related to certain types of foods or fasting.

- History of muscle cramping after exercise can indicate fatty acid oxidation defects.
- The large molecule disorders are typically suspected with a history of developmental delay particularly if there has been regression.
- Family history should include the question of consanguinity and whether there is a history of a sibling or other relatives dying in early childhood with an unexplained illness (sepsis, coma).
- Several of the neurocutaneous syndromes mentioned are inherited in an autosomal dominant fashion, so identifying close relatives or parents with similar skin markings, history of nerve tumors, eye problems, or other types of tumors (heart, kidneys) can be very helpful.
- In patients with new-onset seizures, it is helpful to identify if there are any skin markings, as seizures are a common first presentation of many of the neurocutaneous syndromes.
- Questions about developmental milestones or developmental concerns as well as identification of frequent infections can also be helpful.
- For structural lesions the history should focus on the pregnancy, including any potential toxic exposures, medications used, infections, if prenatal supplements were taken prior to pregnancy, and also problems with prior pregnancies or congenital anomalies of any organ system noted on ultrasound or after birth.
- History should also focus on developmental milestones and symptoms of increased intracranial pressure including lethargy, repetitive vomiting, and abnormal eye movements.

Physical examination
- Head size should be noted, as macrocephaly can indicate certain storage disorders.
- Tone should be noted as it can be decreased in fatty acid oxidation defects, urea cycle disorders, and peroxisomal disorders.
- Peripheral neuropathy or ataxia can be seen in peroxisomal and lysosomal disorders.
- The eyes should be examined for cherry-red spot, cataracts, and retinitis pigmentosa.
- The abdomen should be palpated to identify organomegaly – seen in storage disorders.
- Any unusual odors (fruit, rotten egg, musty) should be noted as they can help identify organic acidurias.
- In any patient where neurocutaneous syndrome is suspected a thorough evaluation of the skin should be done. On the face look for a port-wine stain, which is a capillary malformation and is a blanchable pink or red patch. A brown fibrous plaque on the forehead can indicate tuberous sclerosis, as can angiofibroma (adenoma sebacium), which are acne-like lesions in a malar distribution in the face.
- In the eyes look for Lisch nodules, which are pigmented hamartomatous nodules in the iris.
- In the mouth, gingival fibromas and dental pits can indicate TS.
- In the axilla and groin look for freckling.
- On the body look for CAL spots, which are hyperpigmented macules with regular borders and coloring. Also look for ashleaf spots, which are hypomelanotic macules that can be elliptical and typically present since birth, or a shagreen patch, which is a skin hamartoma that has an orange peel texture, typically occurring in the lumbosacral region.
- Look at the nails for periungual or ungual fibromas, which are growths that may distort the nail, longitudinal nail grooves, or white streaks (leukonychia).
- For structural lesions, examination should include head circumference charting to look for microcephaly or progressive macrocephaly. The face should be examined for hypotelorism, microphthalmia, cleft lip or palate, and single central incisor. The back should be examined for scoliosis.
- In meningomyelocele a defect will be seen over the back along with kyphosis, and there is usually clubbing of the feet and contractures of the legs. There may be flaccid paralysis with absent reflexes.

- Dandy–Walker can be associated with PHACE syndrome (*P*osterior fossa brain malformations, *H*emangioma, *A*rterial lesions, *C*ardiac abnormalities, *E*ye abnormalities) in which children have facial hemangiomas, microphthalmia, and defects in the digits of the hands or feet.

Disease severity classification
Holoprosencephaly is categorized as:
- lobar, which is the mildest, with distinct right and left cerebral ventricles and continuity seen just across the frontal cortex;
- semilobar, which is slightly more severe with only partial separation of the forebrain;
- alobar, which is the most severe with complete failure of separation of the right and left sides.

Laboratory diagnosis
Diagnostic tests for inborn errors of metabolism (Algorithm 29.1)

Disorder	Tests
Hyperammonemia	Serum amino acids, urine organic acids
Hypoglycemia	Serum amino acids, urine organic acids, acylcarnitine profile
Epileptic encephalopathy	Serum amino acids, urine organic acids
Amino acidopathy	Serum amino acids, urine organic acids
Organic aciduria	Serum amino acids, urine organic acids, acylcarnitine profile
Mitochondrial disorder	Serum amino acids, serum/CSF lactate and pyruvate
Fatty acid oxidation defect	Acylcarnitine profile, carnitine status
Congenital disorder of glycosylation	Carbohydrate-deficient transferrins
Lysosomal storage disease	Urine glucosaminoglycans, urine oligosaccharides, skin biopsy, MRI
Peroxisomal disorders	Very-long-chain fatty acids, MRI

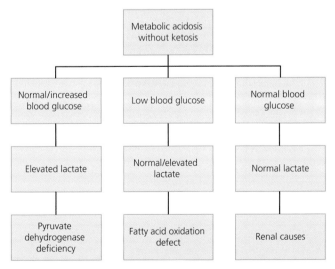

Algorithm 29.1 Evaluation of metabolic acidosis.

Diagnostic tests for neurocutaneous syndromes

- NF1: genetic testing to assess for mutation of NF1 gene used typically to screen family members of a patient with NF1 or in cases where the clinical diagnosis is unclear. The role of routine imaging of the brain and optic nerves is controversial and is generally considered unnecessary. In symptomatic individuals a contrast MRI of the brain and orbits should be done.
- TS: genetic testing is used most frequently in prenatal diagnosis or it can be used in at-risk relatives. MRI should be done in all patients to identify intracranial tumors. Renal ultrasound should be done to identify cysts and angiomyolipomas.
- SW: in a child with facial port-wine stain and seizures, glaucoma, or hemiparesis a MRI with contrast of the brain should be done to confirm presence of the characteristic leptomeningeal angioma. Genetic testing can now be performed.

Diagnostic tests for structural lesions (Algorithm 29.2)

- AFP is ordered in all pregnant women as a prenatal screen for neural tube defects.
- Prenatal ultrasound is done in all pregnant women and may pick up structural malformations of the brain.
- MRI is the most sensitive and definitive test to establish the diagnosis of all structural malformations.

Potential pitfalls/common errors made regarding diagnosis of disease

- Blood for lactate, pyruvate, and ammonia should be collected free flowing from a vein without a tourniquet, sent on ice, and analyzed quickly otherwise values will be falsely elevated.
- Samples should ideally be taken at the onset of a crisis before any hydration has occurred. It is possible for some mild or partial IEM to be missed if testing is done in a period of wellness or if treatment has already begun.

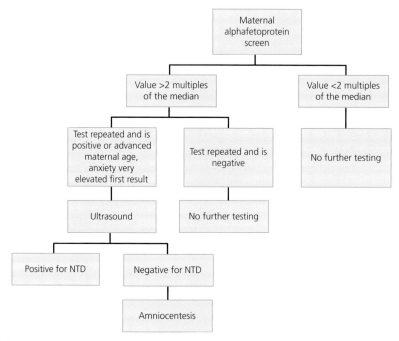

Algorithm 29.2 Investigation of elevated maternal alphafetoprotein.

- In neurocutaneous syndromes, patients with very dark or very light pigmentation markings may be missed, and the use of a Wood's lamp can be very helpful.
- In diagnosing structural lesions, maternal AFP can be low in Down's syndrome, but it may be falsely low with incorrect gestational age, maternal diabetes, or maternal obesity. It can be elevated in abdominal wall defects as well.
- Patients identified with Chiari 1 should have their spine imaged to identify if there is a syrinx present as this may alter management.

Section 4: Treatment
Treatment rationale
IEM
- Principles of treatment depend on controlling accumulation of the toxic substrate by either decreasing accumulation or accelerating its removal.
- The mainstay in most amino/organic acidopathies and urea cycle defects is dietary restriction of amino acids. Patients follow a low-protein diet with supplementation of essential amino acids and trace elements using special formulas.
- In those with fatty acid oxidation defects try to maintain a high-carbohydrate, low-fat diet and avoid fasting.
- In organic acidopathies supplementation with carnitine or glycine can help remove intramito-chondrial accumlation of coenzyme A (CoA)-esters.
- Certain disorders may benefit from specific vitamins or cofactors (B2, B6, B12). In adrenoleu-kodystrophy "Lorenzo's oil" (mixture of glyceryl trioleate and glyceryl trierucate) is thought to competitively inhibit the synthesis of very-long-chain fatty acids. It seems to be useful only in delaying the progression of disease in presymptomatic or mildly affected patients.
- In urea cycle defects medications can be used to remove ammonia; these include sodium ben-zoate and sodium phenylbutyrate as well as lactulose, which binds intestinal ammonia. In some cases arginine and intermittent carnitine should also be supplemented.
- In cases where symptoms are secondary to the deficiency of a product there have been attempts at replacing the product through gene replacement. In certain lysosomal storage disorders (Gaucher's and Pompe's) a synthetic enzyme is made with recombinant DNA technology and infused.
- Gene transfer therapy tries to get around the issue of the blood–brain barrier by using bone marrow transplants to repopulate the macrophage derivative microglial cells in the brain with functioning lysosomal/peroxisomal enzyme. It is the treatment of choice for mucopolysacchari-dosis type 1 before children turn 24 months and/or have a developmental quotient below 70, and for X-linked adrenoleukodystrophy if the disease is presymptomatic.

Neurocutaneous syndromes
- NF1: Surgical resection is used for symptomatic benign and malignant tumors. Chemotherapy is used for optic gliomas that show progression (radiologically or on ophthalmologic examination).
- TS: For infants with infantile spasms and tuberous sclerosis, vigabatrin can be considered along with adrenocorticotrophic hormone (ACTH) as first-line treatment. Vigabatrin is started at 50 mg/kg/day b.i.d. and titrated to 150 mg/kg/day. (Vigabatrin is only available to physicians reg-istered with a distribution program.) For refractory seizures, focal surgical resection of cortical tubers can be helpful. For those with brain tumors causing increased intracranial pressure, hydrocephalus, or with rapid growth, surgical resection is considered. In those patients with SEGAs that are not candidates for surgical resection, everolimus should be considered.

- SW: Seizures are often difficult to control and while medical management should be attempted first, surgical intervention including hemispherectomy or corpus callosotomy may be necessary. Some centers recommend that all patients also be placed on low-dose aspirin to help slow the progression of the hemiparesis from hypoxia-induced neuronal injury.

Structural lesions

- Infants diagnosed with meningomyelocele must be delivered at a center that has a pediatric neurosurgeon. Delivery can be vaginal as long as the infant is head first and does not have a large meningomyelocele. At birth, the defect should be covered with saline-soaked dressing (with plastic if it is large to avoid heat loss). The infant should be placed in a prone or lateral position. Antibiotics are given until the defect is closed. The defect should be closed within the first 72 hours. Serial head ultrasounds should be performed to identify hydrocephalus and, if the infant becomes symptomatic, a ventriculoperitoneal (VP) shunt should be placed. In patients with bladder dysfunction (almost all), parents should be taught to intermittently catheterize the bladder. Bowel dysfunction should be treated with an aggressive bowel regimen of laxatives and enemas. If this is not sufficient, a conduit between the umbilicus and the large intestine can be made surgically to irrigate the colon. Patients should be managed by a multidisciplinary team and be placed in physical therapy to provide adaptive equipment for mobility and to maintain optimal range of motion and posture.
- Fetal surgery to close the defect in the back has been used in infants with myelomeningocele between 18 and 25 weeks of gestation and has shown reversal of the Chiari, reduction in the need for a shunt, improved mental development, and possible improvement in lower limb function. It is offered at specialized centers.
- Symptomatic hydrocephalus in Dandy–Walker should be treated with surgical placement of a ventriculoperitoneal shunt.

When to hospitalize

- IEM patients entering a catabolic state (fasting, infection, surgery) should stop all protein and use a home glucose solution with slow reintroduction of protein to the diet after about 24 hours.
- Patients who cannot maintain oral intake or become increasingly symptomatic despite home treatment should be hospitalized.

Managing the hospitalized patient

- The catabolic state needs to be interrupted and protein intake stopped – high-energy dextrose solution is given intravenously. Parenteral lipids should be given as well if the patient does not have a fatty acid oxidation defect.
- If ammonia is elevated >400 µmol/L, dialysis should be started.

Table of treatment for IEM

Conservative treatment	Protein-restricted diet with amino acidopathies, organic acidurias, and urea cycle defects. Avoidance of fasting/hypoglycemia
Medical	Urea cycle defects: sodium benzoate 250–400 mg/kg/day, sodium phenylbutyrate 250–500 mg/kg/day, lactulose 4–20 g/day
Complementary	Amino acidopathies: carnitine 50–100 mg/kg/day Urea cycle defects: arginine 100–600 mg/kg/day, folic acid 500 µg/day, carnitine 30–50 mg/kg/day
Other	Bone marrow transplant in MPS 1 or adrenoleukodystrophy Gene replacement therapy in Gaucher's and Pompe's

Prevention/management of complications

- IEM: With high dextrose infusion, insulin may be needed to avoid significant hyperglycemia.
- Neurocutaneous syndromes: Vigabatrin causes irreversible bilateral concentric visual loss. This can happen at any time during treatment, but the risk increases with increasing dose and duration. All patients should have baseline visual testing prior to taking vigabatrin and should be monitored with visual testing every 3 months during treatment.
- Structural lesions: Ventriculoperitoneal shunts can malfunction, leading to signs of increased intracranial pressure; this should be managed by revision of the shunt.

CLINICAL PEARLS

- In infants with a presumed metabolic disorder, high-dextrose-containing fluid should be started immediately and all protein intake should stop.
- Dialysis should be considered in cases of significantly elevated ammonia or when cerebral edema is present.
- In neonates with seizures that do not respond to typical treatment, pyridoxine deficiency should be considered and an intravenous or oral pyridoxine challenge should be given.
- Not all patients with meningomyelocele need a VP shunt. Avoiding this procedure by close monitoring of head circumference and ultrasound may prevent multiple surgeries for placement of shunt and revisions.
- Children with meningomyelocele should be managed by a multidisciplinary team of neurologist, neurosurgeon, urologist, and physical and occupational therapists.

Section 5: Special populations

Pregnancy

In pregnant women that have uncontrolled phenylketonuria, the fetus is at risk for severe mental retardation, intrauterine growth retardation, and heart disease.

Section 6: Prognosis

BOTTOM LINE/CLINICAL PEARLS

- Early identification and management for many of the IEM has improved disability, prolonged lifespans, and improved neurodevelopmental outcomes.
- There is a wide variation in disability in IEM, depending on the specific defect and degree of enzymatic deficiency.
- There is a wide variation in severity of the neurocutaneous syndromes even within families.
- Patients need close surveillance to monitor for new tumors and malignant transformation.
- Despite the complicated nature of meningomyelocele the majority of children will be able to complete high school and go on to higher education.

Natural history of untreated disease

For NF1 the overall life expectancy is 15 years less than the general population. Poorer prognosis is associated with CNS tumors outside of the optic pathway or a symptomatic tumor that develops in adulthood. Up to 15% of patients will suffer from a malignant tumor.

Tuberous sclerosis has a very wide range of phenotypes, with some patients having only the dermatologic features and normal life expectancy. Those with CNS disease (intractable seizures or SEGAs) and renal disease have poorer prognoses. In younger patients, the common causes of death include status epilepticus and increased intracranial pressure or hemorrhage from SEGAs. Older patients typically die of renal failure or pulmonary disease.

The prognosis in Sturge–Weber depends on the extent of leptomeningeal involvement. If it is bilateral, seizures are more difficult to control and there is usually profound cognitive delay. In those with hemispheric involvement, up to 60% will have developmental delay. By adulthood, about 50% of patients will have neurologic impairment.

In meningomyelocele, prior to the invention of shunts, survival rate was 10%. Survival is now about 90% to age 30. Around 90% require shunt placement and most need revisions. One-third require tethered cord release.

Holoprosencephaly has a wide variation in morbidity and mortality. Severe forms are not compatible with life. Survival rate beyond 1 year of life in those with cytogenetic abnormalities is 2%, and 30–54% in those without. Dandy–Walker is associated with early death in up to one-quarter of patients typically because of associated malformations, hydrocephalus, or shunt malfunctions, and more rarely sudden death possibly related to brainstem ischemia. Up to 50% of patients have normal development, especially if there are no other associated malformations.

Follow-up tests and monitoring
- TS: MRI of the brain and renal ultrasound should be performed every 1–3 years.
- NF1: Annual dermatologic examination to monitor for progression of existing lesions, blood pressure monitoring for hypertension, screening for skeletal changes, and ophthalmologic screening.

Section 7: Reading list
Key reading sources for this chapter can be found online at www.mountsinaiexpertguides.com

Suggested websites
GeneTests: http://www.genetests.org
National Newborn Screening and Global Resource Center: http://genes-r-us.uthscsa.edu
New England Consortium of Metabolic Programs: http://newenglandconsortium.org
Tuberous Sclerosis Alliance: http://www.tsalliance.org/
Tuberous Sclerosis Association: http://www.tuberous-sclerosis.org/

Section 8: Guidelines

Title	Source	Weblink
Serving the Family from Birth to the Medical Home	Newborn Screening Task Force, American Academy of Pediatrics (AAP); Health Resources and Services Administration (HRSA) (2000) General policies about newborn screening	http://pediatrics. aappublications. org/content/106/ Supplement_2/389.extract
Newborn screening: toward a uniform screening panel and system	American College of Medical Genetics (2006) Recommended panel of genetic and metabolic disorders to test for	http://www.ncbi.nlm.nih. gov/pubmed/16735256
Health Supervision for Children with Neurofibromatosis	AAP (2008)	http://pediatrics. aappublications.org/ content/121/3/633
Tuberous Sclerosis Consensus Conference: recommendations for diagnostic evaluation	National Tuberous Sclerosis Association (1999)	http://www.ncbi.nlm.nih. gov/pubmed/10385849
Neural Tube Defects	American College of Obstetricians and Gynecologists (ACOG) (2003)	http://www.ncbi.nlm.nih. gov/pubmed/14626221

International society guidelines

Title	Source	Weblink
Tuberous Sclerosis Complex Surveillance and Management: Recommendations of the 2012 International Tuberous Sclerosis Complex Consensus Conference	International Tuberous Sclerosis Complex Consensus Group (2013)	http://www.pedneur.com/article/ S0887-8994%2813%2900491-8/ pdf
Tuberous Sclerosis Complex Diagnostic Criteria Update: Recommendations of the 2012 International Tuberous Sclerosis Complex Consensus Conference	International Tuberous Sclerosis Complex Consensus Group (2013)	http://www.pedneur.com/article/ S0887-8994%2813%2900490-6/ pdf

Section 9: Evidence for therapies

Type of evidence	Title and comment	Comment
Randomized controlled trial (RCT)	A randomized trial of prenatal versus postnatal repair of myelomeningocele (2011) **Comment**: Trial stopped early because of efficacy	http://www.nejm. org/doi/full/10.1056/ NEJMoa1014379
Prospective observational study	Hurler syndrome: II. Outcome of HLA-genotypically identical sibling and HLA-haploidentical related donor bone marrow transplantation in fifty-four children. The Storage Disease Collaborative Study Group (1998) **Comment**: Largest trial of BMT in Hurler's disease	http://www.ncbi. nlm.nih.gov/ pubmed/9516162
RCT	Efficacy and safety of everolimus for subependymal giant cell astrocytomas associated with tuberous sclerosis complex (EXIST-1): a multicenter, randomized, placebo-controlled phase 3 trial (2013) **Comment**: Supports the use of everolimus for SEGAs in TS. Suggests it may be disease-modifying in other TS symptoms	http://www.ncbi. nlm.nih.gov/ pubmed/23158522
RCT	Randomized trial of vigabatrin in patients with infantile spasms (2001) **Comment**: First evidence that subset IS patients with TS patients respond favorably to vigabatrin	http://www.ncbi. nlm.nih.gov/ pubmed/11673582

Additional material for this chapter can be found online at:
www.mountsinaiexpertguides.com

This includes a case study, multiple choice questions, and a reading list.

CHAPTER 30

Epilepsy

Madeline C. Fields and Lara V. Marcuse
Icahn School of Medicine at Mount Sinai, New York, NY, USA

OVERALL BOTTOM LINE
- Epilepsy is the fourth most common neurologic disease and affects approximately 1–3% of adults in the USA.
- The most common causes of epilepsy are prenatal injury, head trauma, tumors, stroke, meningitis, encephalitis, dementing illnesses, genetic etiologies, and other structural abnormalities.
- The treatment of epilepsy involves giving appropriate anti-seizure medication taking into account comorbidities as well as identifying appropriate surgical candidates.

Section 1: Background
Definitions
- Seizure: Transient occurrence of signs or symptoms due to hypersynchronous or excessive neuronal activity. The abnormal neuronal activity can affect sensory, motor, and autonomic function; consciousness; emotional state; memory; cognition; or behavior.
- Epilepsy: At least two unprovoked seizures occurring >24 hours apart; or one unprovoked seizure and a likelihood of more than 60% for another seizure based on the etiology; or diagnosis of an epilepsy syndrome such as absence or juvenile myoclonic epilepsy.
- After a single unprovoked seizure, the risk for another is 45% within the first 2 years. However, under certain circumstances some patients after a single seizure are at a much higher risk of future attacks (e.g. a patient with a prior brain injury, EEG with seizure waves, brain imaging abnormality and a nocturnal seizure).

Disease classification
Seizures are classified as being focal or generalized. Focal seizures originate at some point within networks limited to one hemisphere. Generalized seizures rapidly engage bilateral networks. The etiology of epilepsy can be subdivided into three categories: genetic, structural or metabolic, and unknown.

Incidence/prevalence
- About 15,000 adults present per year with an unprovoked first time seizure.
- Around 10% of US citizens will experience a seizure over the course of their lives.

Mount Sinai Expert Guides: Neurology, First Edition. Edited by Stuart C. Sealfon, Rajeev Motiwala, and Charles B. Stacy.
© 2016 John Wiley & Sons, Ltd. Published 2016 by John Wiley & Sons, Ltd.
Companion website: www.mountsinaiexpertguides.com

Table 30.1 Causes of epilepsy.

Etiology	Percentage
Unknown	66
Stroke	10.9
Head trauma	5.5
Neurodegenerative disease	3.5
Encephalopathy (pre- or preinatal origin)	8
Brain tumors	4.1
Infections	2

- Epilepsy affects more than 2 million people in the USA and more than 50 million people worldwide.
- The incidence of epilepsy in the USA and Europe is approximately 55 per 100,000 population.
- The incidence rates are much higher among children under 1 year of age and in individuals over age 60.
- The overall prevalence of epilepsy is 4.7 cases per 1000 persons.

Economic impact
- Epilepsy and seizures affect nearly 3 million US citizens of all ages, at an estimated annual cost of US$17.6 billion in direct and indirect costs.

Etiology and pathogenesis
- Over 50% of epilepsy cases have no identifiable cause (Table 30.1).
- Frequently identified causes include prenatal injury, head trauma, tumors, stroke, meningitis, encephalitis, dementia, genetic causes, and structural abnormalities such as cortical dysplasia or heterotopias.
- The mechanisms of pathogenesis are poorly understood.

Section 2: Prevention and screening

> **BOTTOM LINE/CLINICAL PEARLS**
> - No interventions have been demonstrated to decrease the risk of developing epilepsy.
> - Short-term anti-seizure medications may be used to decrease the immediate occurrence of seizures when they are especially likely or dangerous, such as after trauma, subarachnoid hemorrhage, or neurosurgical procedures, but this has not been shown to affect the long-term risk of developing epilepsy.
> - Anti-seizure medication is used to reduce the risk of subsequent seizure, usually after the occurrence of two unprovoked seizures, or after a single seizure and in someone who has an EEG with seizure waves, brain imaging abnormality, or nocturnal seizure.

Primary prevention
- Possible preventable causes of epilepsy include traumatic brain injury, stroke, and brain infection.

Secondary prevention

• Antiepileptic medication is used to reduce the risk of subsequent seizure.

Section 3: Diagnosis

> **BOTTOM LINE/CLINICAL PEARLS**
> • The diagnosis is made by a combination of history, physical examination, and diagnostic tests.
> • History is crucial to ascertain the patient's subjective experience, if any, prior to loss of consciousness.
> • Certain experiences, like déjà vu or a rising sensation in the epigastrium, are highly suspicious for seizure auras.
> • Seizures are stereotypic. Brief events, particularly experiences on the order of seconds to minutes, are characteristic of seizures. If a patient loses awareness, information from a witness is essential.
> • Urinary incontinence, tongue biting, post-event confusion, and muscle aches are all typical features of a generalized tonic-clonic convulsion. Transient motor weakness after a seizure (Todd paralysis) is a useful sign.
> • A comprehensive physical and neurologic examination should be performed to look for cardiac arrhythmias, cutaneous stigmata, and neurologic deficits. Additionally, ancillary tests such as blood tests, EEG, and MRI are useful.

Differential diagnosis

Differential diagnosis	Features	Examination	Investigations
Syncope	Syncope is often preceded by feelings of lightheadedness, palpitations, and diaphoresis. The syncope itself is typically brief (<20 seconds) without post-ictal confusion. Convulsions may occur at the end of the syncope if hypoperfusion is sustained (convulsive syncope)	The neurologic examination is typically normal	Full blood count, serum electrolytes, renal panel, random blood glucose. EKG. Check for orthostatic hypotension; tilt table testing, if available
Migraine	Typically strong family history of migraine. Progression of symptoms on the order of 15–30 minutes (seizures are briefer). Visual symptoms may be prominent	The neurologic examination is typically normal	May have non-specific white matter lesions on MRI
TIA or stroke	Sudden onset with negative symptoms such as aphasia, weakness, sensory loss. Vascular risk factors including diabetes, hypertension, hyperlipidemia, previous stroke or TIA. TIA and strokes tend not to be stereotyped	Fixed focal neurologic deficit	Check HbA1c, cholesterol, carotid Dopplers, echocardiogram, and MRI

Differential diagnosis	Features	Examination	Investigations
Transient global amnesia	Episode typically lasts for 4–24 hours. No alteration in consciousness. May recur	At the time of the event people suffer from anterograde more than retrograde amnesia. Remote memory remains intact. The patient must not have loss of personal identity or clouding of consciousness. Motor function, speech, and judgment remain intact	MRI brain may show abnormalities in the hippocampal region or may be normal
Sleep disorders	Obstructive sleep apnea (OSA), REM sleep disorders, and hypnic jerks occur at night or right before sleep and must be differentiated from frontal lobe epilepsy. In OSA the patient often has a history of snoring	Neurologic examination typically normal. For OSA the patient may be obese	Sleep study
Panic attack	Feelings of intense fear and imminent doom. Typically lasts longer than a seizure (5–30 min). No loss of consciousness	Tachycardia, diaphoresis, nausea	EKG and EEG should be normal
Psychogenic non-epileptic attacks	Psychiatric history. History of sexual or physical abuse. History of coexisting epilepsy	Eyes tend to be closed during the event. Movements are often bilateral with preserved awareness. Pelvic thrusting common	Capturing the event itself during long-term EEG monitoring followed by clear communication with the patient is often the most effective intervention

Clinical diagnosis

History

- Inquire about premature birth, developmental delay, or febrile seizures that may be relevant to the etiology of epilepsy.
- Consider risk factors such as traumatic brain injury, meningitis, encephalitis, and family history of epilepsy.
- Recurrent feelings of déjà vu, rising epigastric sensations, funny smells or tastes, and feelings of intense fear raise the possibility of temporal lobe epilepsy.
- Ask if the patient has periods of unaccounted time. For example, has he gone from one place to another and not known how he got there?
- Ask if the patient was a "spacey kid" – looking for possible absence seizures.
- Ask about early morning jerks – looking for possible juvenile myoclonic epilepsy (JME).

Physical examination

- Cardiac examination – are there any possible cardiac causes for loss of consciousness (e.g. cardiac arrhythmia, structural heart disease)?
- Skin examination – café-au-lait spots, hypopigmentation, shagreen patches, port-wine stain, and other skin lesions suggest an underlying neurocutaneous disorder.
- General examination – as infection can lower the seizure threshold, each patient should be examined for signs of an underlying infection.
- Neurologic examination – are there any focal neurologic findings to suggest underlying structural brain lesion or brain dysfunction? A funduscopic examination should be performed to look for papilledema from increased intracranial pressure.

Disease severity classification

Around 70% of people with epilepsy are well controlled on one or two anti-seizure medications. However, approximately 30% of individuals continue to have seizures despite medications. These people are considered medically refractory.

Laboratory diagnosis

- Reversible causes
  - Metabolic:
    - Hypo or hypernatremia
    - Hypo or hyperglycemia
    - Hypomagnesemia
    - Hypocalcemia
    - Hypokalemia
    - Liver failure
    - Uremia
    - Altered anti-seizure drug metabolism, bioavailability (protein binding), or non-compliance.
  - Toxic or withdrawal states:
    - Many drugs are epileptogenic, including B-lactam antibiotics specifically penicillin, the cephalosporins and carbapenems, clozapine, phenothiazines, sevoflurane and bupropion.
    - Alcohol withdrawal or intoxication.
    - Cocaine intoxication.
    - Barbiturate or benzodiazepine withdrawal.
    - Phencyclidine, amphetamines, and heroin.
  - Infection:
    - Meningitis or encephalitis.

List of diagnostic tests

- EKG to evaluate for arrhythmia or prolonged QT syndrome.
- CT head.
- MRI brain with and without contrast with high-resolution protocol for the temporal lobes.
- EEG – epileptiform potentials (between events) are an indicator that the event itself may have been a seizure.
- Long-term inpatient or ambulatory video EEG monitoring to capture the actual event is often necessary to clarify the diagnosis. Long-term monitoring is also used to make sure that the patient is no longer having seizures, as seizures can often be subclinical.

- Lumbar puncture if the history or examination are worrisome for meningitis or encephalitis, especially in immunocompromised patients.
- Genetic testing in selected cases as appropriate.

Diagnostic clinical and EEG findings for common seizure types

Common seizure types	Clinical	EEG
Generalized		
Absence seizures	Frequent brief spells of inattention. May be unrecognized or confused with attention deficit disorders. Can sometimes be triggered by hyperventilation	3 Hz spike-and-wave discharges
Juvenile myoclonic epilepsy (JME)	Typically early morning jerks. Facilitated by sleep deprivation and sudden arousal	4.5–5 Hz polyspike-and-wave discharges. 20% triggered by photic stimulation
Generalized tonic clonic convulsion (GTCC)	Stiffening with loss of consciousness typically with a fall to the ground and eyes rolling up. This is followed by contraction and relaxation of the muscles	Generalized spike-and-wave discharges may be seen followed by movement and muscle artifact
Focal seizures		
Temporal lobe	Feelings of fear, déjà vu, rising epigastric sensations, funny smells or tastes. Various automatisms like lip smacking, rubbing hands together	Abnormal evolving discharges over the temporal region
Frontal lobe	Tend to be short (<1 min), occur in clusters, typically out of sleep. Bicycling, pelvic thrusting, screaming, laughing, crying, fencer posturing (one arm extends while the other flexes), difficulty speaking or unresponsiveness	Often normal
Parietal lobe	Numbness, tingling, heat, pressure, electricity, pain. May occur as a jacksonian march	Abnormal evolving discharges over the parietal region
Occipital lobe	Visual hallucinations, decreased vision, blindness, involuntary eye movement	Abnormal evolving discharges over the occipital region

Potential pitfalls/common errors made regarding diagnosis of disease

- TIA, syncope, psychogenic events, and migraine can all mimic seizures as they are all paroxysmal. If there is a persistent diagnostic question, long-term EEG monitoring should be performed in an attempt to document and characterize the episode.
- Metabolic derangements (i.e. hypoglycemia, hyponatremia) can cause seizures but should not be treated with anti-seizure medications.
- A single seizure caused by alcohol withdrawal should not be treated with anti-seizure medications. Long-term anticonvulsants will not prevent seizures during future episodes of alcohol withdrawal. However, alcoholics can have epilepsy and the etiology for their seizures needs careful consideration.

Section 4: Treatment

The goal of treatment with antiepileptic medication is to prevent further seizures. Currently there are over 25 anti-seizure medications available in the USA (Tables 30.2 and 30.3).

The choice of anti-seizure medication depends upon the seizure type as well as the comorbidities of each individual.

- For people with depression, lamotrigine, oxcarbazepine, carbamazepine, and valproic acid are good choices whereas levetiracetam may need to be avoided.
- For those people with comorbid migraine headaches, topiramate, zonisamide, and valproic acid should be considered.
- People who are already on medications that utilize the cytochrome P450 system (e.g. statins, warfarin, steroids, chemotherapy, antiretrovirals) should avoid medications that induce P450 such as phenytoin, carbamazepine, and phenobarbital.
- In women of child-bearing age, valproic acid should be avoided as it is the most teratogenic.
- If a patient is typically non-compliant, a once-a-day drug, for example levetiracetam extended release or lamotrigine extended release, is preferable to medications that require frequent dosing.
- For people who cannot swallow pills, a liquid formulation may be necessary.
- Zonisamide and topiramate should be avoided in people with a history of renal calculi.

  Other treatment options include vagal nerve stimulation (VNS), epilepsy surgery, and responsive neurostimulation (RNS) known as NeuroPace.

- VNS is FDA approved for supplementary treatment of refractory focal epilepsy. The apparatus consists of a pulse generator and a bipolar VNS lead, which is attached to the left vagus nerve in its mid-cervical portion. The lead delivers biphasic current that cycles between on and off periods. Patients wear a magnet bracelet, which when placed over the pulse generator in the chest can change the frequency of stimulation to interrupt a seizure. A new VNS (AspireSR) provides responsive stimulation to heart rate increases that may be associated with seizures.

Table 30.2 Anti-seizure medications.

Carbamazepine (Tegretol)	Oxcarbazepine extended release[a] (Oxtellar XR)
Clobazam[a] (Onfi)	Perampanel (Fycompa)
Eslicarbazepine[a] (Aptiom)	Phenytoin (Dilantin)
Ethosuximide (Zarontin)	Pregabalin[a] (Lyrica)
Ezogabine[a] (Potiga)	Primidone (Mysoline)
Felbamate (Felbatol)	Rufinamide[a] (Banzel)
Gabapentin (Neurontin)	Tiagabine[a] (Gabitril)
Lacosamide[a] (Vimpat)	Topiramate[a] (Topamax)
Lamotrigine[a] (Lamictal)	Topiramate extended release (Qudexy XR)
Lamotrigine extended release[a] (Lamictal XR)	Topiramate extended release[a] (Trokendi XR)
Levetiracetam[a] (Keppra)	Valproic acid (Depakote)
Levetiracetam extended release[a] (Keppra XR)	Vigabatrin (Sabril)
Oxcarbazepine[a] (Trileptal)	Zonisamide[a] (Zonegran)

[a] Denotes newer anti-seizure medications; these may have fewer side effects but may not be superior in efficacy.

Table 30.3 Commonly used anti-seizure medications.

Medication	Starting dose; initial target dose	Adverse effects
Carbamazepine	100 mg q. 12 h; 400 mg q. 12 h	Dizziness, double/blurred vision, ataxia, agranulocytosis, aplastic anemia, hepatic failure, hyponatremia
Clobazam	5 mg q. 12 h; 20 mg q. 12 h	Sedation
Gabapentin	100 mg three times daily; 600 mg three times daily	Sedation, fatigue, dizziness
Lacosamide	50 mg q. 12 h; 100 mg q. 12 h	Ataxia
Lamotrigine	25 mg/day; 200 mg q. 12 h	Insomnia, rash, Stevens–Johnson syndrome, multiorgan failure, ataxia Titration schedule varies depending on interactions with other medications
Levetiracetam	500 mg q. 12 h; 1000 mg q. 12 h	Fatigue, irritability, anxiety, psychosis
Oxcarbazepine	150 mg q. 12 h; 600 mg q. 12 h	Hyponatremia, Stevens–Johnson syndrome
Phenobarbital	30 mg/day; 120 mg/day	Depression, blood dyscrasias, hepatic failure, rash, arthritis
Phenytoin	3–5 mg/kg/day; 300 mg/day	Gingival hyperplasia, blood dyscrasias, rash, hepatic failure, lupus-like syndrome
Topiramate	25 mg q. 12 h; 100 mg q. 12 h	Word-finding difficulty, slowed speech, problems concentrating, anorexia, weight loss, paresthesias, metabolic acidosis, renal calculi, acute glaucoma, heatstroke
Valproic acid	250 mg q. 12 h; 1000 mg q. 12 h	Thrombocytopenia, tremor, hair loss, weight gain, hepatic failure, hyperammonemia, aplastic anemia, pancreatitis
Zonisamide	25 mg q. 12 h; 100 mg q. 12 h	Problems concentrating, irritability, anorexia, weight loss, aplastic anemia, renal calculi

Results with VNS are variable, but data from randomized trials have shown a reduction of seizures by about 30% in the first year with therapeutic stimulation.

- A randomized controlled trial comparing epilepsy surgery for temporal lobe epilepsy versus best medical management was conducted by Wiebe et al. (2001; see Reading list). At 1 year, seizures impairing awareness and quality of life were significantly better in the surgical group than in the medical group. For refractory focal epilepsy, surgical evaluation should be discussed and explored with patients. The pre-surgical workup includes tests to quantify the prognosis for curing the epilepsy surgically and assessing the risks of removing the epileptic focus. The pre-surgical workup may include capturing seizures on long-term EEG monitoring, Wada testing, neuropsychiatric testing, MRI imaging, fMRI, a psychiatric consultation.
- Intracranially placed RNS is also available. NeuroPace provides responsive cortical stimulation via an implanted programmable neurostimulator connected to depth or subdural strip electrodes. These electrodes are placed on the brain according to the seizure focus. The neurostimulator senses electrocorticographic activity and is programmed to provide stimulation in response to

seizure activity. In a randomized, double-blind, multicenter, sham-stimulation controlled study seizures were significantly reduced in 37.9% of treated patients compared to the sham 17.3%.
- Other treatments for epilepsy including diet (e.g. ketogenic diet or modified Atkins diet) have anti-seizure affects. Additionally, medications targeted at inflammation, and laser ablation of epileptic foci are on the horizon.

When to hospitalize
- Status epilepticus – any seizure lasting longer than 5 minutes or two seizures where the person does not return to baseline in between.
- Head trauma.
- New focal neurologic deficits.
- Elective admission with video EEG monitoring to clarify the diagnosis.
- Elective admission with video EEG monitoring to change medication in people with refractory epilepsy who are at risk for uncontrolled dangerous seizures.

Managing the hospitalized patient
- Patients should have an intravenous line.
- Seizure precautions including an order for lorazepam (Ativan) 2 mg i.v. p.r.n. if seizure longer than 5 minutes.
- If possible, all hospitalized epilepsy patients with video EEG should be watched on a screen in real time by a nurse or patient care assistant. This ensures the safety of the patient and allows nursing to assess the patient during any clinical event.

Prevention of complications
- Assess and promote medication compliance.
- Avoid triggers, most commonly stress, lack of sleep, and alcohol.
- Avoid medication interactions.

CLINICAL PEARLS
Initial approach to treatment
- Start treatment after two unprovoked seizures more than 24 hours apart; after one seizure and a high risk of recurrent attacks; or after the diagnosis of an epilepsy syndrome.
- Chose an anti-seizure medication that best suits the patient's comorbidities and current medications.

Section 5: Special populations
Pregnancy
- Supplement women of child-bearing age with at least 0.4 mg of folic acid before and during pregnancy.
- Clinicians should be aware that many anti-seizure medications interfere with oral contraception.
- Ideally, women with epilepsy should be seizure free for at least 9 months prior to pregnancy. This is associated with a high rate (84–92%) of remaining seizure-free during pregnancy.
- Monitor drug levels during pregnancy. Often higher doses of the medication are needed to maintain the same level.
- Try to avoid valproic acid as well as polypharmacy during pregnancy in order to decrease the risk of congenital malformations and poor cognitive outcomes. If possible, avoidance of phenytoin and phenobarbital during pregnancy may be considered to prevent reduced cognitive outcomes.

- Anti-seizure medication is excreted in the breastmilk to a lesser or greater degree depending on the medication. However, given the proven benefits of breastfeeding and the unclear risks, the American Academy of Neurology recommends encouraging breastfeeding in women with epilepsy.

Children

- The neonatal period has the greatest risk of seizure.
- Febrile seizures affect children aged 6 months to 6 years of age. They occur in 2–5% of children. There is a hereditary predisposition. Typical febrile seizures are tonic clonic in nature and occur in the setting of a viral illness with fever.
  - Prolonged febrile seizures have been linked with mesial temporal sclerosis, which is the most common pathology found in patients with temporal lobe epilepsy.
- Valproic acid is avoided, if possible, in the first 2 years of life due to the risk of liver failure and hemorrhagic pancreatitis.
- There are many well-described benign and malignant pediatric epilepsy syndromes.

Elderly

- For adults, the incidence of epilepsy increases over the age of 65.
- Status epilepticus is the presenting seizure type in 70% of the elderly who have not previously suffered from epilepsy.
- The elderly have a higher rate of seizure recurrence (Musicco et al. 1997; see Reading list).
- For those that develop epilepsy, morbidity and mortality are high.
- The elderly typically have slower elimination of drugs (by 20–40%) owing to several factors, including slowed metabolic rate and reduction in renal clearance.
- Elderly patients are typically taking medications fo other medical conditions and are at risk for adverse drug–drug interactions.
- Enzyme-inducing anti-seizure medications such as phenobarbital, phenytoin, and carbamazepine increase the metabolism of many commonly prescribed drugs such as coumadin, statins, and immunosuppressants.

Section 6: Prognosis

> **CLINICAL PEARLS**
> - Most types of epilepsy are not progressive.
> - Progressive epilepsy syndromes include Lafora disease, Unverricht–Lundborg disease, neuronal ceroid lipofuscinoses, sialidosis, myoclonic epilepsy with ragged red fibers, and dentatorubral-pallidoluysian atrophy.

Natural history of untreated disease

- After a first unprovoked seizure, approximately 32% will have a recurrence at 1 year and 46% by 5 years.
- Patients with a history of symptomatic seizures, even in the remote past, have an increased risk of mortality.
- Seizure etiology and the EEG are the strongest predictors of recurrence.

- Seizures in a patient with HIV, or in someone with a meningioma, neurocysticercosis, or stroke, have a risk of recurrence of more than 60%.
- Multiple seizures prior to the initiation of anti-seizure medication are a risk factor for the development of refractory epilepsy.

Prognosis for treated patients

- About 70% of patients with epilepsy will be seizure free on one or two anti-seizure medications; 30% will be refractory.
- Most patients with epilepsy live full and healthy lives. However, overall mortality is higher than for the normal population. Death can occur from the underlying neurologic disorder in individuals with symptomatic epilepsy, accidents during seizures, sudden unexplained/unexpected death in epilepsy patients (SUDEP), medication-related deaths, and status epilepticus. The risk of SUDEP is approximately 1 case for every 370–1100 patients with epilepsy.

Section 7: Reading list

Key reading sources for this chapter can be found online at www.mountsinaiexpertguides.com

Suggested website

International League Against Epilepsy: www.ilae.org

Additional material for this chapter can be found online at:
www.mountsinaiexpertguides.com

This includes advice for patients, a case study, multiple choice questions, and a reading list.

CHAPTER 31

Autonomic Disorders

Jessica Robinson-Papp
Icahn School of Medicine at Mount Sinai, New York, NY, USA

Overall bottom line

- Autonomic disorders can cause a wide array of symptoms, which may mimic the effects of other systemic or organ-specific illnesses.
- Patients with these disorders may experience one or more of the following symptoms: orthostatic dizziness or fainting, nausea or vomiting especially with meals, diarrhea, constipation, dry eyes and mouth, urinary incontinence, sexual dysfunction, and changes in sweating, skin temperature, or color.
- The clinician must attempt to determine if the autonomic disorder is a feature of a neurologic disorder (such as Parkinson's disease or peripheral neuropathy) or if it is an isolated syndrome (such as neurocardiogenic syncope or postural orthostatic tachycardia syndrome (POTS)).
- Autonomic function is usually assessed using a battery of autonomic reflex tests that include cardiovascular reflexes and sweat output.
- Treatment focuses on management of symptoms, and treatment of the underlying cause of the autonomic disorder when possible.

Section 1: Background

Definition of disease

An autonomic disorder is a disease that causes dysfunction of the autonomic nervous system leading to impaired neurologic regulation of one or more of the following:

- control of heart rate (HR) and vasomotor tone;
- gastrointestinal motility;
- production of saliva and tears;
- pupil constriction and dilation;
- urination;
- sexual function;
- thermoregulation.

Symptoms of autonomic dysfunction are similarly diverse, and may include:

- orthostatic dizziness or fainting;
- nausea or vomiting, especially with meals;
- diarrhea or constipation;
- dry eyes and mouth;

Mount Sinai Expert Guides: Neurology, First Edition. Edited by Stuart C. Sealfon, Rajeev Motiwala, and Charles B. Stacy.
© 2016 John Wiley & Sons, Ltd. Published 2016 by John Wiley & Sons, Ltd.
Companion website: www.mountsinaiexpertguides.com

- urinary incontinence;
- sexual dysfunction;
- changes in sweating, skin temperature, or color.

Disease classification

Autonomic disorders can be classified in the following categories:

- Neurodegenerative autonomic disorders arise from degeneration of autonomic structures, which can be subclassified as disorders of the central nervous system (CNS) (e.g. multiple system atrophy) or of the peripheral nervous system (PNS) (e.g. autonomic neuropathy associated with diabetes).
- Syndromic or "benign" autonomic disorders are not associated with any known neurodegeneration or structural lesions, but still cause autonomic symptoms (e.g. neurocardiogenic syncope or postural orthostatic tachycardia syndrome (POTS)).
- Medication-induced autonomic dysfunction.
- Traumatic injury that affects autonomic function (e.g. spinal cord injury).
- Surgically induced autonomic dysfunction.
- Autoimmune and parainfectious autonomic dysfunction.

Incidence/prevalence

- Approximately 30% of patients with Parkinson's disease have some autonomic dysfunction, although it usually is more prominent late in the course of disease.
- Multiple system atrophy and pure autonomic failure are rare.
- The most common cause of autonomic neuropathy in the USA is diabetes. It is estimated that 73% of type 2 diabetics have at least mild autonomic neuropathy.
- The prevalence of POTS is estimated to be at least 170/100,000 in the general population.
- Neurocardiogenic syncope is extremely common, with an estimated prevalence of 22% in the general population.

Etiology

- Autonomic dysfunction in Parkinson's disease is caused by neurodegeneration in the CNS (brainstem autonomic nuclei) and in the PNS (autonomic ganglia). In contrast, autonomic dysfunction in multiple system atrophy is attributed to the CNS only and pure autonomic failure to the PNS only.
- Autonomic neuropathy is most commonly caused by diabetes. Other causes include amyloidosis (either inherited or acquired), HIV, and autoimmune disease.
- The benign syndromic autonomic disorders such as POTS and neurocardiogenic syncope typically do not have a specific underlying etiology. However, POTS is sometimes post-viral and in this setting may be autoimmune.

Pathology/pathogenesis

- Autonomic dysfunction associated with Parkinson's disease and pure autonomic failure is associated with the deposition of Lewy bodies. Multiple system atrophy is associated with the deposition of α-synuclein.
- Autonomic neuropathy in diabetes is likely caused by direct axonal injury due to hyperglycemia, autoimmune mechanisms, and altered fatty acid metabolism and also ischemic injury due to microvascular compromise.

Section 2: Prevention and screening

Not applicable for this topic.

Section 3: Diagnosis

BOTTOM LINE/CLINICAL PEARLS

- Orthostatic intolerance, i.e. fainting or dizziness or lightheadedness on standing, may be a symptom of an autonomic disorder. The clinician should inquire whether there are symptoms of autonomic dysfunction in other organ systems, e.g. gastrointestinal or genitourinary. Such symptoms may be subtle and the patient may not realize that they could be related to orthostatic intolerance.
- Signs of an underlying neurologic disease should be sought on examination, in particular signs of peripheral neuropathy or parkinsonism. Orthostatic vital signs should be measured. Features of peripheral neuropathy include paresthesias, neuropathic pain, decreased sensation, and diminished deep tendon reflexes in a distal distribution. Features of parkinsonism include tremor, muscular rigidity, and slowed movements.
- Investigation into the autonomic disorder begins with an autonomic reflex screen, which is a non-invasive laboratory-based test of cardiovascular reflexes and sweat output. Further investigations depend on the suspected cause of the autonomic dysfunction. Electromyography may be indicated if peripheral neuropathy is suspected, whereas MRI of the brain may be performed if the neurologic examination reveals parkinsonism.

Differential diagnosis for fainting and episodic dizziness (see also Chapter 5)

Differential diagnosis	Features
Medication-induced orthostasis	Antihypertensives and medications with anticholinergic side effects can cause orthostatic hypotension (OH)
Isolated primary autonomic disorders: Neurocardiogenic syncope	Prodrome of faintness, typically during micturition, pain, stress. Brief loss of consciousness. Transient bradycardia, hypotension (easy to miss, may be followed by sympathetic overdrive). Absence of associated findings
Postural orthostatic tachycardia syndrome (POTS)	Typically occurs in young healthy women. Complaints of palpitations, fatigue, lightheadedness. Increase in heart rate (HR) without significant change in blood pressure on standing
Neurodegenerative disorders: Multiple system atrophy (Shy–Drager syndrome)	Parkinsonian features, profound orthostatic intolerance, may have other systems involved (cerebellar, corticospinal)
Parkinson's disease	Orthostatic hypotension is common and may be worsened by levodopa or dopamine agonists
Autonomic neuropathy	Common in diabetes, also in amyloidosis and post-infectious. May be prominent in Guillain–Barré (acute inflammatory demyelinating polyneuropathy)
Primary cardiac disease	Usually in the setting of vascular risk factors
Seizures	Can also cause episodic loss of consciousness, can be confused with syncope
Vestibular dysfunction	An alternative cause of dizziness, usually a sense of motion rather than lightheadedness

Typical presentation

The presentations of autonomic disorders are variable, but easily recognized when severe. Patients can have features of the causative neurologic disease (e.g. peripheral neuropathy) in conjunction with marked orthostatic intolerance, and many of the other autonomic symptoms described above. In patients with milder disease, the presentation depends on which autonomic functions are impaired. Patients may have severe symptoms in one organ system (e.g. gastrointestinal) and few or absent symptoms in others, or they may experience more diffuse and milder symptoms. Patients with the syndromic or "benign" autonomic disorders typically have orthostatic intolerance without other autonomic symptoms.

Clinical diagnosis

History

Autonomic disorders often cause orthostatic intolerance, which patients commonly report as dizziness. Dizziness is a non-specific complaint, but certain features suggest an autonomic etiology. Symptoms should be positional, occurring while standing but not while supine. Symptoms may be exacerbated by heat or after eating. The dizziness may be described as lightheadedness, weakness, or fatigue, which may be accompanied by darkening of vision, muffling of hearing, tremulousness, nausea, sweating, or pallor. Patients typically do not experience a sense of motion.

Physical examination

The examination begins with a complete neurologic examination to determine if there are signs of a neurologic disease associated with autonomic dysfunction. Particular attention should be paid to signs of peripheral neuropathy (decreased distal sensation and reflexes) and signs of parkinsonism (slowed movements, rigidity, tremor). Patients with a syndromic benign autonomic disorder typically have a normal neurologic examination. Blood pressure (BP) and HR should be measured supine and standing (Figure 31.1). Orthostatic hypotension is defined as a decrease of 20 mmHg in systolic BP or 10 mmHg in diastolic BP. Patients with preserved cardiovagal function will have a compensatory tachycardia. Cold feet with blue or purple discoloration can be a sign of vasomotor changes. Very dry hands and feet can be a sign of anhidrosis or sweating deficits.

Laboratory diagnosis (Algorithm 31.1)

List of diagnostic tests

An autonomic reflex screen should be performed. A typical screen contains the following tests:

- Quantitative Sudomotor Axon Reflex Test. In this test a small disposable capsule that releases acetylcholine under computer control is placed on the skin and sweat output is quantified. This is a measure of the functional integrity of sympathetic fibers innervating sweat glands in the skin.
- The following three tests are measures of cardiovascular autonomic reflexes. They are performed while HR, BP, and respirations are monitored continuously and non-invasively.
  - HR response to deep breathing. The patient is instructed in a standardized, slow, rhythmic breathing exercise. The variability in HR is measured, which reflects parasympathetic (vagal) function.
- Valsalva maneuver. The patient forcibly exhales to a pressure of 40 mmHg for 15 seconds. Changes in HR and BP are measured and reflect both sympathetic and parasympathetic function.
- Tilt table testing. The patient is monitored for OH and heart rate changes associated with changes in body position from supine to upright.

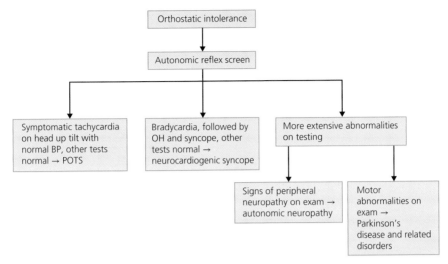

Algorithm 31.1 Diagnostic algorithm for orthostatic intolerance.

Further workup will be determined by the type of autonomic dysfunction detected on the autonomic reflex screen and the findings on neurologic examination.

Potential pitfalls/common errors made regarding diagnosis of disease

- Autonomic disorders may be mistaken for disease of the affected organ system itself. For example, gastric outlet obstruction can cause symptoms similar to gastroparesis due to autonomic dysfunction. The presence of symptoms in multiple organ systems may be a helpful clue.
- Postural orthostatic tachycardia syndrome may be associated with chronic fatigue and chronic pain syndromes, and so symptoms of dizziness in these patient populations should not be dismissed.
- Autonomic disorders should always be considered in symptomatic patients with peripheral neuropathy or parkinsonism. Medication side effects may also be a cause of autonomic symptoms in these patients.

Section 4: Treatment (Algorithm 31.2)
Treatment rationale
Treatment of the underlying disorder should be instituted when applicable, for example hyperglycemia in diabetic autonomic neuropathy. First-line treatment of orthostatic intolerance is to discontinue any aggravating medications when possible (e.g. antihypertensives and medications with anticholinergic side effects) and increasing fluid and salt intake. Other conservative measures are summarized in the Table of treatment. Fludrocortisone, midodrine, and recently approved droxidopa are used to increase BP when conservative measures are insufficient. Other agents such as desmopressin, beta-blockers, and pyridostigmine are often used in the treatment of POTS.

There are various interventions for other symptoms of autonomic dysfunction. Prokinetic agents (e.g. metoclopramide) can be used for nausea and vomiting due to gastroparesis. Loperamide may be used for diarrhea, with a course of antibiotics added if bacterial overgrowth is suspected. Behavioral therapies such as timed voiding, avoidance of caffeine, and biofeedback may be used as first-line treatments for urinary symptoms. Anticholinergics (tolterodine, oxybutynin) are used

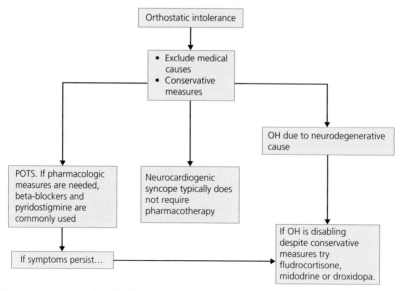

Algorithm 31.2 Treatment algorithm for orthostatic intolerance.

for detrusor overactivity. In more severe cases of urinary dysfunction, intermittent self-catheteriza-tion may be needed. Phosphodiesterase inhibitors (e.g. sildenafil) can be used for erectile dysfunction.

When to hospitalize
• Autonomic disorders rarely necessitate hospitalization. The exception is in the setting of unsta-ble vital signs, such as markedly fluctuating HR and BP, which may occur in the setting of acute neurologic syndromes such as Guillain–Barré syndrome.

Managing the hospitalized patient
• Orthostatic intolerance occurs frequently in hospitalized patients due to deconditioning. Specific treatment other than minimization of fall risk, and gradual reinstitution of physical activity, is usually not required.

Table of treatment

Conservative treatment Conservative treatment is indicated for all patients with orthostatic intolerance, even if medical therapy is also being given	• Discontinue medications with autonomic effects when possible (e.g. antihypertensives, anticholinergics) • Increase salt and fluid intake • Avoid large meals in favor of multiple small meals • Avoid exposure to excessive heat • Compression garments (stockings, abdominal binders) • Elevation of the head of the bed • Lower extremity strengthening • Slow assumption of the upright position Physical counter-maneuvers to prevent fainting: lying down when possible, squeezing the lower extremities with squatting or leg crossing, sitting with the head lowered.

(Continued)

Medical	Fludrocortisone and midodrine are used in OH. Beta-blockers and pyridostigmine are used in POTS. • Fludrocortisone 0.1–0.3 mg daily • Midodrine 5–10 mg 3 times/day • Beta-blockers (dosage varies depending on particular agent) • Pyridostigmine 30–60 mg t.i.d. • Droxidopa 100–600 mg t.i.d.

Prevention/management of complications

- Both fludrocortisone and midodrine may cause hypertension, particularly supine hypertension. This may be mitigated by sleeping with the head of the bed elevated. Fludrocortisone may also cause hypokalemia and peripheral edema.
- Beta-blockers are usually well tolerated at low doses, but may cause fatigue at higher doses in POTS patients.
- Pyridostigmine can cause gastrointestinal side effects, such as nausea and diarrhea.

CLINICAL PEARLS
- Conservative treatment (see Table of treatment) is first line for all patients. If the response is inadequate, pharmacotherapy is added.
- Pharmacotherapy for OH includes midodrine, fludrocortisone, and droxidopa.
- For POTS, often a low-dose beta-blocker or pyridostigmine is tried first, followed by midodrine and fludrocortisone if necessary.

Section 5: Special populations

Pregnancy

Pregnant women may be more prone to syncope because of decreased venous return due to compression of the inferior vena cava by the expanding uterus and decreased peripheral vascular resistance. Specific treatment is not required in most women.

Children

The neurodegenerative causes of autonomic dysfunction do not generally occur in children. However, children can experience POTS or neurocardiogenic syncope. In addition there are rare genetic autonomic disorders, the familial dysautonomias, that may present in childhood.

Elderly

The elderly are at increased risk of syncope. In the absence of signs of neurologic disease, this is often due to medication side effects or deconditioning.

Section 6: Prognosis

BOTTOM LINE/CLINICAL PEARLS
- Prognosis varies considerably based on the underlying cause of autonomic dysfunction.
- Most of the neurodegenerative disorders (e.g. multiple system atrophy) are progressive.
- Although POTS and neurocardiogenic syncope are not expected to alter lifespan, they can reduce quality of life and can cause disability in severely affected patients.

Follow-up tests and monitoring

Repeat autonomic reflex screens may be useful to monitor the effects of therapy. Serum chemistries may be needed to monitor certain medications (e.g. fludrocortisone).

Section 7: Reading list

Key reading sources for this chapter can be found online at www.mountsinaiexpertguides.com

Suggested websites

National Institute of Neurological Disorders and Stroke Dysautonomia information page. This page from the National Institutes for Health also provides links to the websites of several patient advocacy groups: http://www.ninds.nih.gov/disorders/dysautonomia/dysautonomia.htm

Section 8: Guidelines

Not applicable for this topic.

Section 9: Evidence for therapies

Type of evidence	Title and comment	Weblink
RCT	Acetylcholinesterase inhibition improves tachycardia in postural tachycardia syndrome (2005) **Comment**: Pyridostigmine reduces tachycardia in POTS	http://www.ncbi.nlm.nih.gov/pubmed/15911704
RCT	Propranolol decreases tachycardia and improves symptoms in the postural tachycardia syndrome: less is more (2009) **Comment**: Low-dose beta-blockers are helpful for POTS	http://www.ncbi.nlm.nih.gov/pubmed/19687359
Controlled trial	The effects of water ingestion on orthostatic hypotension in two groups of chronic autonomic failure: multiple system atrophy and pure autonomic failure (2004) **Comment**: Drinking water prior to standing helps maintain BP	http://www.ncbi.nlm.nih.gov/pubmed/15548493
RCT	A double-blind, dose-response study of midodrine in neurogenic orthostatic hypotension (1998) **Comment**: Midodrine improves OH	http://www.ncbi.nlm.nih.gov/pubmed/9674789
RCT	Nonpharmacological treatment, fludrocortisone, and domperidone for orthostatic hypotension in Parkinson's disease (2007) **Comment**: Fludrocortisone improves OH	http://www.ncbi.nlm.nih.gov/pubmed/17557339
RCT	Effect of physical countermaneuvers on orthostatic hypotension in familial dysautonomia (2006) **Comment**: Shows the effectiveness of physical movements, such as squatting, on OH	http://www.researchgate.net/publication/7663309_Effect_of_physical_countermaneuvers_on_orthostatic_hypotension_in_familial_dysautonomia

Section 10: Images

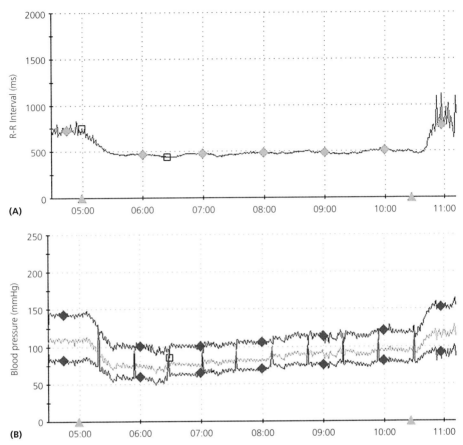

(A)

(B)

Figure 31.1 Continuous heart rate (HR) (A) and blood pressure (BP) (B) recordings in a patient with syncope reveals orthostatic hypotension (OH) on upright tilt associated with increased HR (shown here as decreased R-R interval). Abnormalities reverse when the patient is returned to the supine position (indicated by the second arrow along the time axis).

Additional material for this chapter can be found online at:
www.mountsinaiexpertguides.com

This includes advice for patients, a case study, multiple choice questions, and a reading list.

CHAPTER 32

Peripheral Neuropathies

Rajeev Motiwala
Icahn School of Medicine at Mount Sinai, New York, NY, USA

OVERALL BOTTOM LINE

- Distinguish peripheral neuropathies from other disorders of the central nervous system and other peripheral disorders such as radiculopathy, neuromuscular junction disorder, or muscle disease.
- Determine the specific pattern of involvement:
  - Polyneuropathy – relatively symmetric distribution of symptoms, distal greater than proximal
  - Mononeuropathy – isolated involvement of a single peripheral nerve.
  - Mononeuropathy multiplex – involvement of more than one individual peripheral nerve not in anatomically contiguous locations.
  - Autonomic neuropathy – involvement of autonomic nerves with or without other features of somatic nerve damage.
- Search for clues in history for causes such as diabetes mellitus, alcohol use, or family history.
- In acute cases, identify conditions like Guillain–Barré syndrome (GBS), which may warrant urgent treatment.
- In more chronic cases, look for treatable or correctable conditions such as vitamin deficiency, a toxic agent, or inflammatory conditions, which may respond to treatment.

Section 1: Background
Definition of disease
Conditions affecting peripheral nerves resulting in pain, impaired sensation, and weakness (typically with greater distal involvement).

Disease classification
See Algorithm 32.1.

Incidence/prevalence
- Polyneuropathy: Prevalence in general population was 3.4–3.6% in a study from Italy and 2.4% in a study from India.
- Diabetic neuropathy: A large study showed that 66% of insulin-dependent diabetes mellitus (IDDM) patients had some form of neuropathy and it was symptomatic in 15%. Amongst non-insulin-dependent diabetes mellitus (NIDDM) patients, 59% had some form of neuropathy and it was symptomatic in 13%.

Mount Sinai Expert Guides: Neurology, First Edition. Edited by Stuart C. Sealfon, Rajeev Motiwala, and Charles B. Stacy.
© 2016 John Wiley & Sons, Ltd. Published 2016 by John Wiley & Sons, Ltd.
Companion website: www.mountsinaiexpertguides.com

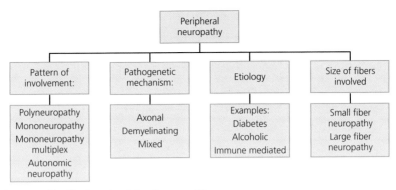

Algorithm 32.1 Classification of peripheral neuropathies.

- Guillain–Barré syndrome: 0.81–1.89 per 100,000 person years, 20% increase with every 10 years increase in age.
- Chronic inflammatory demyelinating neuropathy: A large study showed a prevalence rate of 4.77 per 100,000 population using 2006 European Federation of Neurological Societies/ Peripheral Nerve Society (EFNS/PNS) criteria, and 1.97 per 100,000 using 1991 AAN criteria. Annual incidence rate was 0.70 per 100,000 population in the preceding 3 years.
- Charcot–Marie–Tooth disease (CMT): Prevalence 1 per 2500 population.
- HIV-related neuropathies: Prevalence of peripheral neuropathy was 32.1%, and that of symptomatic peripheral neuropathy was 8.6% in a large population.

Etiology
- Hereditary: examples include Charcot–Marie–Tooth disease, hereditary neuropathy with tendency for pressure palsy, metachromatic leukodystrophy, and Fabry's disease.
- Acquired:
  - Diabetes.
- Other systemic conditions: renal failure, hypothyroidism, vitamin B12 deficiency, amyloidosis, malignancy (paraneoplastic), porphyria.
- Immune-mediated: Guillain–Barré syndrome (GBS), chronic inflammatory demyelinating polyneuropathy (CIDP), other antibody-mediated (e.g. GM1 antibody-related motor neuropathy with multifocal conduction block, demyelinating neuropathy associated with myelin-associated glycoprotein antibody (MAG)).
- Associated with inflammatory disorders: vasculitis, rheumatoid arthritis, Sjögren's syndrome, SLE, systemic sclerosis, sarcoidosis.
- HIV, hepatitis C, leprosy, Lyme disease, diphtheria, rarely syphilis.
- Toxins: alcohol, chemotherapy and other neurotoxic medications, heavy metals.
- Associated with paraproteinemia.
- Critical illness neuropathy.

Pathology/pathogenesis
- Distal axonopathy or dying back neuropathy: distal axon affected first though the neuron or cell body is affected by the toxic process.
- Segmental demyelination or myelinopathy.
- Wallerian degeneration distal to the site of trauma to the peripheral nerve.

Section 2: Prevention and screening

> **BOTTOM LINE/CLINICAL PEARLS**
> - Prevention of worsening of diabetic neuropathy and reduction in rate of foot ulceration and amputation may be facilitated by tighter glycemic control.
>
> It has been recommended that one of the three simple tests (10-g Semmes–Weinstein monofilament examination (SWME), superficial pain, and vibration testing by the on-off method) can be confidently used for annual screening of diabetic neuropathy in both diabetes and primary care clinics.

Section 3: Diagnosis

> **BOTTOM LINE/CLINICAL PEARLS**
> - Symptoms include pain, paresthesia, and weakness in the distal lower extremities.
> - Examination may reveal distal weakness, distal sensory loss, and absence or diminution in deep tendon reflexes. Patients with small fiber neuropathy may have a decrease in pain and temperature perception, hyperalgesia, and allodynia in feet.
> - Investigations include serologic tests for detection of common metabolic abnormalities and possible evidence of immune-mediated neuropathies, electrodiagnostic studies, skin biopsy for epidermal nerve fiber density, CSF examination, and nerve and muscle biopsy.

Differential diagnosis

Differential diagnosis	Features
Myopathy Motor neuron disease Myelopathy Neuromuscular junction disorder Other pain syndromes (e.g. fibromyalgia) Central causes	Refer to Chapter 15: Muscle Weakness and Paralysis

Typical presentation

Presentation depends on the type of neuropathy and the duration (acute, subacute, or chronic).
- Diabetic neuropathy presents insidiously with burning pain and numbness in the feet with subsequent spread of symptoms to the legs and hands. Unsteady gait and weakness develop later. Diabetic amyotrophy presents with acute onset of asymmetric proximal muscle weakness in the lower extremities.
- Guillain–Barré syndrome is a relatively acute condition that presents with weakness that may progress rapidly and can involve respiratory muscles and cranial nerves.
- Chronic inflammatory demyelinating neuropathy presents with progressive or recurrent motor weakness, which can be proximal and distal. Sensory symptoms vary. Motor neuropathy with multifocal conduction block can cause asymmetric weakness, which often starts in one upper extremity.

Clinical diagnosis

History

- Ask about duration of symptoms, sensory, motor and autonomic complaints, and distribution of symptoms.
- Check for history of diabetes, alcohol use or other toxin exposure, preceding infectious illness or immunizations, nutritional state, underlying malignancy or connective tissue disorders, foreign travel, exposure to infectious agents, and use of prescription and non-prescription medications. Certain chemotherapeutic agents such as cisplatin, vincristine, and paclitaxel are known to cause neuropathy.

Physical examination

- Confirm if there are physical signs to support the diagnosis of neuropathy – weakness, atrophy, absent reflexes, sensory loss, signs of autonomic insufficiency.
- Rule out other neurologic disorders (see Differential diagnosis).
- Determine the pattern of neuropathy; confirm if neuropathy is mixed, pure sensory, or pure motor.
- Look for skeletal deformities, skin rash, enlarged peripheral nerves or arthritis.

Laboratory diagnosis (Algorithms 32.2, 32.3, 32.4, and 32.5)

List of diagnostic tests

- Blood tests – these should be used selectively and choice to be determined by the pattern of neuropathy and clinical assessment:
  - Most useful screening tests: blood glucose, B12 level with additional testing of methylmalonic acid and homocysteine if level is in the low range, and serum protein immunofixation electrophoresis.
  - Thyroid function tests, RPR, HIV antibody, hemoglobin A1C level, and oral glucose tolerance test in selected cases.
  - ESR, antinuclear antibody, rheumatoid factor, Sjögren antibodies, Lyme serology, hepatitis B and C screening, urine and blood for heavy metals if there is a clinical suspicion for specific conditions.
  - Urine immunofixation, myelin-associated glycoprotein antibody (MAG) in demyelinating neuropathy, GM1 antibody in multifocal motor neuropathy, paraneoplastic antibodies (particularly anti-Hu antibody) in subacute sensory neuropathy.
- Electrodiagnostic studies – see Chapter 3: Neurophysiologic and Other Neurodiagnostic Tests.
- Skin biopsy – skin biopsy can determine epidermal nerve fiber density and in a few cases help look for presence of amyloidosis and vasculitis. Useful in cases suspected to have small fiber neuropathy.

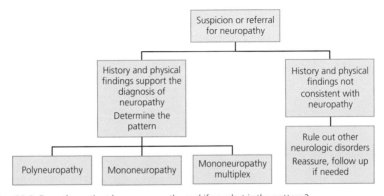

Algorithm 32.2 Does the patient have neuropathy and if so what is the pattern?

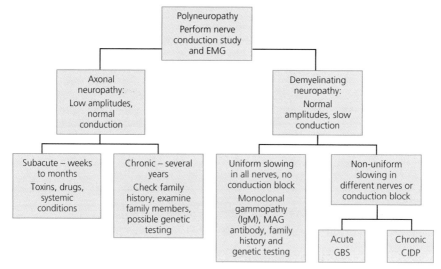

Algorithm 32.3 If polyneuropathy.

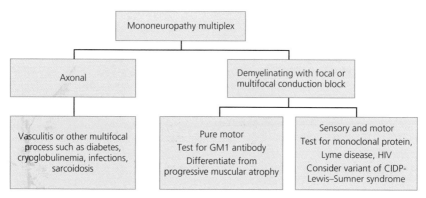

Algorithm 32.4 If mononeuropathy multiplex.

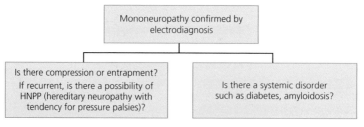

Algorithm 32.5 If mononeuropathy.

- CSF examination:
  - Elevated protein is seen in demyelinating neuropathies (albuminocytologic dissociation) – GBS, CIDP. Presence of increased numbers of cells should suggest infection (HIV, Lyme disease) or malignancy.
  - Lyme antibody and evidence of intrathecal antibody synthesis in Lyme radiculoneuropathies.

- Nerve and muscle biopsy – useful to diagnose vasculitic neuropathy, amyloidosis; can help confirm diagnosis of demyelinating neuropathy when other tests are not conclusive and treatment decisions are dependent on a more definitive diagnosis (e.g. use of steroids or intravenous gamma-globulin therapy).
- Autonomic function testing – useful in cases suspected to have autonomic neuropathy and in patients with distal sensory neuropathy (see Chapter 31: Autonomic Disorders).
- Genetic testing – appropriate testing needs to be considered based on the type of neuropathy, other clinical features such as associated skeletal deformities, and presence or absence of obvious family history. Testing should focus on the most common abnormalities which are PMP22 duplication/mutation in CMT1A, Cx32 (GJB1) in X-linked CMT1X, MPZ in CMT1B and MFN2 mutation screening (CMT2A). This can be guided by clinical and electrodiagnostic data.
- Imaging techniques:
  - MR neurography can demonstrate diffuse thickening of nerves, abnormal focal nerve signal or swelling, loss of continuity, masses, and distortion of nerve at entrapment points.
  - Peripheral nerve ultrasound can show nerve lesions with respect to their location, anatomic course, continuity, and extent, and allow assessment of nerve entrapment and presence of tumors.

Potential pitfalls/common errors made regarding the diagnosis

- Patients with subjective complaints of pain and sensory symptoms are too frequently diagnosed with polyneuropathy when they have other conditions like fibromyalgia and non-specific chronic pain disorders.
- A shotgun approach to evaluation of neuropathy patients with extensive serologic testing, nerve biopsy, and genetic testing is arduous and expensive and has a low yield. Therefore a more thoughtful and selective approach to the evaluation is warranted.
- Patients with prominent symptoms localized only to the lower extremities may have unrecognized vertebral or spinal cord disease.

Section 4: Treatment (Algorithm 32.6)

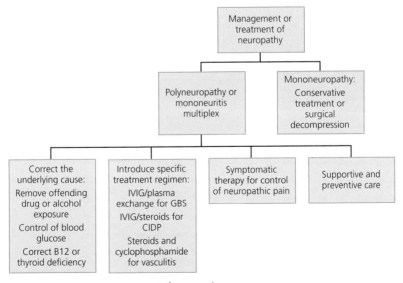

Algorithm 32.6 Management or treatment of neuropathy.

Treatment rationale

- The first priority is to identify those patients who need hospitalization and urgent intervention, for example the patient with Guillain– Barré syndrome and progressive symptoms.
- Treatment should aim at providing specific treatment if possible, preventing progression, utilizing various means of symptomatic relief, and preventing secondary complications of the disease.
- Reducing exposure to the offending agent such as alcohol and toxic medications, correcting vitamin deficiency, good control of blood sugar in patients with diabetic neuropathy, or thyroid supplementation in hypothyroidism are important steps.
- Demyelinating neuropathies have more specific treatment options with immunomodulation.
- Symptomatic and supportive treatment is often the mainstay of therapy.

When to hospitalize

In selected situations where urgent intervention is required, for example, patient with GBS with progressive symptoms.

Managing the hospitalized patient

Beyond the scope of this discussion.

Table of treatment

Condition	Treatment
Idiopathic neuropathies, hereditary neuropathies, and those with residual symptoms after previous toxic exposure	Conservative treatment Supportive treatment, symptom relief, and observation
Guillain–Barré syndrome	Equal efficacy for IVIG 0.4 g/kg/day for 5 days and 4–6 plasma exchanges. No role for steroids or advantage of sequential treatment with IVIG and plasma exchange
Chronic inflammatory demyelinating neuropathy	IVIG or oral steroids for predominantly motor form of CIDP, plasma exchange if no response to IVIG or steroids, other immunosuppressive agents in refractory patients IVIG induction dose is 2 g/kg and maintenance dose may vary Prednisone dose is variable. Typical regimen: 1 mg/kg daily for 6 weeks followed by a slow taper Weekly high-dose steroids have been used as well
Diabetic neuropathy	Control of hyperglycemia Symptomatic treatment of painful diabetic neuropathy: • Pregabalin: 150–600 mg/day • Gabapentin: 900–3600 mg/day • Valproic acid: 500–1400 mg/day • Duloxetine: 60–120 mg/day • Venlafaxine: extended release 75–225 mg/day • Amitriptyline: 30–150 mg/day • Opioids and related drugs: dextromethorphan, tramadol, morphine sulfate, controlled release oxycodone • Topical treatments: 5% lidocaine patch, capsaicin ointment • Non-pharmacologic: transcutaneous nerve stimulation No documented efficacy for surgical treatment, electromagnetic stimulation, Raiki therapy, or low-intensity laser Preventive therapy: foot care, orthotics, aids for ambulation

Condition	Treatment
Neuropathies associated with monoclonal gammopathy and other immune-mediated syndromes	Neuropathy associated with antibody against myelin associated globulin (MAG): recent data indicate efficacy with use of rituximab. There have been reports of partial response to fludarabine, cyclophosphamide, and chlorambucil Multifocal motor neuropathy with or without antibody to GM1: IVIG and if necessary addition of cyclophosphamide, fludarabine, chlorambucil, or rituximab Neuropathies associated with IgG and IgA monoclonal gammopathies: short-term benefit from use of plasma exchange Treatment of underlying myeloma, other plasma cell dyscrasias, and lymphoproliferative diseases is important
Vasculitic mononeuritis multiplex	Oral prednisone 1–2 mg/kg/day or i.v. methylprednisolone 1 g/day followed by oral prednisone 1–2 mg/kg/day for 6–8 weeks followed by a gradual taper and oral cyclophosphamide 2 mg/kg/day or i.v. cyclophosphamide 500 mg/m² every 4–6 weeks
Common compression neuropathies: • Carpal tunnel syndrome • Ulnar neuropathy	Conservative management with bracing, use of anti-inflammatory agents, local injections, and surgical decompression

Prevention/management of complications

Major complications of distal neuropathies are foot ulcers, which have an eventual risk of amputation and falls. Ulcers are particularly concerning in patients with diabetic neuropathies.

- Bedside and formal gait evaluation, referral for physical therapy, use of orthotics, ankle support, and ambulation assistive devices can help prevent falls.
- Skin ulceration and amputation risk can be reduced by self-foot examination, use of a foot mirror, podiatric consultation, wide-based shoes and loose-fitting socks, proper nail cutting, adequate care of bunions and calluses, and prompt treatment of ulcers if they do occur.

CLINICAL PEARLS
- Try to identify the cause and address it when possible.
- Introduce specific therapy early during the course when available.
- Provide optimal symptomatic treatment even if specific etiology is not evident.
- Prevent complications of neuropathy.

Section 5: Special populations

Not applicable for this topic.

Section 6: Prognosis

BOTTOM LINE/CLINICAL PEARLS
- Prognosis depends on whether the condition is self-limited, treatable, or if the underlying cause can be corrected.
- Immune-mediated or inflammatory neuropathies respond to immunomodulatory therapy but the response may not be complete. Natural remissions can occur.
- Treatment of diabetes mellitus does not reverse existing neuropathic signs and symptoms but can help halt or slow down disease progression.

Section 7: Reading list

Key reading sources for this chapter can be found online at www.mountsinaiexpertguides.com

Suggested websites

American Diabetes Association: www.diabetes.org
National Institute of Neurological Disorders and Stroke: http://www.ninds.nih.gov/

Section 8: Guidelines

Title	Source	Weblink
Practice parameter: Evaluation of distal symmetric polyneuropathy: Role of autonomic testing, nerve biopsy, and skin biopsy (an evidence-based review)	American Academy of Neurology (AAN), American Association of Neuromuscular and Electrodiagnostic Medicine (AANEM), and American Academy of Physical Medicine and Rehabilitation (AAPR), online: December 2008; in print: January 2009	http://www.neurology.org/content/72/2/177.full.html
Practice parameter: Evaluation of distal symmetric polyneuropathy: Role of laboratory and genetic testing (an evidence-based review)	AAN, AANEM, and AAPR, online: December 2008; in print: January 2009	http://www.neurology.org/content/early/2008/12/03/01.wnl.0000336370.51010.a1.full.pdf
Practice parameter: Immunotherapy for Guillain-Barré syndrome	AAN, September 2003, reaffirmed August 2008	http://www.ncbi.nlm.nih.gov/pubmed/14504313
Evidence-based guideline: Treatment of painful diabetic neuropathy	AAN, AANEM, and AAPR, online: April 2011; in print: May 2011	https://www.aan.com/Guidelines/home/GetGuidelineContent/480
Guideline on management of chronic inflammatory demyelinating polyradiculoneuropathy: report of a joint task force of the European Federation of Neurological Societies and the Peripheral Nerve Society	European Federation of Neurological Societies and the Peripheral Nerve Society, online: February 2010; in print: March 2010; correction: April 2011	http://static1.squarespace.com/static/53e0d272e4b0ea4fa48a8d40/t/53f1d8d7e4b0058ebcdcd1fe/1408358615476/GuidelinesCDP.pdf
Evidence-based guideline: Intravenous immunoglobulin in the treatment of neuromuscular disorders	Report of the Therapeutics and Technology Assessment Subcommittee of the AAN; endorsed by: the AANEM, February 2012	http://www.ncbi.nlm.nih.gov/pubmed/22454268

Additional material for this chapter can be found online at:
www.mountsinaiexpertguides.com

This includes advice for patients, a case study, multiple choice questions, and a reading list.

CHAPTER 33

Myopathy

Lan Zhou
Icahn School of Medicine at Mount Sinai, New York, NY, USA

OVERALL BOTTOM LINE
- Myopathies are structural and functional skeletal muscle disorders (also sometimes involving heart muscle) caused by muscle inflammation, genetic defect, or myotoxin exposure.
- Myopathies may present with weakness, exercise intolerance, myalgias, and changes in muscle bulk.
- Common types of myopathies include inflammatory myopathies, muscular dystrophies, metabolic myopathies, muscle channelopathies, and toxic myopathies.
- Diagnostic evaluation of a myopathy consists of thorough history taking, physical examination, blood tests (serum creatine kinase (CK) level, myositis antibodies, and genetic testing), electromyogram (EMG), and muscle biopsy.
- Treatment of a myopathy is directed towards the underlying cause, symptom management, and rehabilitation.

Section 1: Background
Definition of disease
Myopathies are a group of diseases that cause structural and functional impairment of skeletal muscle.

Disease classification
- Inflammatory myopathies can be either idiopathic or associated with connective tissue diseases (overlap syndrome). Idiopathic inflammatory myopathies (IIM) consist of polymyositis (PM), dermatomyositis (DM), inclusion body myositis (IBM), and immune-mediated necrotizing myopathy (IMNM).
- Muscular dystrophies mainly include Duchenne or Becker muscular dystrophy (DMD, BMD), myotonic dystrophy, facioscapulohumeral muscular dystrophy (FSHD), limb-girdle muscular dystrophy (LGMD), and congenital muscular dystrophies (CMD).
- Metabolic myopathies chiefly comprise McArdle's disease with myophosphorylase deficiency, acid maltase deficiency, Tarui disease with phosphofructokinase deficiency, lipid storage myopathies, and mitochondrial myopathies.
- Channelopathies consist mainly of periodic paralysis, myotonia congenita, and paramyotonia congenita.
- Toxic myopathies include myopathies induced by myotoxic drugs and alcohol.

Mount Sinai Expert Guides: Neurology, First Edition. Edited by Stuart C. Sealfon, Rajeev Motiwala, and Charles B. Stacy.
© 2016 John Wiley & Sons, Ltd. Published 2016 by John Wiley & Sons, Ltd.
Companion website: www.mountsinaiexpertguides.com

Incidence/prevalence

- The annual incidence of idiopathic inflammatory myopathy (IIM) is approximately 1 in 100,000.
- DMD affects 1 in 3500 live male births.
- Statin myopathy is the most common drug-induced toxic myopathy. Over 36 million Americans are candidates for statin therapy, and up to 20% of statin users develop muscle symptoms, such as myalgia, fatigue, or muscle weakness.

Etiology

- Inflammatory myopathies are caused by autoimmune damage of skeletal muscle.
- Muscular dystrophies are caused by genetic defects that lead to progressive skeletal muscle dysfunction and weakness.
- Metabolic myopathies are caused by genetic defects in skeletal muscle energy metabolism, which often lead to exercise intolerance.
- Muscle channelopathies are caused by genetic defects in muscle cell membrane ion channels, which can lead to cramps, periodic paralysis, or impaired muscle relaxation (myotonia).
- Toxic myopathies are due to exposures to myotoxins, such as certain medications or alcohol, which lead to muscle damage.

Pathology/pathogenesis

- Inflammatory myopathies are caused by endomysial inflammatory cell infiltration, which leads to muscle fiber degeneration, necrosis, and regeneration.
  - PM is a cell-mediated autoimmune muscle disorder. The inflammatory infiltrate is predominantly composed of macrophages and CD8+ T lymphocytes.
  - DM is considered a humorally mediated microangiopathy mainly affecting muscle and skin. The inflammatory infiltrate is predominantly composed of macrophages, B cells, and CD4+ cells. Deposition of the CD5b-9 or membrane attack complex is also detected around small blood vessels. A viral infection may trigger autoimmune attacks in DM based on the upregulation of interferon alpha- and beta-inducible genes.
  - Although IBM is still listed as an inflammatory myopathy, it is largely considered as a degenerative muscle disorder due to its poor response to immunosuppressive therapy and abnormal accumulation of "Alzheimer-characteristic proteins" in vacuoles of muscle fibers, including beta-amyloid protein, hyperphosphorylated tau protein, and neurofilament heavy chain.
  - IMNM displays minimal inflammatory infiltrate and can be triggered by viral infections, medications such as statins, and neoplasms.
- Muscular dystrophies are due to mutations in muscle structural genes involved in the dystrophin-glycoprotein complex, sarcolemma, sarcomere, and nuclear envelope, or in regulatory genes involved in glycosylation of α-dystroglycan, RNA splicing, and other enzyme activities.
- Metabolic myopathies result from mutations in genes involved in glycogen and glucose catabolism, lipid catabolism, or mitochondrial function. These mutations can cause glycogen storage diseases, lipid storage diseases, or mitochondrial myopathies. The major functional defect in metabolic myopathies is inadequate generation of the energy molecule, adenosine triphosphate (ATP), to meet energy demands during exercise.
- Muscle channelopathies are caused by mutations in muscle membrane ion channels, which lead to aberrant muscle cell membrane depolarization or repolarization, with consequent periodic muscle paralysis or impaired muscle relaxation.

- Toxic myopathies are the consequence of exposure to myotoxins, which affect lysosome function (chloroquine and hydroxychloroquine), impair polymerization of microtubules (colchicine), impair protein synthesis and degradation (steroids), or damage mitochondria (zidovudine). The precise mechanisms underlying the myotoxic effect of statin drugs remain elusive.

Risk factors

- Certain HLA alleles, especially HLA-DQA1*0501 and HLA-DRB1*0301, have been associated with and may confer the susceptibility to IIM. Viral infections may trigger immune dysregulation and induce IIM in genetically susceptible hosts.
- Consanguinity and positive family history are risk factors for genetic myopathies.

Section 2: Prevention and screening

> **BOTTOM LINE/CLINICAL PEARLS**
> - Modification of exercise and diet and avoidance of triggers are important to reduce symptoms in metabolic myopathies and muscle channelopathies.
> - Identification and discontinuation of causative and contributory myotoxic substances is key to preventing and treating toxic myopathies.

Primary prevention

- In susceptible patients, it is prudent to avoid myotoxic drug exposure if possible.

Secondary prevention

- Identifying and discontinuing myotoxins is essential to prevent toxic myopathy progression and to allow recovery of damaged muscle. However, in some cases it may be sufficient to reduce the dose, especially with a myopathy related to statin use, if the myopathy is mild and stable and if the offending drug offers a great benefit in a particular patient. It is important to involve the patient and the prescribing physician in reaching a management decision.
- Recurrent rhabdomyolysis is common in patients with metabolic myopathies; it can cause acute renal failure. Patients should be instructed to modify diet and exercise to prevent rhabdomyolysis.
- Patients with some muscle channelopathies can take preventative medications (acetazolamide), and patients with periodic paralysis can reduce episodes by avoiding triggers.

Section 3: Diagnosis

> **BOTTOM LINE/CLINICAL PEARLS**
> - When evaluating a patient with a myopathy, note the age of symptom onset, the rate of symptom progression, the pattern of muscle involvement, and any associated systemic symptoms or conditions, family history, ethnic background, consanguinity in parents, or myotoxic drug exposure.
> - Examination often shows symmetrical proximal limb weakness. Some types of myopathies may affect distal limb, ocular, respiratory, or cardiac muscles. The presence of scapular winging, lumbar hyperlordosis, and calf hypertrophy suggests chronic myopathies, and these are mostly seen with muscular dystrophies.
> - Diagnostic investigation of myopathies consists of blood tests (serum CK level, myositis antibodies, and genetic testing), electromyogram (EMG), and muscle biopsy.
> - CK level is often elevated in a myopathy, but normal CK does not exclude a myopathy.
> - EMG often shows polyphasic motor unit potentials of short duration and low amplitude and increased insertional and spontaneous activity with fibrillation potentials, positive waves, and repetitive discharges. A normal EMG does not exclude a myopathy.

- Muscle biopsy is essential to confirm the diagnosis of inflammatory myopathies, metabolic myopathies, and some muscular dystrophies.
- Many causative genes have been identified and can be tested by commercial labs for genetically determined myopathies. One may proceed with gene testing without muscle biopsy if a patient's phenotype and family history suggest a specific genetic myopathy.

Differential diagnosis

Disease mimicking myopathy	Features
Myasthenia gravis	Weakness is fatigable, predominantly affecting ocular muscles. CK is normal. AChR-Ab and MuSK-Ab can be positive. EMG shows no myopathic motor unit potentials. 3 Hz repetitive nerve stimulation may show characteristic decremental response, and single fiber EMG shows increased jitter
Motor neuropathy, neuronopathy	Weakness is usually asymmetrical, accompanied by muscle atrophy and fasciculations. Patients with amyotropic lateral sclerosis also show brisk deep tendon reflexes and pathologic reflexes. CK can be elevated; however, EMG shows neurogenic changes in recruitment and motor unit potentials
Polymyalgia rheumatica	Morning pain and stiffness in shoulder, neck, and hip muscles, may be associated with temporal arteritis
Chronic fatigue syndrome	Complaints of weakness and fatigue with normal muscle mass and strength
Benign muscle cramps, cramp-fasciculation syndrome	Isolated muscle cramps with normal muscle strength (may have associated fasciculations) are not indicative of nerve or muscle disease

Myopathy	Clinical features	Diagnostic features
Inflammatory myopathies		
Polymyositis	Mainly affects adults, more common in women, subacute onset of proximal limb weakness, may be associated with interstitial lung disease and connective tissue disease	CK is elevated. EMG shows irritable myopathy. Muscle biopsy shows primary endomysial inflammation
Dermatomyositis	Can affect adults or children, subacute onset of proximal limb weakness; skin rash; can be associated with malignancies; may have interstitial lung disease	CK is elevated or normal. EMG shows myopathy. Muscle biopsy shows perifascicular atrophy and perifascicular and perivascular inflammation
Inclusion body myositis	Mainly affects men above 50 years of age; subacute or chronic proximal and distal limb weakness; knee extensors and finger flexors most affected; may have dysphagia	CK is elevated or normal. EMG may show both myopathic and neurogenic changes. Muscle biopsy shows primary endomysial inflammation, red rimmed vacuoles and tubulofilamentous inclusion bodies

Myopathy	Clinical features	Diagnostic features
Muscular dystrophies		
Dystrophinopathies	This group includes Duchenne muscular dystrophy (DMD), Becker muscular dystrophy (BMD), and X-linked dilated cardiomyopathy (XLDC). DMD boys develop proximal limb weakness around age 3–5 years, become non-ambulatory around age 12, and die around age 20 from respiratory and cardiac muscle weakness. BMD has a broad clinical spectrum; it is less severe than DMD, and the incidence of dilated cardiomyopathy is high. XLDC shows no obvious skeletal myopathy but cardiomyopathy with rapid progression to congestive heart failure in males around age 20. It may also affect manifesting female carriers	CK is markedly elevated. EMG shows an irritable myopathy. The disease can be confirmed by the dystrophin gene test. Muscle biopsy may not be needed; if done, it shows dystrophic changes, including myofiber degeneration, regeneration, necrosis, endomysial inflammation, fibrosis, and reduced or absent dystrophin
Myotonic dystrophy	Most common muscular dystrophy seen in adults. Autosomal dominant. A multisystem disease commonly associated with diabetes mellitus, cholecystitis, cataracts, cardiac conduction defect, and testicular failure. DM1 has earlier onset (infant to young adult), distal muscle weakness and myotonia, facial weakness, and mental retardation. DM2 has adult onset of myalgia, fatigue, and proximal limb weakness. These patients often show long facies, frontal balding, and temporal hollowing	CK is often mildly elevated. EMG shows myopathy with myotonic discharges. The disease can be confirmed by gene tests, which show trinucleotide CTG expansion in 3′-UTR of the *DMPK* gene (chromosome 19) in DM1, and tetranucleotide CCTG expansion in the first intron of the *ZFP9* gene (chromosome 3) in DM2. Muscle biopsy is not needed; but if done, it shows no dystrophic changes, but type 1 fiber atrophy or predominance, increased central nuclei, and presence of pyknotic nuclear clumps
FSHD	Autosomal dominant. Age of onset varies from the first to the sixth decades. It more affects facial, shoulder girdle, abdominal, and foot extensor muscles with signs of scapular winging, Beevor's sign (movement of navel towards head when attempting to flex the neck), and foot drop. The weakness can be asymmetrical. Cardiac and respiratory muscles are usually spared and lifespan is usually normal	CK is elevated. EMG shows myopathic features. The disease can be confirmed by genetic testing, which shows a deletion of 3.3 kb repeats (D4Z4) in the subtelomeric region of chromosome 4q (4p35). Muscle biopsy is not needed; if done, it can show myopathic and inflammatory changes
LGMD	Genetically and phenotypically heterogeneous. LGMD1 is autosomal dominant while LGMD2 is autosomal recessive. Predominantly affects limb and girdle muscles; some may also affect cardiac and respiratory muscles. Proximal limb weakness, scapular winging, lumbar hyperlordosis, waddling gait, and calf hypertrophy are common signs	CK is elevated. EMG shows a myopathy. Muscle biopsy shows dystrophic changes. Special immunostains of biopsy specimen and gene panel testing may lead to specific genetic diagnoses in some cases

(Continued)

Myopathy	Clinical features	Diagnostic features
Channelopathies		
Periodic paralysis	Episodes of muscle weakness, often precipitated by specific triggers such as starvation, high carbohydrate diet, exercise or rest after heavy exercise, stress, cold exposure, and thyrotoxicosis. May develop fixed weakness	Serum potassium can be abnormal during episodes. EMG may show myotonic discharges in hyperkalemic periodic paralysis. Gene tests confirm specific diagnosis. Muscle biopsy is not needed; but if done it may show vacuolar myopathy with tubular aggregates
Myotonia congenita	Complaints of muscle stiffness and difficulty initiating movements. Repeated muscle contractions alleviate muscle stiffness. Myotonia and muscle hypertrophy are often detected on exam. Autosomal dominant or autosomal recessive	EMG shows myotonic discharges. *CLCN1* gene test confirms the diagnosis
Paramyotonia congenita	Muscle stiffness brought on by repeated contractions and worsened by cold exposure. Autosomal dominant	Cold-induced myotonia can be observed on EMG. *SCN4A* gene test confirms the diagnosis
Metabolic myopathies		
McArdle's disease	Most common metabolic myopathy. Defect in glycogen metabolism. Symptoms typically start in adolescence. Extreme muscle fatigue and pain occur shortly after strenuous physical activity and improve after continuous activity at a slow pace (second wind phenomenon). May develop recurrent rhabdomyolysis with exercise. Exam between attacks can be normal or show mild fixed proximal limb weakness	CK fluctuates with physical activity, ranging from mild to marked elevation. EMG often shows myopathy with myotonic discharges. Muscle biopsy shows subsarcolemmal glycogen accumulation with absent myophosphorylase staining
Acid maltase deficiency	Progressive proximal limb, paraspinal, and respiratory muscle weakness in adults. Pompe disease with cardiac and hepatic involvement in children	CK is usually mildly to moderately elevated. EMG shows myopathy with myotonic discharges. Muscle biopsy shows myopathic changes with autophagic vacuoles and abnormal glycogen accumulation. Acid alpha-glucosidase (GAA) deficiency detected by dried blood spot test confirms the diagnosis
Lipid storage myopathy	Exercise intolerance with extreme muscle pain, fatigue, and weakness after prolonged strenuous activity. May develop rhabdomyolysis. May also have progressive proximal limb weakness	CK can be normal or mildly elevated between attacks of rhabdomyolysis. EMG may show myopathy. Muscle biopsy shows abnormal lipid accumulation. Biochemical analysis of muscle tissue may reveal deficiency of carnitine or enzymes involved in fatty acid oxidation

Myopathy	Clinical features	Diagnostic features
Mitochondrial myopathy	Progressive ophthalmoplegia and proximal limb weakness. Often associated with short stature, hearing loss, pigmentary retinopathy, cardiac conduction blocks, or cardiomyopathy. May also develop encephalopathy, epilepsy, or stroke episodes. Can be maternally inherited or autosomal dominant or recessive depending on whether the mutant gene is a mitochondrial or nuclear gene	CK and lactate levels are often elevated. EMG can be normal or show mild non-irritable myopathy. Muscle biopsy often shows ragged red fibers, COX-negative fibers, or mitochondrial structural abnormalities with crystalline inclusions. Genetic testing may reveal specific genetic causes
Toxic myopathies		
Statin myopathy	Ranges from more common mild toxic myopathy with myalgia, fatigue, and subjective proximal limb weakness to severe immune-mediated necrotizing myopathy and rhabdomyolysis. Symptoms typically develop shortly after statin exposure or dose escalation. The symptoms usually resolve shortly after statin withdrawal but may linger beyond 1 year	CK is markedly elevated in rhabdomyolysis and immune-mediated necrotizing myopathy. CK is mildly elevated or normal in mild toxic myopathy. EMG shows myopathy but can be normal in mild toxic myopathy. There are no specific pathologic features for mild toxic myopathy induced by statin drugs
Steroid myopathy	Mild proximal limb muscle weakness and fatigue after steroid exposure. Usually dose and duration related	Steroid myopathy does not cause CK elevation or abnormal spontaneous changes (fibrillation potentials and positive waves) on EMG. Muscle biopsy shows type 2 fiber atrophy but no inflammation
Plaquenil myopathy	Progressive proximal limb weakness after Plaquenil (hydroxychloroquine) exposure. Symptoms improve or resolve shortly after discontinuation of the drug	CK is elevated. EMG often shows irritable myopathy. Muscle biopsy shows a vacuolar myopathy
Colchicine myopathy	Proximal limb weakness after chronic exposure in gout patients. May also develop neuropathy	CK can be normal or elevated. EMG shows myopathy. Muscle biopsy shows a vacuolar myopathy
Zidovudine myopathy	Proximal limb weakness in patients with chronic HIV infection treated with zidovudine	CK is usually mildly elevated. EMG often shows myopathy. Muscle biopsy shows myopathic changes and many COX-negative fibers
Other myopathies		
Critical illness myopathy	ICU stay with exposure to high-dose steroids and neuromuscular blockade. Profound weakness, which improves relatively quickly after withdrawal of offending agents	CK is often elevated and EMG often shows irritable myopathy. Muscle biopsy is not needed; if done, it shows loss of myosin with vacuoles in myofibers stained with ATPase
Myopathy associated with endocrinopathies	Muscle fatigue and weakness in patients with thyroid diseases, Cushing's disease, osteomalacia, or parathyroid disorders. Symptoms improve or resolve after controlling underlying endocrinopathy	CK is often normal, but elevated in hypothyroidism. EMG may show myopathy. Muscle biopsy is not needed; if done, it shows type 2 fiber atrophy
Muscle wasting in cachexia of chronic diseases	Associated with many chronic diseases, including cancer and chronic infections. Prominent weight loss, muscle atrophy, and diffuse weakness	CK is normal. EMG is normal or may show mild non-irritable myopathy. Muscle biopsy is not needed; if done, it shows type 2 fiber atrophy

Typical presentation

Myopathies typically present with symmetrical proximal limb weakness and neck flexor weakness. Several types of myopathies, such as inclusion body myositis, some muscular dystrophies, and mitochondrial myopathies, may display prominent distal limb, ocular, facial, bulbar, respiratory, or cardiac muscle weakness. Metabolic myopathies may or may not have fixed muscle weakness, and they mainly manifest exercise intolerance associated with recurrent episodes of rhabdomyolysis. The symptoms typically start in adolescence when patients become more athletic. Periodic paralysis presents with episodes of flaccid limb muscle weakness, which can be associated with abnormal serum potassium levels. Myotonia and paramyotonia congenita present with difficulty relaxing muscles.

Clinical diagnosis

History

The history should include the following key questions:
- Which muscle symptoms does the patient have: weakness, pain, cramps, spasms, difficulty relaxing, dark colored urine?
- Which muscles are affected?
- When and how did the muscle symptoms start?
- How did the muscle symptoms progress?
- Are the muscle symptoms constant or episodic? If episodic, what are the triggers?
- Are there any other neurologic or systemic symptoms or associated conditions?
- Is there a family history of a similar condition? If yes, what is the inheritance pattern?
- What is the patient's ethnic background?
- Is there consanguinity in the patient's family?
- Is there a history of myotoxin exposure?

Physical examination

The physical examination should address the following key questions:
- Which muscles are affected: limb, torso, facial, bulbar, ocular, respiratory, or cardiac?
- What is the pattern of muscle weakness – distal, proximal, symmetrical, or asymmetrical?
- Are there any other associated findings, such as skin rash, joint contractures, spine scoliosis, scapular winging, calf hypertrophy, lumbar hyperlordosis, or facial dysmorphism?
- Are there any fasciculations, sensory findings, brisk reflexes, or pathologic reflexes to suggest a motor neuron disease, other neuromuscular disorder, or a CNS disorder?

Disease severity classification

The severity of a myopathy is usually judged by the severity of muscle weakness, functional impairment, and CK elevation.

Laboratory diagnosis

List of diagnostic tests

- CK, CBC, comprehensive metabolic panel, rheumatologic markers (ESR, ANA, ENA, and RF), and thyroid function tests (TSH and free T4) should be ordered in all patients with myopathies.
- EMG should be ordered in nearly all patients with a suspected myopathy. EMG not only confirms a myopathy but also helps to target a muscle for biopsy.
- MRI often shows signal changes in affected muscles in IIM, which may help to choose a muscle or muscle site for biopsy and to follow up treatment response.
- Muscle biopsy should be ordered in all patients with suspected inflammatory myopathies and metabolic myopathies and in some patients with muscular dystrophies and toxic myopathies.

- Genetic testing should be ordered in patients with a suspected genetic myopathy for which the gene test is available.
- Serum myositis specific antibodies should be ordered in subsets of patients with inflammatory myopathies. Jo-1 (histidyl t-RNA synthetase) antibody should be ordered in patients with PM, DM, and IMNM, because 50% of Jo-1 antibody-positive patients either have or will develop interstitial lung disease (ILD). In these patients methotrexate should be avoided due to its pulmonary side effects. Signal recognition particle (SRP) antibody should be ordered in patients with severe fulminant PM or IMNM, because the presence of this antibody is associated with a severe phenotype and marked cardiac involvement, and indicates the need for aggressive immunosuppressive therapy.
- EKG, echocardiogram, and chest CT should be ordered in all patients with IIM to evaluate for potential cardiac and pulmonary involvement.
- Malignancy screening should be ordered in all patients with DM. Evaluation includes CT of chest, abdomen, and pelvis, mammogram and pelvic examination in women, testicular and prostate examinations in men, and colonoscopy in men and women over 50 years of age. If the primary screening is negative, screening should be repeated at periodic intervals.

Potential pitfalls/common errors made regarding diagnosis of disease

- CK elevation does not always indicate a myopathy; it can be seen in motor neuropathies or motor neuronopathies with active denervation, as well as following trauma, immobilization, or prolonged muscle compression.
- Marked CK elevation does not always indicate an inflammatory myopathy; recurrent rhabdomyolysis is common in metabolic myopathies.
- Inflammation on muscle biopsy does not always indicate an inflammatory myopathy; endomysial inflammation can also be seen in muscular dystrophies and necrotizing myopathies.

Section 4: Treatment
Treatment rationale

- A multidisciplinary approach is often needed to manage patients with myopathies. Depending on the disease manifestations, the treatment team may include a neurologist, rheumatologist, dermatologist, cardiologist, pulmonologist, physical therapist, speech therapist, and orthopedic surgeon.
- All patients with fixed muscle weakness from myopathies should undergo physical therapy early in the disease course, as well as orthotics when needed, to avoid or slow down joint contractures and muscle atrophy and to maximize muscle function.
- For PM, DM, and IMNM, the initial therapy is high-dose corticosteroids with prednisone initiated at 0.5–1 mg/kg/day for 2–4 weeks followed by slow tapering. For DM, IVIG can be used initially if there are contraindications to prednisone, such as diabetes or a history of GI bleeding. Maintenance drugs may be needed, and include methotrexate (15–25 mg weekly), azathioprine (2 mg/kg/day in two divided dose), mycophenolate (1000 mg b.i.d.), and IVIG. These may be started concurrently with steroids to reduce or spare steroid use. Other treatments used for severe refractory cases include intravenous high-dose methylprednisolone, cyclophosphamide, rituximab, ciclosporin (cyclosporine), and tacrolimus.
- For IBM, any benefit of steroids is usually transient, and if this diagnosis is firmly established steroids are best avoided. If dysphagia is present, IVIG may be tried based on anecdotal reports. No therapy has been shown to stop IBM disease progression.

- The treatment of muscular dystrophies remains supportive. DMD patients over 5 years of age should be treated with prednisone 0.75 mg/kg/day; the dose may be reduced to 0.5 or 0.3 mg/kg/day if side effects (weight gain, GI symptoms, behavioral changes, etc.) are severe. The treatment can prolong independent ambulation, but the effect is modest and inducing osteoporosis is a major concern.
- No specific treatment is available for most metabolic myopathies. Exceptions are enzyme replacement for acid maltase deficiency, carnitine deficiency, and CoQ10 deficiency. A diet rich in complex carbohydrates combined with regular aerobic exercise may be beneficial, and sucrose or fructose (40 g) ingestion before exercise may improve exercise intolerance in patients with McArdle's disease.
- For myotonia associated with dystrophic or non-dystrophic myotonic disorders, antiarrhythmic (mexiletine) and antiepileptic (phenytoin and carbamazepine) medications may be used to control the symptoms.
- In periodic paralysis, the potassium level should be checked and corrected, and acetazolamide should be tried in addition to avoidance of triggers to reduce attacks.

When to hospitalize
- Hospitalization is indicated in patients who have rhabdomyolysis, severe limb weakness, dysphagia, or difficulty breathing, or who require intravenous hydration or medications, feeding tube placement, or inpatient rehabilitation.

Prevention/management of complications
- Prolonged steroid use can cause significant serious side effects, including central obesity, hypertension, diabetes, bone loss, gastric ulcer bleeding, and infections. Patients requiring maintenance corticosteroids should have blood pressure, HbA1C (at baseline and every 6 months), and periodic bone density measurements (dual-energy X-ray absorptiometry (DEXA, DXA)).
- They should also take calcium, vitamin D, bisphosphonate (for postmenopausal women and for patients with osteoporosis), proton pump inhibitors (for gastrointestinal bleeding prevention), and sulfamethoxazole/trimethoprim in selected cases (for *Pneumocystis* prophylaxis).

Section 5: Special populations
Not applicable for this topic.

Section 6: Prognosis

BOTTOM LINE/CLINICAL PEARLS
- Among inflammatory myopathies, PM and DM usually have a favorable response to immunosuppressive therapies. IMNM is relatively difficult to treat. IBM typically has a poor response to treatment.
- There is no specific effective therapy for muscular dystrophies. The management remains supportive. DMD patients usually die by their 20s from cardiomyopathy and respiratory weakness.
- With diet and exercise modification, rhabdomyolysis can usually be avoided in metabolic myopathies.
- Periodic paralysis and myotonia can be controlled by medications and avoidance of triggers.
- Symptoms from statin myopathy usually resolve shortly after statin withdrawal, but may linger for more than a year.

Section 7: Reading list

Key reading sources for this chapter can be found online at www.mountsinaiexpertguides.com

Suggested websites

GeneTests: www.genetests.org
Muscular Dystrophy Association: www.mda.org
The Myositis Association: www.myositis.org

Additional material for this chapter can be found online at:
www.mountsinaiexpertguides.com

This includes advice for patients, a case study, multiple choice
questions, and a reading list.

CHAPTER 34

Neuromuscular Junction Disorders

Mark A. Sivak

Icahn School of Medicine at Mount Sinai, New York, NY, USA

OVERALL BOTTOM LINE
- The majority of neuromuscular junction diseases are autoimmune in nature, affecting either pre- or post-synaptic membrane structures.
- Myasthenia gravis (MG) is the most common neuromuscular junction disease and results from a post-synaptic defect, most often due to antibodies against the acetylcholine receptor complex, and less frequently against MUscle Specific tyrosine receptor Kinase (MuSK).
- While most patients with MG have mild to moderate disease, some patients experience severe disease, necessitating prolonged and intense hospitalization.
- With advances in intensive care and disease management, the majority of patients, even with severe myasthenic exacerbations, can return to normal function.
- Autoimmune attack against pre-synaptic P/Q calcium channels causes Lambert–Eaton myasthenic syndrome (LEMS), which is often associated with neoplasms, particularly small cell lung carcinoma.
- Congenital myasthenias are rare structural diseases due to genetic abnormalities of the pre- or post-synaptic structures. These will not be included in this chapter.

Section 1: Background
Definition of disease
- Myasthenia gravis (MG) is an autoimmune disease directed at the post-synaptic neuromuscular junction characterized by fluctuating weakness and fatigability.
- Lambert–Eaton myasthenic syndrome (LEMS) is an autoimmune disease affecting the presynaptic neuromuscular junction causing weakness of the limbs.

Disease classification
According to the Myasthenia Gravis Foundation of America (MGFA), the clinical classification of MG encompasses the following:
- Class I (ocular muscle or eye closure weakness only).
- Classes II–IV (II – mild, III – moderate, and IV – severe weakness of muscles beyond ocular muscle involvement).
- Classes II–IV are further subclassified by minimal oropharyngeal and respiratory muscle involvement (IIa–IVa) or predominantly oropharyngeal and respiratory muscle involvement (IIb–IVb).
- Class V crisis (requiring intubation for airway maintenance or ventilation support).

Mount Sinai Expert Guides: Neurology, First Edition. Edited by Stuart C. Sealfon, Rajeev Motiwala, and Charles B. Stacy.
© 2016 John Wiley & Sons, Ltd. Published 2016 by John Wiley & Sons, Ltd.
Companion website: www.mountsinaiexpertguides.com

Incidence/prevalence
- The prevalence of MG is 14–20 individuals per 100,000.
- The annual incidence of LEMS in the USA is about 4/100,000 per year, and the prevalence is 25 per 100,000.

Etiology
- MG and LEMS are both autoimmune diseases.
- The exact triggers of these diseases remain unknown.
- There is a strong association of these diseases with tumors, especially thymoma for MG (10–15% of cases) and small cell lung cancer for LEMS (60% of cases; in two-thirds the cancer is known or detected at time of presentation and in one-third the cancer is detected within several years).

Pathology/pathogenesis
- In MG there are autoantibodies directed against the acetylcholine receptors (ACHR) in the post-synaptic membrane. The binding of the various types of ACHR antibodies (binding, blocking, and modulating antibodies) may inactivate the receptors, and can induce destruction of the receptors and neuromuscular endplate by the recruitment of complement.
- The autoimmune process leads to a functional or structural insufficient density of ACHRs for continued and reliable transmission of the nerve signal to the muscle, which manifests as fatigue-induced weakness.
- Thymoma and thymus hyperplasia are associated with the development of anti-ACHR antibodies and MG.
- In LEMS, autoimmune-mediated inactivation of the pre-synaptic binding of acetylcholine vesicles to the pre-synaptic membrane is caused by antibodies against P/Q type voltage-gated calcium channels or synaptotagmin. This results in the failure of sufficient release of acetylcholine into the synaptic cleft to allow nerve signals to be transmitted to the muscle.
- With continued activation over seconds to minutes in LEMS, there is opening of enough non-specific ion channels to increase calcium influx, acetylcholine release, and increased muscle contraction.
- Small cell lung cancer may be associated with the development of pre-synaptic neuromuscular junction antibodies and LEMS.

Section 2: Prevention and screening

> **BOTTOM LINE/CLINICAL PEARLS**
> - There are no treatments or interventions known to prevent disease onset of MG or LEMS.

Screening
As MG and LEMS may be associated with tumors (MG with thymoma or thymic hypertrophy; LEMS with small cell carcinoma of the lung) adequate screening for these tumors with chest CT or MRI is essential. This is especially true in older patients.

Secondary prevention
Myasthenia gravis
While proper medication doses will keep MG patients doing well, disease recurrence may happen despite this. Prompt attention to or avoidance of known triggers for disease worsening is important.

- Infection should be addressed promptly and effectively with careful attention to choice of antibiotics (see below).
- Avoid drugs that can interfere with neuromuscular transmission such as aminoglycoside and fluoroquinolone antibiotics, quinine, and quinine-containing compounds. For a complete list, see the MGFA website.
- Pre-surgical optimization of MG is mandatory. This may include plasmapheresis.
- Proper choice of anesthetics and muscle relaxants is crucial. Occasionally there may be difficulty extubating the patient following surgery. Careful observation with monitoring pulmonary function prior to extubation is essential in these patients.
- MG can worsen during emotional stress and the post-partum period. Close monitoring and medication adjustment is important for managing these transient exacerbations.

Lambert–Eaton myasthenic syndrome

LEMS may respond to effective treatment of the underlying malignancy in cancer-associated cases.

Section 3: Diagnosis

BOTTOM LINE/CLINICAL PEARLS

Myasthenia gravis

- The history should focus on determining whether symptoms show a large degree of variation in severity, with attention to visual disturbances, blurred or double vision up close or at a distance, alterations in articulation and swallowing, as well as proximal arm and leg weakness especially during activities such as stair climbing, or blow-drying hair. Attention should be focused on the time of day when these changes are most severe or likely to occur and on how symptoms change with persistent or repeated activity. .
- Worsening of symptoms is particularly common in the evening or at night, with mildly elevated body temperature (e.g. during warm weather), with illness, fatigue, or stressful situations.
- The examination may show disconjugate extraocular movements (EOM), especially evident during slow, tracking eye movements, and fatigable ptosis with prolonged upgaze. There may be facial weakness and proximal arm and neck muscle weakness worsened with repetitive effort against resistance. Reflexes are normal to brisk.
- The edrophonium test and ice-pack test (see Physical examination, below) are useful bedside diagnostic tools for MG.
- Electrophysiologic (repetitive stimulation) studies may show characteristic decremental response, and single fiber studies can show characteristic increased variability (jitter) and blocking.
- Serology may detect confirmatory anti-ACHR or anti-MuSK antibodies.
- Chest CT or MRI should be done to look for possible thymic pathology.

Lambert–Eaton myasthenic syndrome

- History and examination show characteristic proximal muscle weakness that in contrast to MG improves with activity, and loss of deep tendon reflexes.
- Autonomic signs and symptoms are common, for example dry mouth, orthostatic hypotension.
- Oculomotor abnormalities are uncommon.
- Electrophysiology shows marked increase in the response size with rapid repetitive stimulation or immediately following brief forceful exercise.
- Serology may detect antibodies to voltage-gated calcium channels.

Differential diagnosis

Differential diagnosis	Features
Other causes of ptosis, diplopia, and dysphagia	
Guillain–Barré syndrome	Loss of reflexes, diffuse weakness, abnormal nerve conduction studies (prolonged F wave and H reflex latencies), elevated CSF protein
Miller Fisher syndrome	Miller Fisher variant (ophthalmoparesis, ataxia, areflexia) usually has GQ1b antibody
Botulism	Dilated sluggish or fixed pupils, cranial nerve motor weakness, rapidly descending paralysis, autonomic involvement
Mitochondrial myopathy	Chronic diffuse weakness, may have external ophthalmoplegia
Posterior communicating artery aneurysm	Usually an abrupt-onset diplopia with headache. Abnormal CT angiogram or MR angiogram
Multiple sclerosis, neuromyelitis optica (NMO)	Disseminated CNS symptoms and signs. Brain and spinal cord MRI show characteristic changes
Structural brainstem lesions: tumor, infarct, cerebral vasculitis	Multiple brainstem findings, abnormal imaging studies
Lyme disease	Multiple cranial nerves, may have history of rash, tick bite, arthralgias, positive Lyme serology
Thyroid disease	Never causes ptosis, but may cause EOM changes with diplopia and lid retraction (stare). Abnormal thyroid function tests
Myotonic dystrophy	Associated with myotonia in muscles with distal weakness. Typical facies, cardiac conduction disease, and positive family history
Diabetes mellitus	Sudden onset of painless oculomotor palsy. Abnormal glucose
Chronic progressive external ophthalmoplegia (Kearns–Sayre)	Gradual onset with eventually complete loss of EOMs. Patient is usually thin, and has a long history of weakness. Commonly have short stature, hearing loss, cardiac disease, and positive family history
Oculopharyngeal dystrophy	Gradually worsening over months with swallowing difficulties. Patient is usually thin, with long history of weakness
Other causes of arm and neck weakness	
Cervical stenosis with radiculopathy	Pain, sensory and reflex changes. Muscle atrophy. Abnormal cervical spine MRI; weakness follows radicular pattern
Inflammatory myopathies	Proximal weakness in upper and lower extremities, systemic features, elevated creatine kinase (CK) level, may have muscle pain and tenderness
Becker's dystrophy (late onset)	Abnormal CK, and slowly progressive. Legs are usually involved first. Abnormal dystrophin
Adult-onset acid maltase deficiency	Slow progression with abnormal CK and diffuse proximal weakness, especially in legs. Lymphocytes contain PAS-positive vacuoles. Prominent chronic respiratory difficulties
Hypo- and hyperthyroidism	No ptosis. CK elevation, Abnormal thyroid tests and antibodies

Typical presentation

MG commonly presents with ptosis and diplopia. Initially symptoms may occur in episodes, particularly at the end of the day, in hot environments, or with illness and fever. Proximal arm weakness may also be noted, which worsens with continued activity. The arms are typically more affected than the legs. Speech difficulties with worsening articulation due to tongue weakness or nasal speech may occur with prolonged speaking. As the symptoms are commonly produced with prolonged activity, they may be difficult to reproduce during an office visit. Occasionally, fatigue-induced shortness of breath may develop. Over weeks to months, the symptoms tend to recur more frequently, last longer, and may fail to resolve.

Clinical diagnosis

History

- Inquire about double vision, drooping eyelids, and weakness of the arms or legs.
- Does the patient show muscle fatigue with use (e.g. difficulties combing or drying hair) or worsen with overheating or stress? Is there a reduction in endurance or shortness of breath with prolonged speaking or moderate exertion?
- What is the daily pattern of symptoms? Is there worsening by the end of the day?
- Do the symptoms tend to vary in intensity and have the episodes worsened over time?
- Are there difficulties with head control (sensation of a "heavy head"), speech, or swallowing? Does the patient choke?
- Note that LEMS typically presents with progressive proximal weakness affecting the legs and arms, with the legs being more commonly affected as compared to MG. In contradistinction to MG, eye muscle and bulbar muscle dysfunction are relatively rare in LEMS.
- Does the patient have known lung cancer, weight loss, a persistent cough, or shortness of breath? Patients with LEMS often have a known lung cancer, but sometimes LEMS may precede detection of the cancer.
- Does the patient have a dry mouth, swallowing difficulty, constipation, impotence (in males), and orthostatic dizziness? LEMS patients without an underlying malignancy commonly have autonomic symptoms.
- Does the patient have difficulty climbing stairs or getting out of a chair or sofa; does it get better or worse with activity? Proximal muscle fatigue that improves with activity is characteristic of LEMS.

Physical examination

- Myasthenia gravis:
  - The cranial nerve examination, especially the ocular motor system is important. Look for fatigue-induced ptosis, diplopia (red glass or Maddox rod testing is helpful), and facial weakness (especially eyelid closure) with normal sensation. Tongue strength and mobility may be decreased. Articulation, especially with prolonged speaking, is also commonly involved, with nasal and lingual dysarthria.
  - Look for weakness and fatigue on appendicular muscle strength assessment. The proximal arm muscles are usually more affected than distal muscles. Arm muscles are usually affected more often than leg muscles and more severely. Fatigue may be induced by having the patient repetitively use a muscle group against strong resistance. Muscle bulk and reflexes are not affected by MG.
  - An edrophonium test may provide significant help in confirming the diagnosis of MG. It is important to identify an obvious and reproducible sign of muscle weakness, such as ptosis or eye movement abnormalities, which can be used to gauge improvement. This test is only

positive with a strong repair of function, which gradually returns to the pre-test level over 4–6 minutes.
- Application of an ice pack on the eyelid for 1–2 minutes, which improves ptosis, is a diagnostic sign. There must be a robust improvement to be judged positive.
- Lambert–Eaton myasthenic syndrome:
  - Ptosis may be seen, but diplopia is uncommon.
  - Characteristically there is marked proximal weakness in the arms and legs with the initial test, and the legs are usually more significantly affected than the arms.
  - A useful bedside equivalent of the EMG repetitive stimulation test for LEMS can be performed. Select a proximal muscle that is weak. Have the patient isometrically activate the muscle against gradually increasing resistance for 30–40 s. Retest the muscle immediately after the exercise; a positive test will produce significantly greater strength in the muscle; the prior level of weakness returns in 1–2 min.
  - There may be significant orthostasis, and dry mouth or eyes. There may also be sensory abnormalities on examination.
  - As the disease progresses there may be worsening shortness of breath due to the cancer as well as the disease.

Disease severity classification: MGFA classification for MG

There is no classification system currently in use for LEMS. Cases are characterized by whether or not they are associated with a neoplasm.

Class I	Any ocular muscle weakness May have weakness of eye closure All other muscle strength is normal
Class II	Mild weakness affecting other than ocular muscles May also have ocular muscle weakness of any severity
IIa	Predominantly affecting limb, axial muscles, or both May also have lesser involvement of oropharyngeal muscles
IIb	Predominantly affecting oropharyngeal, respiratory muscles, or both May also have lesser or equal involvement of limb, axial muscles, or both
Class III	Moderate weakness affecting other than ocular muscles May also have ocular muscle weakness of any severity
IIIa	Predominantly affecting limb, axial muscles, or both May also have lesser involvement of oropharyngeal muscles
IIIb	Predominantly affecting oropharyngeal, respiratory muscles, or both May also have lesser or equal involvement of limb, axial muscles, or both
Class IV	Severe weakness affecting other than ocular muscles May also have ocular muscle weakness of any severity
IVa	Predominantly affecting limb and/or axial muscles May also have lesser involvement of oropharyngeal muscles
IVb	Predominantly affecting oropharyngeal, respiratory muscles, or both May also have lesser or equal involvement of limb, axial muscles, or both
Class V	Defined by intubation, with or without mechanical ventilation, except when employed during routine postoperative management. The use of a feeding tube without intubation places the patient in class IVb

Laboratory diagnosis

List of diagnostic tests

- Tests for suspected MG
  - Blood tests (confirmatory):
    - Acetylcholine binding, modulating, and blocking antibody
    - Anti-MuSK antibody
  - Blood tests to eliminate other disease:
    - CPK elevation
    - Thyroid testing
    - Lyme titers
    - ANA
  - EMG testing (refer to Chapter 3 for further information):
    - Repetitive stimulation looking for decremental response. Post-activation studies may help yield a positive test.
    - Single fiber testing.
  - Radiologic testing:
    - CT of the chest with and without contrast for thymoma (MG).
    - Chest MRI is useful in young women to reduce breast tissue radiation exposure, although anatomy not as clearly defined as with CT. MRI anatomy is not sufficient for surgical planning.
    - MRI of the brain to rule out aneurysms or tumors affecting cranial nerves III, IV, or VI, or detect changes characteristic of multiple sclerosis.
- Tests for suspected LEMS
  - Blood tests (confirmatory):
    - P/Q-type VGCC (voltage-gated calcium channel) antibodies
    - Anti-synaptotagmin antibodies
  - Blood tests to eliminate other diseases:
    - CPK
    - Acetylcholine receptor antibody testing
  - Radiologic testing:
    - CT/MRI of chest for lung tumors
  - EMG testing (refer to Chapter 3 for further information):
    - Repetitive stimulation with post-activation studies.
    - Small CMAP amplitudes on standard motor conduction studies with improvement of more than 100% following strong muscle volitional activation, or rapid repetitive stimulation are characteristic.

Potential pitfalls/common errors made regarding diagnosis of disease

Myasthenia gravis

- Patients may appear normal when tested in the office setting as they are usually well rested. Fatigue with continued effort is characteristic of MG, which is difficult to reproduce in the examination room.
- Avoid false positive edrophonium tests. Minimal changes are not considered positive.

Lambert–Eaton myasthenic syndrome

- The characteristic incremental response of the CMAP amplitude with activation must increase by more than 100% to be considered positive.

Section 4: Treatment
Treatment rationale
Myasthenia gravis

The treatment of MG should be tailored to the severity and rate of progression of the disease. MG patients may present with varying degrees of involvement, ranging from isolated mild eye movement changes to severe respiratory problems developing shortly after disease onset.

- MG patients with more mild symptoms may be treated initially with 30–60 mg pyridostigmine every 4 hours. This may be all that is needed to correct the patient's problems.
- If the response is inadequate, the patient is usually treated with prednisone at doses ranging from 10 to 80 mg daily. Care must be taken with this drug to avoid worsening weakness, which can result from large doses or rapid dose escalation.
- When higher prednisone doses are needed, consider hospitalizing the patient for concomitant plasmapheresis (PLEX) to blunt the worsening of the MG by steroids. Prednisone takes many weeks to reach its full potential, and will cause side effects, which have to be managed.
- Immunosuppressive medications may be used for their steroid-sparing effect, or to assist in disease control in more severely affected patients. These drugs take many months to become effective, and have no place in the acute setting. The most commonly used drugs at present are azathioprine or mycophenolate mofetil. Other agents, including ciclosporin (cyclosporine) and rituximab, appear to work more quickly, taking weeks to become effective, but entail more complex dosing risks, side effects, and monitoring requirements.
- The use of prednisone or immunosuppressive medications for MG is complex. These medications have serious side effects and are best used by clinicians with significant experience in the diagnosis and management of MG.
- Other treatments for quick responses are intravenous immune globulin (IVIG) and PLEX. These treatments are invasive and complex. Their onset is usually rapid, but of limited duration (weeks). These treatments are used in acute settings or as a bridge to another therapy that takes longer to take effect.
- Thymectomy is used in all patients with increased thymic tissue for age suspicious for thymoma. It is also used for disease control in patients with generalized MG. The benefit of thymectomy can take years to appear, and it is not useful for acute exacerbations.

Lambert–Eaton myasthenic syndrome

Symptomatic therapy for the treatment of LEMS is limited.

- In cancer-related disease, the treatment is directed at the underlying cancer.
- Occasionally, pyridostigmine may cause some improvement in weakness.
- In non-cancer-related disease, the use of 3,4-diaminopyridine (amifampridine) may provide improvement in strength and endurance.
- Immunosuppressive medications are sometimes successful in controlling the disorder.
- Occasionally, in severe rare cases, bone marrow transplant may be effective, but this treatment has a high rate of severe complications.

When to hospitalize

MG patients with severe symptoms such as swallowing or breathing difficulties may need to be hospitalized immediately and stabilized. Indications include:

- Shortness of breath, especially with speaking or eating. Monitor vital capacity, negative inspiratory force, positive expiratory force, and respiratory rate.
- Difficulty swallowing, prominent throat clearing, especially while eating or drinking.
- Choking while eating or on saliva.

Other possible indications for hospitalization include:
- Disease worsening with severe bulbar, arm, or leg weakness.
- Initiation of steroid therapy.
- Infection with disease worsening, or monitoring of infection and response to treatment.
- Preparation for surgery.

LEMS patients with associated cancer may need care of the tumor or its consequences. LEMS patients without associated tumor rarely require hospitalization.
- Rarely, non-tumor LEMS patients with such severe disability that they are unable to stand or walk may need hospitalization for safety and to administer intensive treatment focused on the immune system, possibly including bone marrow transplant.

Table of treatment for myasthenia gravis

Conservative	Patients with minimal ocular (e.g. mild ptosis) or other mild symptoms may require only monitoring without any medication
Oral medications	
• Pyridostigmine bromide (Mestinon: 60 mg tablet)	30–150 mg every 3–4 hours, usually while awake
• Pyridostigmine bromide (Mestinon time span: 180 mg tablet)	90–180 mg at bedtime
• Prednisone	Varying doses up to 80 mg daily
• Azathioprine (Imuran: (50 mg tablet)	Varying doses based on weight from 2 to 3 mg/kg/day, or smaller in some maintenance situations
• Mycophenolate mofetil (CellCept: 500 mg tablets)	Usually 1 g twice daily, but may be smaller or higher doses as tolerated **(not for women of childbearing potential without adequate contraception)**
• Ciclosporin (cyclosporine)	Effective but highly toxic drug rarely used today
Intravenous treatments	
• IVIG	Doses up to 400 mg/kg/day, with the initial treatment of 5 consecutive days. This may be repeated as a single day dose monthly or other schedules as needed
• Plasmapheresis (PLEX for plasma exchange)	For crisis, exchanges of approximately one plasma volume are done every other day until patient is stable (usually 5–6 times total). For maintenance, treatment is continued every few weeks. The process lowers fibrinogen, and cannot be done the day prior to, or following, surgery
• Rituximab (Rituxan)	Dosing based on surface area, usually once a week for 4 weeks
Surgical treatment	
• Thymectomy	This may be done by various techniques including the classic sternal split with total thymectomy including neck dissection, video assisted thymectomy (VATS) via an endoscope, and, more recently, robotic thymectomy. There is no clear "best" method currently. The role of thymectomy in non-thymomatous MG is currently being studied. Historically this has been a necessary part of the care of patients with generalized MG
Symptomatic surgical therapy	
• Tracheostomy	In patients with prolonged respiratory failure
• Percutaneous gastrostomy (PEG)	In patients with prolonged severe dysphagia
Radiotherapy	
• With thymoma	In some cases of invasive thymoma this is useful for tumor treatment or palliation

Prevention/management of complications

- Pyridostigmine (Mestinon) complications:
  - Diarrhea and abdominal pain may be treated with diphenoxylate and atropine or similar drugs as needed.
  - Drug-induced muscle cramping may respond to lowering the dose.
- Prednisone:
  - Weight gain is a common problem. Patients should be forewarned of the hunger caused by prednisone, and to use non-fattening foods such as vegetables or rice cakes or similar choices. Exercise should be encouraged when possible.
  - Glucose metabolism is significantly impacted and diabetes can be precipitated. Patients with pre-existing diabetes need careful management of their medications with the assistance of their diabetologist. Dividing the dose into smaller uniform doses to be used throughout the day may make the adjustments of medication for the diabetes easier.
  - Steroids can induce hypertension or exacerbate underlying hypertension, and may require careful management. Dietary salt restriction should be encouraged. Persistently elevated blood pressure should be treated.
  - Some patients become anxious and agitated with the use of steroid medications, which can be very disturbing to the patient as well as to family and colleagues. This condition may interfere with sleep, as well as work and concentration. This may be helped with a gentle sleep aid, but it may occasionally become disruptive and require the use of stronger medications and the assistance of a psychiatrist.
  - GI upset may be handled with the use of H2 receptor blockers or similar drugs. These should be used prophylactically if prednisone use is protracted.
  - Calcium metabolism changes and bone loss may be treated with supplemental calcium and vitamin D. This should be monitored with bone density studies, and the use of bisphosphonate drugs and endocrinologic consultation may be needed.
  - Glaucoma develops in 10–15% of patients chronically taking steroids. Patients on chronic steroids require an ophthalmologic examination 2–3 times yearly. Normal eye pressure does not guarantee that glaucoma will not develop later with continued steroid use. If elevated intraocular pressure develops, treatment is required.
  - Cataracts develop in many patients taking steroid medications. These should be monitored and treated by an ophthalmologist.
  - Other problems with no specific treatment include the easy bruising that many patients experience, weight gain, and hair loss. These may be helped with reassurance that these will remit when the prednisone dose is lowered.
- Immunosuppressive drugs:
  - Monitor CBC and metabolic panels to check for anemia, abnormalities in liver function, abnormal WBCs, and pancreatic dysfunction (especially with azathioprine).
  - Each agent has its own side effects, and these should be monitored as indicated. Some agents have specific effects on the fetus (e.g. mycophenolate), and proper birth control methods need to be practiced in women of childbearing potential, if those agents are used. Teratogenic drugs should be discontinued for the interval required (depending on the drug) in patients who are planning to have a child. Obstetric consultation is very helpful as pregnant patients with myasthenia are considered high-risk.

CLINICAL PEARLS
- Infection, the most common reason for disease worsening, should always be investigated and treated promptly. Prompt treatment may avoid crisis.
- Rapid changes in steroid doses in either direction may precipitate severe disease worsening. These patients need close monitoring.
- Respiratory impairment may worsen rapidly. Patients with respiratory insufficiency should always be monitored in an ICU setting.
- Atelectasis may lead to A/V shunting through the lung, and rapid onset of respiratory crisis. Active chest PT as well as the frequent use of an incentive spirometer and suctioning is paramount in avoiding crisis.
- Patients who complain of severe excess saliva may be having severe swallowing problems, placing them at high risk for aspiration; they need close monitoring, and possibly intubation.
- Edrophonium tests are only considered positive if there is a marked rapid response (within a minute) and gradual reversion to pretest level in 5–7 minutes.
- Pregnancies in myasthenic women are high-risk pregnancies and need appropriate prenatal and obstetric care. There is a 20% risk for the newborn to have transient neonatal myasthenia.

Section 5: Special populations

Pregnancy
- During pregnancy MG usually does well, with remission of symptoms and reduced medication need. This may change abruptly with the onset of labor or during the immediate or later post-partum period.

Children
- Approximately 20% of babies born of myasthenic mothers may have transient neonatal MG. This generally resolves spontaneously, but sometimes requires medical therapy.
- The incidence of MG in children is about 4–6 patients per million population. The medications used are similar to adults, but doses are adjusted to age and weight.

Elderly
- MG is underdiagnosed in the elderly, since symptoms and signs such as ptosis and proximal arm weakness may be ascribed to age-related decline in function. Also of importance is the increasing incidence of thymic tumors in older populations.
- LEMS is often missed in the elderly in the presence of lung cancer or other cancers as the weakness is considered to be part of the debilitation of the cancer.

Others
- Diabetes or hypertension is exacerbated by prednisone.

Section 6: Prognosis

BOTTOM LINE/CLINICAL PEARLS
- With proper care MG patients should live normal full lives.
- Despite severe complications of MG, recovery to normal is usual with proper care.
- LEMS, as it is often associated with cancer, has a poor prognosis.
- In LEMS without underlying cancer, the patients generally do relatively well, although there may be significant weakness and debility in some severely affected patients. The current treatments are of limited benefit. In patients with antibody-mediated LEMS, bone marrow transplant, while rarely performed, has sometimes been effective.

Natural history of untreated disease

Occasionally the course of MG may be self-limited or the symptoms remain mild. In such cases, medication may be of little practical value, especially if it involves significant side effects. However, mild cases of MG usually worsen, making effective treatment necessary.

Untreated, LEMS is variably progressive. Severe worsening may occur over time in both cancer-associated and idiopathic LEMS.

Prognosis for treated patients

- With few exceptions MG patients achieve a normal level of function for routine activities. The exceptions are sustained heavy physical activity and competitive sports. Most patients require medication, and the doses of medication may vary as the circumstances dictate. There are rare patients with very severe disease who are relatively refractory to treatment. These patients often have MuSK antibody.
- With cancer-related LEMS, there is usually significant worsening of the disease as the cancer progresses.
- In the LEMS cases without cancer, the disease usually progresses despite treatment. There may be responses to various forms of immunosuppression. Some patients achieve prolonged remission, while others have significant disability.

Follow-up tests and monitoring

Follow-up frequency of MG patients is based on clinical status. Even with prolonged remission, there is always the possibility of disease recurrence, which may be severe.

LEMS patients require close follow-up. Most patients will need lifelong immunosuppression, and must be followed for complications of the disease and the effects of the drugs. Most patients have significant disability, and many require assistance with walking.

Section 7: Reading list

Key reading sources for this chapter can be found online at www.mountsinaiexpertguides.com

Suggested websites

- Myasthenia Gravis Foundation of America: myasthenia.org
  An extensive site with educational and support information, and information about ongoing research. This is a patient oriented site.
- Muscular Dystrophy Association: mda.org
  Provides a good source of information about the disease and some information about research. This is a patient oriented site.
- Neuromuscular Disease Center of Washington University, St Louis, MO: neuromuscular.wustl.edu
  An excellent site for information about the disease, both clinical and basic science information with clear explanation of terminology. This is a sophisticated source for information about myasthenia gravis and virtually all diseases of the neuromuscular systems. This is a site with information for patients as well as physicians.

Section 8: Guidelines
National society guidelines

Title	Source	Weblink
Myasthenia gravis: recommendations for clinical research standards. Task Force of the Medical Scientific Advisory Board of the Myasthenia Gravis Foundation of America	Myasthenia Gravis Foundation of America (2000)	http://www.ncbi.nlm.nih.gov/pubmed/10921745

Section 9: Evidence for therapies

Type of evidence	Title and comment	Comment
RCT	Preliminary results of a double-blind, randomized, placebo-controlled trial of cyclosporine in myasthenia gravis (1987) **Comment**: Demonstrated efficacy of cyclosporine in the treatment of MG	http://www.ncbi.nlm.nih.gov/pubmed/3547126
Systematic review	Practice parameter: Thymectomy for autoimmune myasthenia gravis (an evidence-based review) Report of the Quality Standards Subcommittee of the American Academy of Neurology (2000) **Comment**: Review of prior studies on success with thymectomy versus non-thymectomy for clinical outcome. This is the basis for a current study to evaluate the benefit of thymectomy in non-thymoma-associated MG as an RCT	http://www.ncbi.nlm.nih.gov/pubmed/10891896

Additional material for this chapter can be found online at:
www.mountsinaiexpertguides.com

This includes advice for patients, a case study, multiple choice questions, and a reading list.

CHAPTER 35

Motor Neuron Disease

Mark A. Sivak

Icahn School of Medicine at Mount Sinai, New York, NY, USA

OVERALL BOTTOM LINE

- Amyotrophic lateral sclerosis (ALS, motor neuron disease, Lou Gehrig's disease) is a neuro-degenerative disease usually of unknown cause, although a small number of cases are hereditary and familial.
- Aside from the mild symptomatic help provided by riluzole, there are no effective disease-specific treatments.
- Patients typically succumb to respiratory failure and pulmonary complications.
- Timely and appropriate supportive care can significantly extend life and improve its quality.
- Patients and their families are most efficiently and effectively treated by a team of specialists at a multidisciplinary ALS center.
- ALS was previously thought to preserve cognitive function, but cognitive deficits are increasingly recognized in ALS. There may be a link between ALS and fronto-temporal dementia, with several mutations identified that cause both diseases.
- Patients participating in clinical research generally do better than those not enrolled in clinical trials.

Section 1: Background
Definition of disease

The motor neuron diseases cause progressive reduction in the control of voluntary muscle. The cell bodies of motor neurons involved in voluntary muscle control anywhere in the body can be affected, with the specific symptoms depending on the predominant pattern of cell loss.

Disease classification

The term motor neuron disease generally refers to variants of ALS, an adult-onset disease of motor neurons. Another category of motor neuron diseases includes childhood-onset hereditary motor neuron disorders, the spinal muscular atrophies (SMA).

Clinically, the most common motor neuron diseases are variants of ALS and are divisible into three main groups – progressive muscular atrophy, primary lateral sclerosis, or classical amyotrophic lateral sclerosis – depending on the predominant localization of the affected motor neurons:

- Progressive muscular atrophy (PMA) affects only lower motor neurons, which directly contact appendicular or bulbar muscles. PMA is characterized by weakness, fasciculations, muscle atrophy, reduced or absent reflexes, reduced muscle tone, and a relatively slow rate of progression.
- Primary lateral sclerosis (PLS) affects only upper motor neurons. PLS is characterized by increased tone, brisk and pathologic reflexes, and mild muscle atrophy, usually late in the disease course.

Mount Sinai Expert Guides: Neurology, First Edition. Edited by Stuart C. Sealfon, Rajeev Motiwala, and Charles B. Stacy.
© 2016 John Wiley & Sons, Ltd. Published 2016 by John Wiley & Sons, Ltd.
Companion website: www.mountsinaiexpertguides.com

- ALS most commonly consists of a mixture of upper and lower motor neuron involvement and deficits, and shows a rapid rate of progression.
- Additional forms of ALS have been described when bulbar involvement is the prominent or presenting feature (bulbar palsy with LMN features and pseudobulbar palsy with UMN features). Bulbar involvement is often present in the commonest form of ALS.
- Familial ALS is often considered a separate category. Several mutations have been identified, which account for less than 10% of cases of ALS, including mutations in the genes *SOD1*, *TDP43*, and *C9orf27*.
- "ALS plus" syndromes are the combination of motor neuron diseases with other neurodegenerative disorders, such ALS-Parkinson's and ALS-fronto-temporal dementia.

Spinal muscular atrophy (SMA) types I, II, and III belong to a group of hereditary diseases that cause weakness and wasting of the voluntary muscles in infants and children. The disorders are caused by an abnormal or missing gene known as the survival of motor neuron gene 1 (*SMN1*), which is responsible for the production of a protein essential to motor neurons. The type of SMA (I, II, or III) is determined by the age of onset and the severity of symptoms. These disorders will not be discussed further in this chapter.

- Type I (also known as Werdnig–Hoffman disease, or infantile-onset SMA) is evident at birth or within the first few months.
- Type II (the intermediate form) usually begins between 6 and 18 months of age.
- Symptoms of type III (also called Kugelberg–Welander disease) appear between 2 and 17 years of age.

Incidence/prevalence

In Europe and North America the incidence of ALS is 0.8–1.5/100,000 individuals, with a disease prevalence of 2–7/100,000 individuals in the population.

Etiology

- Most cases of ALS are idiopathic and sporadic; their etiology is not yet established.
- 5–10% of cases of ALS are familial and genetic in etiology. Autosomal dominant genes found to cause ALS include *SOD1* (superoxide dismutase 1), *TDP43* (TAR DNA binding protein 43), and *C9orf72* (chromosome 9 open reading frame 72). These and other disease-causing mutations can be found in some sporadic cases of ALS.
- *TDP43* and *C9orf27* have been identified both in cases of ALS and of fronto-temporal dementia (FTD). The increasing recognition of cognitive dysfunction in ALS and the presence of ALS-FTD syndromes suggest an etiologic relationship between the two diseases.
- Several systemic diseases can induce clinical syndromes that mimic motor neuron diseases and are potentially treatable. These include:
  - anti-Hu antibody syndrome;
  - breast cancer-associated PLS-like syndrome;
  - subacute motor neuronopathy of lymphoma, which has a PMA-like presentation;
  - HIV infection-associated ALS syndrome.

Pathology/pathogenesis

The hallmark of motor neuron diseases is the relatively selective loss of motor neurons in the cerebral cortex, brainstem, and spinal cord with secondary degeneration of corticobulbar tracts, corticospinal tracts (the origin of the term lateral sclerosis), and peripheral motor axons. The pathology is notable for the relative lack of reactive astrocytosis, cellular infiltration, and inflammatory responses. Degenerating motor neurons typically have inclusion bodies, which may be TDP43 positive.

Predictive/risk factors

- Advanced age and positive family history are the two best-established risk factors. This is based on a single article that is a records review of all cases of MND reported in the UK over several years looking for other diagnoses in the patients' charts.

Section 2: Prevention and screening

BOTTOM LINE/CLINICAL PEARLS
- No interventions have been demonstrated to decrease the risk of disease onset.
- While testing of family members of a proband having a genetic cause of ALS is feasible this is not performed due to ethical concerns.

Section 3: Diagnosis

BOTTOM LINE/CLINICAL PEARLS
- The history should focus on the complaints of painless progressive weakness, evolving over weeks to months, often beginning in one area with associated muscle atrophy.
- Other areas, either in the same or opposite side of the body, may also become affected. This may also include problems with articulation and swallowing.
- Unexplained weight loss, muscle cramping in unusual sites, such as in the neck with head turning, or in the upper abdomen, and gradual reduction of stamina are important features.
- The classical hallmark is a combination of UMN and LMN signs in the same body segment. The examination should be directed at looking for presence of focal weakness with or without muscle atrophy (amyotrophy), fasciculations, abnormal muscle tone, and relative hyperreflexia.
- Changes in speech prosody and articulation may be noted.
- There may be changes in swallowing, especially with water or saliva.
- Slowing of tongue movement, and atrophy may be noted.
- Gait may be spastic.
- Changes in sensory systems, special sensation (e.g. vision), or other findings such as ptosis or extraocular muscle weakness are not associated with ALS and other diagnoses should be considered.
- MRI examination of brain and cervical spine is performed to exclude masses, compressive, vascular, or other structural lesions.
- Workup also involves electromyography including:
  - motor and sensory conduction studies;
  - needle studies to demonstrate diffuse changes involving muscles supplied by cranial nerves (tongue, face, jaw), cervical, thoracic, and lumbosacral roots.
- Pulmonary function studies are useful to demonstrate subclinical respiratory involvement, and the degree of compromise.
- Swallowing studies (modified barium swallow) may demonstrate the presence and degree of swallowing changes, which may not be clinically evident.

Differential diagnosis

Differential diagnosis	Features
Cervical myelopathy	No abnormalities above neck, and normal jaw jerk, with hyperreflexia below. May have sensory level below the face or upper neck. Abnormal cervical spine MRI
Syringomyelia cervical cord	May have sensory dissociation (impaired pin-prick and temperature with preserved light touch, vibration, and proprioception) below the shoulders in cape-like distribution. Syrinx detected on MRI of the cervical cord, brainstem may also be involved
Multifocal motor neuropathy	Distally preponderant weakness affecting arms more than legs, usually asymmetric, with absent reflexes and no UMN signs. Focal slowing on EMG with conduction block in non-entrapment locations. GM1 antibody titer elevated in 50% of patients
Inclusion body myositis	Unusual weakness pattern sparing finger extensors with severe weakness of finger flexors, prominent involvement of the quadriceps
Brainstem tumors	Cranial neuropathies, long tract signs, detected by MRI with contrast
Chronic inflammatory demyelinating polyradiculoneuropathy	Absent deep tendon reflexes (DTRs), may have sensory findings, bulbar findings rare. Abnormal nerve conduction studies
Lymphoma motor neuronopathy with paraproteinemia	Abnormal immunofixation with monoclonal protein. Systemic disease or abnormal bone marrow. May be presenting complaint
Monoclonal gammopathies	Abnormal immunofixation with monoclonal protein. Sensory complaints and findings in addition to weakness common
Monomelic amyotrophy	Process remains confined to one limb, usually upper limb. Most common in young men
Sarcoidosis with myelopathy and neuropathy	Abnormal spine MRI and abnormal EMG and conduction studies. May have abnormal ACE titer. CSF may be abnormal with elevated protein

Typical presentation

The symptom onset in motor neuron disease is quite variable.

- This may begin with changes in speech or swallowing, handgrip, pincer strength, or foot drop.
- Painless, progressive changes is the clinical feature that best distinguishes this disease. Initially, symptoms may be intermittent, typically being more evident when the patient is fatigued or at the end of the day. With time the symptoms become more constant, and gradually worsen in degree. Symptoms typically worsen gradually in an affected area and also appear in previously unaffected regions, spinal or bulbar segments.
- The presenting features depend on the location of the pathologic process within the nervous system, with both upper and lower motor neuron signs being present. Relatively brisk reflexes are often noted in the same areas with muscle atrophy or weakness. With time the symptoms gradually spread widely, and become symmetrical.
- Other non-specific symptoms commonly develop such as fatigue, weight loss, and reduced endurance. Cramp also is a common problem, and occurs in "exotic" areas such as across the chest or upper abdomen, or in the neck with head turning.
- Significant abrupt changes usually indicate other disorders.

Clinical diagnosis

History

The following historical features are characteristic:

• Progressive painless difficulty with hand or arm use.
• Progressive changes in articulation, speech prosody, or slowing of speech.
• Coughing while drinking especially with water or other thin liquids.
• Progressive gait changes with stiffness or slowness.
• Bowel and bladder functions are preserved.
• Difficulty lying supine.
• Cramping.
• Unexplained weight loss.
• Reduced endurance, especially with continued effort.
• Excessive emotional responses, such as crying or laughing inappropriately (pseudobulbar affect).

Physical examination

• Exaggerated emotional responses.
• Cranial nerve findings:
  • Slowed tongue movements, with or without atrophy (scalloping of the tongue) and fasciculations.
  • Slow, slurred speech, commonly with a monotonous prosody.
  • Lingual, pharyngeal or nasal dysarthria, which worsens with prolonged speaking.
  • Exaggerated gag reflex, brisk jaw jerk.
  • Slow saccadic extraocular movements or fixed stare in some patients.
• Motor examination:
  • Focal limb muscle atrophy, fasciculations.
  • Weakness either proximal or distal.
  • Fine motor clumsiness, slowed rapid alternating movements, may be asymmetric.
• Reflexes are disproportionately brisk, extensor plantar responses are relatively rarely found (in PMA type reflexes may be absent).
• Sensory examination including special sensory functions (vision, hearing, etc.) is normal.
• Impaired cognitive or executive function may be subtle but is increasingly recognized.

Disease severity classification

No disease severity classification is used in ALS and other motor neuron diseases. The ALS-FRS (Functional Rating Scale) is a tool developed in ALS research to track the patient's course over time.

Laboratory diagnosis

List of diagnostic tests

• No tests are entirely specific for the diagnosis of ALS or other motor neuron diseases.
• Common diagnostic testing used for the diagnosis of ALS and exclusion of other diseases includes:
  • EMG and nerve conduction studies to demonstrate the diffuse spontaneous activity and ongoing motor involvement. EMG findings supportive of motor neuron disease include evidence of active and chronic neurogenic changes in three body segments including the head as a segment, without sensory involvement (see Guidelines, below).

- MRI of brain and cervical spine to eliminate cord compressive lesions, vascular diseases, tumors, or other diseases such as MS or CJD, spinal AV-dural fistulas, and so forth. May show signal abnormalities along corticospinal and corticobulbar tracts.
- MR spectroscopy of brain in selected cases to demonstrate cerebral motor neuron loss.
- Laboratory tests may include:
  - GM1 antibody to differentiate multifocal motor neuropathy from PMA.
  - Immunofixation (lymphoma and other paraproteinemias), TSH, and thyroid antibodies.
  - Lyme titers.
  - ACE levels (sarcoidosis).
  - Methylmalonic acid and homocysteine levels to assure normal B12 and folate metabolism.
  - Rheumatoid factor, anti-Ro/SSA, anti-La/SSB to eliminate vasculitides.
  - CPK to demonstrate muscle involvement. This is commonly elevated in ALS up to about 5–7 times normal levels. Higher levels suggest other diseases.
  - Muscle MRI of symptomatic muscle area to select a site for biopsy to eliminate myopathies (e.g. inclusion body myositis) is required very infrequently.
  - CSF oligoclonal bands and IgG synthesis rate tests (e.g. in primary progressive multiple sclerosis).

Potential pitfalls, common errors made regarding diagnosis of disease

- Fasciculations alone in the absence of weakness do not indicate ALS. Fasciculations are common in normal individuals who seek attention or are referred for possible ALS. They may be observed and detected on EMG. When fasciculations are seen on EMG, they must be accompanied by other changes (fibrillations and positive waves, abnormal appearing motor units) to be considered an abnormal finding.
- Cervical stenosis with myelopathy may evolve in a slowly progressive course with minimal sensory symptoms, leading to an erroneous diagnosis of motor neuron disease.
- The combination of cervical and lumbar spine disease causing LMN findings in the limbs and long tract signs can be difficult to distinguish from ALS.
- Patients with inclusion body myositis (IBM) may have reflex changes and unusual weakness patterns, which may lead to an erroneous diagnosis of motor neuron disease. These patients have marked weakness of the finger flexors with preservation of the finger extensors, associated with forearm atrophy. This unusual symptom complex is pathognomonic for IBM.

Section 4: Treatment
Treatment rationale

- While riluzole is the only FDA-approved treatment to slow ALS progression, its efficacy is limited.
- The use of symptomatic treatment depends on the patient's wishes, especially mechanical ventilation and artificial feeding. Supportive and symptomatic areas to address may include:
  - Nocturnal non-invasive ventilation, tracheostomy, and long-term ventilator use.
  - Nasogastric tube or feeding gastrostomy to maintain nutrition and reduce the risk of aspiration when swallowing is affected significantly.
  - Spasticity may be painful and troublesome interfering with activities of daily living. This may be helped with oral baclofen, or tizanidine. In rare cases with severe painful leg spasticity, intrathecal baclofen may be helpful for improved function and pain control.

- Cramp is a common and troublesome problem for patients. Previously quinine provided great relief, but is no longer on the market in the USA. There are no good substitutes currently available.
- Pain management becomes a severe problem as the disease becomes more advanced. With the loss of muscle, tendons are stretched by the weight of the bones, particularly at the shoulders and hips. This causes severe pain. Skin ischemia in severely immobile patients also produces severe pain, as does falling of the head either forward or backward, due to the weakness of neck muscles. Most pain medications suppress respiration, which is usually already compromised by disease. Careful positioning with mechanically assisted bed devices to shift patient position is often valuable in improving patient comfort. These measures have to be adjusted to the needs of each patient on an ongoing basis.

When to hospitalize

- While there are guidelines (see below) that help determine timing of a specific intervention, it is critical to individualize the approach based on the patient's goals of care, wishes, and ethical concerns.
- There are generally two disease-related reasons for hospitalization:
  - worsening of swallowing causing inadequate nutrition or problems with aspiration;
  - respiratory insufficiency.
- Patients with ALS who become systemically ill with other diseases may require hospitalization for those causes as well. These issues may precipitate ALS disease worsening.

Managing the hospitalized patient

- Typically nutritional concerns become important:
  - when the patient has lost about 6–8% of their body weight from their previous healthy state, or
  - when eating has become unacceptably prolonged or dangerous with recurring near aspiration.
- A modified barium swallow test may be of value in gauging the appropriate time to consider PEG (percutaneous endoscopic gastrostomy).
- Spirometry may be a useful tool to measure impending respiratory insufficiency. This is also important in assessing the safety of doing a PEG procedure in patients with compromised respiratory function. The vital capacity (Vc) should be greater than 20 mL/kg and the negative inspiratory force (NIF) should be greater than −40 mmH$_2$O or the positive expiratory force greater than +50 mmHg.

Table of treatment

Conservative	Nutrition, physical therapy, orthotics, and related supportive measures are the mainstay of current treatment
Medical: • Riluzole • Quinidine/ dextromethorphan • Amitriptyline • Glycopyrrolate • Antidepressants and anxiolytics	Riluzole has been reported to delay onset of ventilator dependence or need for tracheostomy in selected patients and may prolong survival by 3–5 months Quinidine/dextromethorphan preparation reduces pseudobulbar symptoms Amitriptyline is of use in pain control, reducing secretions and sedation without respiratory compromise Glycopyrrolate reduces excessive salivation Judicious use of antidepressants and anxiolytics may help with coping

(Continued)

Conservative	**Nutrition, physical therapy, orthotics, and related supportive measures are the mainstay of current treatment**
Surgical: • Gastrostomy (PEG) • Tracheostomy • External diaphragm pacemaker	These procedures are of value for patients who desire these types of supportive life-extending interventions Placement of an external diaphragm pacemaker supplements diaphragm strength with electrical stimulation via electrodes implanted into the diaphragm with a laparoscopic procedure
Radiological	MRI of brain and cervical spine to investigate potential other causes for the symptoms mimicking ALS
Psychological	Counseling and therapy can be beneficial for patients and family members

Prevention/management of complications

- Tracheostomy, while preserving breathing, is profoundly life altering, usually making the patient home and bed bound.
- In some patients without significant bulbar and facial weakness, non-invasive ventilation is possible with resultant better quality of life.
- Generally riluzole and quinidine/dextromethorphan combination have no significant complications.
- Amitriptyline used to control excessive salivation, may also produce sedation, usually without affecting ventilation, which is an added benefit. This may be especially useful at night. The drug may also provide mild antidepressant benefit as well.

CLINICAL PEARLS
- Nutrition may be helped with the use of a PEG tube when eating becomes problematic due to aspiration risk, or too slow for the patient to tolerate.
- Breathing may be supplemented with non-invasive ventilation (NIV, BiPAP) in patients with good bulbar function. Invasive ventilation is a significant life-altering measure.
- Before these measures are considered, a thorough discussion with the patient and family members is crucial for their clear understanding of the expected benefits and anticipated change in the quality of life. Many patients elect not to use invasive ventilation.
- Diaphragm pacing may provide some assistance in suitable patients. The usefulness is temporary as the diaphragm becomes more involved with the disease process and stops responding to external pacing.
- Patients with ALS who become systemically ill with other diseases may require hospitalizations for those causes as well. These issues may precipitate ALS disease worsening.

Section 5: Special populations

Not applicable for this topic.

Section 6: Prognosis

BOTTOM LINE/CLINICAL PEARLS
- Most patients with ALS die within 5 years.
- While the rates of progression vary significantly with the type of involvement, all forms of the disease are progressive. PLS and PMA progress very slowly.
- Bulbar onset disease implies poorer prognosis. Nutritional concerns and risk of aspiration affect the prognosis adversely as the disease progresses.
- The onset of measurable changes in respiratory function heralds the end stage of the disease in the absence of mechanical ventilation.

Natural history of untreated disease

- ALS and the other motor neuron diseases are unrelentingly progressive with no specific disease-modifying therapy. Most patients with ALS die within 3–5 years from the symptom onset, but 10% survive for 10 years or longer.
- Any volitionally controlled muscle may be involved, but the order, degree of involvement, and progression rates are variable.
- Patients tend to progress at uniform rates of change, with some patients having more aggressive disease than others.
- More recently, changes in mentation, behavior, language, and executive functions have been recognized as being present in larger numbers of patients. These features need to be recognized and monitored to assist in patient care and decision-making.

Prognosis for treated patients

While there are no effective treatments that influence the outcome of the disease, various palliative therapies may provide significant improvement in quality of life, and to some extent, the duration of life as well. These include nutritional support, treatment of spasticity, judicious pain medication when appropriate, and non-invasive ventilation such as BiPAP at night.

Follow-up tests and monitoring

- Tests of speech and swallowing (modified barium swallow) and respiratory function (spirometry) yield data useful in plotting the disease progression, and in the timing of interventions such as diet modification and respiratory assistance.
- Respiratory function is the most vital of these, as it is of paramount prognostic importance.
- Significant abrupt changes usually indicate other processes developing, and these need to be fully and rapidly evaluated.
- Findings of slow saccadic EOMs, fixed stare, and exaggerated emotional responses suggest development of features of concomitant fronto-temporal dementia. These patients need special attention for non-motor difficulties as well.

Section 7: Reading list

Key reading sources for this chapter can be found online at www.mountsinaiexpertguides.com

Suggested websites

ALS Association: http://www.alsa.org/

Section 8: Guidelines

Title	Source	Weblink
El Escorial World Federation of Neurology criteria for the diagnosis of amyotrophic lateral sclerosis	Subcommittee on Motor Neuron Diseases/Amyotrophic Lateral Sclerosis of the World Federation of Neurology Research Group on Neuromuscular Diseases and the El Escorial "Clinical limits of amyotrophic lateral sclerosis" workshop contributors (1994)	http://dx.doi.org/ 10.1016/0022-510X(94) 90191-0

(Continued)

Title	Source	Weblink
Good practice in the management of amyotrophic lateral sclerosis: clinical guidelines. An evidence-based review with good practice points. EALSC Working Group	European ALS Consortium (EALSC; 2007)	http://www.tandfonline.com/doi/abs/10.1080/17482960701262376?journalCode=iafd19
ALS Functional Rating Scale-Revised (ALSFRS-R)	BDNF ALS Study Group (1999) A tool to chart disease progression	http://www.ncbi.nlm.nih.gov/pubmed/10540002
Awaji criteria for the diagnosis of ALS	de Carvalho M, Dengler R, Eisen A, et al. (2008) Allows earlier diagnosis particularly in patients with bulbar symptoms, allows inclusion of fasciculation as an indicator of lower motor neuron involvement	http://www.ncbi.nlm.nih.gov/pubmed/18164242

Section 9: Evidence for therapies

Type of evidence	Title and comment	Weblink
RCT	A controlled trial of riluzole in amyotrophic lateral sclerosis **Comment**: Initial evidence of usefulness of riluzole. Effect modest	http://www.ncbi.nlm.nih.gov/pubmed/8302340
RCT	Treatment of pseudobulbar affect in ALS with dextromethorphan/quinidine: a randomized trial **Comment**: Good effect with improved quality of life (QOL). No survival change	http://www.ncbi.nlm.nih.gov/pubmed/15505150
Systematic review of two RCTs	Mechanical ventilation for amyotrophic lateral sclerosis/motor neuron disease [Review] **Comment**: Good evidence of improved QOL with less invasive therapy in selected patients	http://www.ncbi.nlm.nih.gov/pubmed/23543531

Additional material for this chapter can be found online at: www.mountsinaiexpertguides.com

This includes advice for patients, a case study, multiple choice questions, and a reading list.

CHAPTER 36

Metabolic Encephalopathy, Hypoxic-Ischemic Encephalopathy, and Brain Death

Mandip S. Dhamoon
Icahn School of Medicine at Mount Sinai, New York, NY, USA

> **OVERALL BOTTOM LINE**
> - The treatment of metabolic encephalopathy is tailored to the specific etiology, with the goal of correcting the metabolic disturbance and thereby the encephalopathy.
> - Improvement of metabolic encephalopathies may have a delay of several hours to days after the correction of the metabolic abnormality.
> - Treatment of hypoxic-ischemic encephalopathy may include induced hypothermia to reduce neurologic injury in addition to cardiovascular support and management.
> - Brain death is established according to local criteria. It is a condition of irreversible loss of hemispheric and brainstem function.

Section 1: Background

Definition of disease

- Encephalopathy is a general term referring to global brain dysfunction, particularly involving impaired arousal, inattention, and confusion, due to processes that affect brain regions diffusely.
- Metabolic encephalopathy (also called "toxic-metabolic encephalopathy") is due to metabolic derangements, not a structural brain abnormality.
- Hypoxic-ischemic encephalopathy is caused by diffuse brain damage, particularly cortical, that results from a prolonged period of impaired blood flow to the brain.
- Brain death is the irreversible loss of cortical and brainstem function.

Disease classification

- Metabolic encephalopathy is classified by the causative metabolic derangement.
- The severity of hypoxic-ischemic encephalopathy depends on the extent of brain involvement, which is proportional to the degree and duration of cerebral blood flow reduction.
- Although brain death may be caused by a number of conditions, its determination is independent of its etiology and it is diagnosed when specific criteria are met (discussed further below).

Incidence and prevalence

Accurate data on the incidence and prevalence of these disorders are lacking. Metabolic encephalopathy occurs most commonly in critical care settings and in a variety of acute medical conditions such as hepatic or renal disease.

Mount Sinai Expert Guides: Neurology, First Edition. Edited by Stuart C. Sealfon, Rajeev Motiwala, and Charles B. Stacy.
© 2016 John Wiley & Sons, Ltd. Published 2016 by John Wiley & Sons, Ltd.
Companion website: www.mountsinaiexpertguides.com

Etiology

- Metabolic encephalopathy: hepatic dysfunction, sepsis, renal failure, hyponatremia, hypernatremia, hypercalcemia, hypocalcemia, hypomagnesemia, thiamine deficiency, hyperglycemia,
  hypoglycemia, medications.
- Hypoxic-ischemic encephalopathy: shock of any cause, drug overdose, head trauma.
- Brain death is caused by the irreversible cessation of key neuronal function, usually due to the
  interruption of cerebral perfusion. It has many causes, including cardiac arrest, head trauma,
  hemorrhagic or ischemic stroke, and other conditions leading to cerebral edema and irreversible intracranial hypertension.

Pathology and pathogenesis

The pathophysiology of metabolic encephalopathy differs by etiology.

- In hepatic dysfunction, for example, circulating neurotoxic substances, originating from nitrogen-
  containing compounds in the gastrointestinal tract that the healthy liver eliminates, accumulate
  in the bloodstream. While the causative neurotoxic substances have not been definitively identified, ammonia, endogenous benzodiazepines, and false neurotransmitters (such as octopamine)
  are the leading candidates. This build-up is due to shunting of blood flow from the portal vein to
  the systemic circulation and reduced detoxification of portal blood due to dysfunction and death
  of hepatocytes. In advanced hepatic encephalopathy, cerebral edema may develop.
- Encephalopathy due to sepsis is thought to result from systemic inflammation, altered blood–
  brain barrier permeability, and microcirculatory dysfunction.
- In renal failure, there are multiple derangements in the balance of electrolytes, acids, bases,
  and water in the body; the most likely causes of encephalopathy are elevated levels of organic
  acids and increased brain calcium.
- Since sodium is an osmole and influences the movement of water into and out of cells, hyponatremia produces brain edema and hypernatremia produces cerebral dehydration. In each case,
  the severity of the encephalopathy is proportional to the rapidity of the change in serum
  sodium level.
- Calcium is involved in presynaptic neurotransmitter release and in the stabilization of neuronal
  membranes along with magnesium, and disturbances in serum levels alter these functions in
  the brain.
- Thiamine deficiency results in dysfunction of the periaqueductal and periventricular gray matter, thalami, and mammillary bodies due to altered adenosine triphosphate synthesis.
- In hyperglycemia, intravascular hyperosmolality results in cerebral dehydration.
- Hypoglycemia causes reduced cerebral access to sufficient glucose, especially in states of high
  cerebral metabolic rate, and results in neuronal dysfunction. The brain, more than other body
  organs, is dependent on a constant supply of glucose as a source of energy. Other factors may
  also contribute to brain dysfunction in hypoglycemia, including the accumulation of metabolic
  by-products of alternate energy pathways and altered levels of neurotransmitters.
- Various classes of medications may contribute to encephalopathy, especially sedatives, psychotropic medications, and anticholinergic medications.

Any condition resulting in cerebral hypoperfusion may lead to hypoxic-ischemic encephalopathy due to neuronal dysfunction and damage from reduced oxygen and glucose delivery to the
cerebrum as well as from impaired waste removal. A common example is cardiac arrest due to
arrhythmia, which results in cardiogenic shock and reduced cerebral perfusion.

Brain death can be caused by a number of conditions whose common features include irreversible damage to the brain resulting in permanent loss of cerebral and brainstem function. For

example, a large middle cerebral artery ischemic stroke may cause neuronal death and progressive cytotoxic edema in the area of the ischemia, resulting in increased intracranial pressure and uncal herniation. The increased intracranial pressure prevents cerebral perfusion, leading to progressive diffuse cerebral neuronal death.

Section 2: Prevention and screening

BOTTOM LINE/CLINICAL PEARLS
- Apart from treatment or avoidance of the specific etiologies discussed above, there is no general preventive or screening strategy for these conditions. For example, in an individual with chronic renal failure dependent on hemodialysis, regularly scheduled dialysis will prevent the development of uremic metabolic encephalopathy.
- With regard to hypoxic-ischemic encephalopathy, the likelihood of cardiac arrest in an individual with increased risk of coronary artery disease can be reduced by regular cardiologic care and management of vascular risk factors.

Section 3: Diagnosis

BOTTOM LINE/CLINICAL PEARLS
- In patients with altered sensorium and a non-focal examination causing suspicion of metabolic encephalopathy, the history can confirm the presence of a predisposing cause such as renal failure (uremic encephalopathy) or uncontrolled diabetes (hyperglycemia).
- For hypoxic-ischemic encephalopathy, a history of an inciting event causing systemic hypoperfusion, such as cardiac arrest, shock, or arrhythmia is relevant, and a past medical history involving cardiac disease may be informative.
- For brain death, a history of a catastrophic event causing irreversible brain damage would be helpful, such as massive intracerebral hemorrhage or significant head trauma.
- Typical examination findings of encephalopathy include impaired arousal, inattention, and confusion while other features may be specific to the cause, such as jaundice in hepatic encephalopathy.
- Supportive investigations differ according to the presumed cause of the encephalopathy, such as neuroimaging in the case of suspected stroke or intracerebral hemorrhage, but a general approach includes a broad chemistry panel, brain imaging, and EEG.

Differential diagnosis

Differential diagnosis	Features
Partial seizures or post-ictal state	History of epilepsy; witnessed seizure; electroencephalogram suggestive of seizure
Dementia with superimposed acute delirium	History of progressive cognitive decline, with superimposed acute episodes not suggestive of seizure. Often caused by minor concurrent illness (e.g. bladder infection) or medication toxicity

Typical presentation
- Metabolic encephalopathy typically presents with subacute to acute onset of impaired arousal, inattention, and confusion in the presence of medical diseases, commonly in a hospital or critical care setting.
- Hypoxic-ischemic encephalopathy becomes evident following a catastrophic circulatory event such as cardiac arrest, and manifests as new global cerebral deficits.
- Brain death presents after a major event causes irreversible damage to the brain with absent brain and brainstem function.

Clinical diagnosis
History
- For metabolic encephalopathy, a history of a predisposing condition should be sought, such as hepatitis C cirrhosis or diabetic nephropathy.
- A history of an infection or immunodeficiency may predispose to sepsis.
- Sodium disorders may be suggested by the use of diuretics, fluid resuscitation, heart failure, or renal failure.
- Calcium disorders may be suggested by parathyroid hormone dysregulation, such as is seen with renal failure, by the use of certain medications including antineoplastic agents and diuretics, and by malignancy itself, particularly with bone metastases.
- Thiamine deficiency occurs with nutritional deficiency, especially in alcoholics, or with bariatric surgery, and may be precipitated by intravenous glucose administration without concomitant thiamine.
- A history of diabetes, especially without appropriate medical management or compliance, raises the possibility of hypoglycemia or hyperglycemia.
- The use of sedative, psychotropic, and anticholinergic medications is consistent with medication-induced encephalopathy.
- Diagnosis of hypoxic-ischemic encephalopathy may be supported by a history of cardiac disease or prior arrhythmia with evidence of an acute coronary event, trauma with blood loss, or hypovolemia and hypotension.
- Brain death requires a history of an irreversible insult to the brain; an unknown cause of coma and lack of brainstem reflexes is not sufficient since the cause may be reversible, such as opiate drug overdose.

Physical examination
Encephalopathy involves global brain dysfunction, manifesting as impaired arousal, inattention, and confusion. Various classifications exist to quantify or define the degree of impaired arousal, such as the Glasgow Coma Scale (see Chapter 41: Trauma), but because there is no consensus about terminology, these are not a satisfactory substitute for recording a careful examination (Table 36.1).
- It is imperative to describe the individual's response to specific stimuli. For example, instead of stating that an individual is "stuporous," one should state that he opens his eyes and turns toward the examiner upon a loud vocal stimulus, but closes his eyes after 10 seconds in the absence of further stimulation. Inattention can be tested by tasks requiring continuous focus on a challenging mental or physical task, such as subtracting 7 serially from 100. The task should be tailored to patient's cognitive level.
- Confusion will be evinced by disorientation, language disturbance, and apraxia.
- The general examination will show other evidence supporting specific metabolic and toxic causes; for example, an individual with hepatic encephalopathy will show stigmata of advanced liver disease such as jaundice, hepatomegaly, and ascites.

Table 36.1 Features of the general and neurologic examination for encephalopathy and brain death.

	Encephalopathy	Brain death
General examination	Specific features may identify cause, for example: • hepatic encephalopathy: jaundice, hepatomegaly, ascites • uremic encephalopathy: generalized edema	Specific features may identify cause of brain injury, such as: • trauma • cardiac disease: e.g. pitting edema, elevated jugular pressures, extra heart sounds, cardiomegaly
Neurologic examination	Impaired arousal, inattention, and confusion Severity may vary based on cause and may fluctuate	Absence of cerebral function Absence of brainstem function Absent respiratory drive (apnea test)

- Brain death is diagnosed according to locally established criteria that share certain core features. In general, prerequisites include: a known irreversible cause and the absence of hypothermia, recent sedative administration, and metabolic derangements. The examination must verify the absence of cerebral and brainstem function including respiratory drive, which is evaluated by an apnea test.

Laboratory diagnosis
List of diagnostic tests
Laboratory tests are essential to diagnose the etiology of metabolic encephalopathy.
- A comprehensive metabolic panel and liver function tests would identify the most common derangements, but other specific testing is required if suspected, for example toxicology screen or ammonia. In the case of glucose disorders, a fingerstick glucose test should be used to exclude hypoglycemia, which would cause ongoing brain damage if not corrected immediately.
- For hypoxic-ischemic encephalopathy, an electrocardiogram and tests of cardiac enzymes would identify an acute coronary syndrome as a cause of arrhythmia or cardiogenic shock. For blood loss or hypovolemia, testing should be tailored to the suspected medical cause. Imaging with CT or MRI of the brain would assist in identifying the brain regions affected by the ischemia, which classically would involve the "watershed" areas of the brain.
- Several ancillary studies may be required if brain death is suspected, but the diagnosis can be established by history and physical examination alone. Some countries require particular ancillary studies. These ancillary studies include brain blood flow studies, including radionuclide studies, transcranial Dopplers, perfusion MRI and CT, and cerebral angiography, which are not affected by confounders such as sedatives but depend upon adequate systemic blood pressure. After ensuring adequate systemic blood pressure and excluding conditions that lower intracranial pressure (e.g. trauma, brain surgery, ventricular drain, open cranial sutures), the absence of cerebral blood flow is consistent with brain death. Other ancillary studies include electroencephalography and evoked potentials.

Potential pitfalls/common errors made regarding diagnosis of disease
- Brain death can be mimicked by several reversible conditions.
- Guidelines attempt to safeguard against misdiagnosis by establishing strict criteria for brain death, including the absence of medical confounders such as hypotension (shock), severe metabolic disturbance, sedative drug use, or hypothermia.

Section 4: Treatment
Treatment rationale

- The treatment of metabolic encephalopathy is tailored to the specific etiology, with the goal of correcting the metabolic disturbance and thereby the encephalopathy, which may improve after a delay of several hours to days after the correction of the metabolic abnormality.
- With hepatic failure, prevention of hepatic encephalopathy is central to the care of those with known liver failure and cirrhosis, through maintenance of nutrition and renal function, and by reducing ammonia production and absorption in the colon. The dosage of lactulose and other cathartics is titrated to 2–3 bowel movements per day, and enteral rifaximin may be used to suppress bacteria in the colon that produce urea and other nitrogenous waste compounds. Protein restriction and adequate vitamin supplementation is important in general. End-stage liver failure can be reversed with a liver transplant.
- In encephalopathy due to renal failure, therapy is directed at addressing the renal defect and should be tailored to the chronicity of the dysfunction and clinical characteristics of the patient. Options include continuous veno-venous hemofiltration, peritoneal dialysis, hemodialysis, and renal transplant.
- In hyponatremia, symptoms and complications are more severe with more rapid reduction in sodium levels; however, correction of sodium should not exceed 8 mEq/L in a 24-hour period in order to avoid central pontine myelinolysis. Correction should be tailored to the cause of hyponatremia and may range from discontinuing a diuretic, to water restriction in heart failure, to hypertonic saline infusion in critical care settings.
- Hypocalcemia is corrected with either oral or intravenous calcium supplementation, and correction of hypercalcemia may include intravenous fluids and furosemide if severe.
- Hypoglycemia requires emergent intravenous administration of glucose bolus followed by a continuous infusion in most cases, and hyperglycemia mandates a combination of continuous insulin administration, fluids, and repletion of potassium with monitoring of glucose and electrolytes.
- Treatment of hypoxic-ischemic encephalopathy due to cardiac arrest may include, in addition to cardiovascular support and management, induced hypothermia with a goal core temperature of 32–34°C for several hours in order to reduce neurologic injury. Patients are potential candidates for therapeutic hypothermia if they are not following commands or showing purposeful movements. Although the optimal timing and degree of hypothermia are not established, guidelines generally recommend a core temperature of between 32 and 34°C to be achieved within 6 hours and maintained for 12–24 hours. Institutional protocols specify the means of achieving hypothermia and controlling shivering and other possible complications, such as coagulopathy and arrhythmia.

Prevention and management of complications

- Severe hepatic encephalopathy may cause cerebral edema, which requires intracranial pressure monitoring and medical management of edema with mannitol or hypertonic saline.
- Hyponatremia, if corrected too quickly, may cause osmotic myelinolysis that typically involves the central pons.

CLINICAL PEARLS

- A metabolic encephalopathy has an identifiable cause, and treatment of the cause is the means of treating the encephalopathy. Improvement of the cognitive symptoms may be delayed after initiation of therapy.
- Neurologic injury after cardiac arrest may be mitigated by induced hypothermia.
- Brain death must be diagnosed according to institutional protocol, since the implications are profound and significant local variations exist in its definition.

Section 5: Special populations
Not applicable for this topic.

Section 6: Prognosis

BOTTOM LINE/CLINICAL PEARLS

- The prognosis of metabolic encephalopathy is good if the metabolic derangement can be corrected before structural brain damage occurs. The time course of optimal correction varies by etiology: for example, immediate correction is required for hypoglycemia, but slow correction over several weeks is appropriate for mild chronic hyponatremia.
- In hypoxic-ischemic encephalopathy, poor prognosis is associated with the presence of certain features: absent pupillary or corneal reflexes at 3 days, absent somatosensory evoked responses bilaterally at 24 to 72 hours, and biomarkers such as elevated serum neuronal-specific enolase. The accuracy of these criteria in those treated with induced hypothermia is unknown and an area of current investigation.

Section 7: Reading list
Key reading sources for this chapter can be found online at www.mountsinaiexpertguides.com

Section 8: Guidelines
National society guidelines

Title	Source	Weblink
Evidence-based guideline update: Determining brain death in adults. Report of the Quality Standards Subcommittee of the American Academy of Neurology	American Academy of Neurology (AAN), 2010 Reviews updated evidence for diagnosis of brain death	http://www.guideline.gov/content.aspx?id=23852
Practice Parameter: Prediction of outcome in comatose survivors after cardiopulmonary resuscitation (an evidence-based review)	AAN, 2006 Reviews the evidence for predicting neurologic outcome after cardiopulmonary resuscitation	http://www.neurology.org/content/67/2/203

Local Mount Sinai policy

Title	Source	Weblink
GPP-310 Definition of Brain Death	Mount Sinai Hospital, revised December 2012	http://icahn.mssm.edu/

Additional material for this chapter can be found online at:
www.mountsinaiexpertguides.com

This includes advice for patients, a case study, multiple choice questions, and a reading list.

CHAPTER 37

Pain Disorders

Charles B. Stacy
Icahn School of Medicine at Mount Sinai, New York, NY, USA

> **OVERALL BOTTOM LINE**
> - Pain disorders constitute the most frequent medical and neurologic presentations.
> - Addressing pain issues should be a goal of all physicians, who must develop the appropriate skill sets.
> - Always empathetically, supportively, and non-judgmentally listen to the patient's complaints of pain. Avoid negative reactions to embellishment – this is part of pain syndromes.
> - Proper management depends on determining the relationship between how the patients describe their pain to what they experience and the underlying cause.
> - Understanding the role of the nervous system in pain enables effective treatment.
> - Pain is not only a major indicator of disease, but also its most troublesome symptom.
> - The diagnosis and effective treatment of neuropathic pain disorders are complex and the neurologist is typically the practitioner best able to care for these patients.
> - For information on headache, which will not be addressed in this chapter, please refer to Chapter 8 (Headache) and Chapter 38 (Migraine and Other Headache Disorders).

Section 1: Background
Definition of disease

- Pain is "an unpleasant sensory and emotional experience associated with actual or potential tissue damage, or described in terms of such damage" (International Association for the Study of Pain, IASP).
- At the present time there is no objective substitute for the patient's assertion of pain and estimate of its magnitude, though recent studies with functional MRI suggest objective measures can be found.
- Pain is not simply the sensation, but its impact on attention, aversion, and function.
- The patient's experience of pain may contain emotional components of varying degrees. It is up to the clinician to intuit to what extent the patient's complaint reflects the direct experience of a physiologic nociceptive event.
- Acute pain is associated with an immediate stimulus, while in chronic pain the connection is less direct.

Mount Sinai Expert Guides: Neurology, First Edition. Edited by Stuart C. Sealfon, Rajeev Motiwala, and Charles B. Stacy.
© 2016 John Wiley & Sons, Ltd. Published 2016 by John Wiley & Sons, Ltd.
Companion website: www.mountsinaiexpertguides.com

Disease classification
- Pain occurs in diseases of all categories.
- Pain may be due to a primary pain disorder or secondary to other disease processes.

Incidence/prevalence
- Pain is the single most common complaint that brings patients to the doctor.
- The values for incidence and prevalence differ widely among pain disorders, but also depend on methods of ascertainment.
- For most disorders there is a distinct age effect, and women outnumber men.
- In the case of low back pain, for example, lifetime prevalence is estimated between 58 and 84%, while the 1-year prevalence is between 18 and 50%, peaking around age 60. There is a significant effect of the workplace, partly attributable to mechanical factors, and partly to job dissatisfaction.

Economic impact
- According to surveys, the burden of chronic pain is greater than that of diabetes, heart disease, and cancer combined, affecting over 70 million Americans.
- The cost in 1998 was estimated at US$100 billion annually related to medical management and lost productivity, and in 2008 US$86 billion was attributed to low back pain alone.

Etiology
- Pain disorders include all categories of disease etiology.
- The mechanisms of pain can be broadly divided into nociceptive and neuropathic, depending whether the pain systems are responding to a noxious stimulus or whether dysfunction of the nociceptive apparatus itself gives rise to pain.

Pathology/pathogenesis
- Pain is the conscious experience accompanying activation of nociceptive circuits whose role is to signal tissue damage.
- Pain depends ultimately on the pattern of activation in the nervous system, whether from nociceptors reacting to tissue damage or from aberrant signals in defective nerves.

Section 2: Prevention and screening

BOTTOM LINE/CLINICAL PEARLS
- Prevention of acute pain is applicable to the surgical setting and to illness in which episodic pain is anticipated (migraine, shingles, gout, etc.).
- Preoperative instruction, intraoperative analgesia, and postoperative patient controlled analgesia (PCA) are several keys to pain prevention in the surgical setting.
- When the patient has a condition in which pain is expected, providing the patient with the autonomous pain control methods (such as PCA or medications) and encouraging their use early in the development of pain are much more effective than having the patient experience increasing pain that requires outside help.
- The prevention of chronic pain is very difficult to study. In particular instances (e.g. phantom limb pains) there is strong evidence that pre-emptive analgesia reduces the occurrence. In some models, repeated and uncontrolled exposure to acute pain predisposes to chronic pain.

Screening

A familial predisposition exists for the development of chronic pain. Besides a genetic role in many painful diseases (e.g. migraine, osteoarthritis, complex regional pain syndrome (CRPS)), risk factors can be identified in the personal histories of pain sufferers. Particularly problematic are a history of past substance abuse, especially opioids; sexual or physical abuse; depression; multiple surgical procedures; and previous pain disorders.

Primary prevention

* Preparation in the form of accurate information about what types of pain the patient may expect and management techniques reduces the impact of pain.
* Prompt and adequate treatment of acute pain often reduces overall requests for analgesics.
* Patients' confidence in their ability to control pain eliminates panic and overreaction.
* Coping strategies can be taught in advance.

Secondary prevention

* A detailed pain history illuminates present pain problems.
* Knowing the patient's analgesic tolerance as well as limiting side effects allows targeted efforts.

Section 3: Diagnosis

> **BOTTOM LINE/CLINICAL PEARLS**
> * History: delineate features – location, radiation, intensity, time course, sensory descriptors, exacerbating and relieving factors, impact on function.
> * Examination: tenderness, sensitivity to palpation, manipulation, or stimulation; reproduction of pain; accompanying signs of nerve dysfunction such as sensory disturbance, motor or reflex impairment, autonomic activation.
> * Investigations: imaging to define local pathology, electrical studies to define peripheral nerve involvement, and therapeutic trials to define response.

Differential diagnosis: the various types of deep somatic, visceral, neuropathic, and oncologic pains and their differences in presentation

Pain disorder	Presentation	Findings
Traumatic	Immediate or delayed a few days, even longer; mechanical, but possibly multifocal	Evident injury; clear relationship of pathology to pain
Postoperative	As operative anesthesia wears off; may be complicated by confusion	Monitor by rise in BP, HR, and RR; evolves rapidly
Spinal	Immobility, spasm, with or without radiation	Intense and reflexive guarding of spinal motion; palpable spasm
Visceral	Nauseating; poorly localized; marked autonomic features; wavelike in case of GI or GU, respiratory link if chest, crushing if cardiac	Guarding of area; altered organ function
Arthritic	Mono- or polycentric, highly mechanical, deep	Swelling, spasm, pain on manipulation

(Continued)

Pain disorder	Presentation	Findings
Soft tissue	Aches and fatigue; referred pain Consider: if localized, myofascial pain syndrome; if generalized, fibromyalgia syndrome, myositis, inflammatory conditions	Tenderness to palpation, sometimes very specific sites
Orofacial	Hard to localize source as may be referred; many pain-sensitive structures – dental, jaw, sinus, intracranial, ocular, auricular, trigeminal, glossopharyngeal	Tenderness or sensitivity may be highly specific
Cancer-related	Incremental, seldom abates; multiple mechanisms – bone, viscera, nerve infiltration	Known disease; often visible on radiologic studies, infiltration of nerves or meninges may be difficult to detect
Neuropathic	Focal or centrifugal, along nerve pathways, shock-like, jabbing, burning, dysesthetic	Deficits in sensory, motor, reflex, or sympathetic function; induced dysesthesias
Radiculopathic	Combined neuropathic and spinal mechanical symptoms; radiating pain may be dermatomal, myotomal, or sclerotomal	Combined spinal mechanical, nerve stretch, and neuropathic signs
Myelopathic	Band-like, hyperpathic, with mechanical features, as most are from epidural disease	Evolving signs of motor, sensory, and reflex dysfunction, plus mechanical at site
Central	Regional (hemi-corporeal) bizarre and deeply affective pain; may begin instantly or months after cerebral event	Accompanied by evidence of sensory deficit, though not necessarily profound, and radiologic evidence of lesion
Sympathetically mediated	Pain following injury that escalates and becomes hypersensitive; in a region, not necessarily following peripheral nerve boundaries	Hypersensitivity to all stimuli in the region; signs of autonomic dysfunction, both excessive and variable; eventual irreversible tissue changes

Typical presentation

- Pain that is expected and self-limited (minor trauma, dental, etc.) tends not to elicit anxiety or referral to the specialist.
- Pain with high intensity or prolonged duration demands immediate help either because it interferes with mechanical function (e.g. walking) or becomes unbearable.
- Pain from which there is no respite is the most threatening, and even the lowest level pains grow unendurable with persistence.
- Pain evokes fear and imagination, as well as desperation, which is communicated to the clinician with the greatest urgency.
- Acute pain is often accompanied by autonomic signs of bodily stress, the reactions to injury or immune invasion, and the behavioral patterns of defense or preservation. These features, which predominate in the presentation of acute pain, are distorted or absent in patients with chronic pain.
- In chronic pain, the relationship between adequate stimulus and response is complicated and may appear disproportionate. The cues that we instinctively employ to judge the veracity of suffering may not serve us as well.

Clinical diagnosis

History

The history should elucidate the context in which the pain appeared, its impact on function, associated medical conditions, and responses to treatment. It is important to develop a sense of what the pain means to the patient.

Specific areas of detailed questioning are:

- Pain descriptors – see above.
- Previous pain experiences.
- Pain intensity, expressed by rating scales – numerical, visual analog, faces.
- Pain dimensions – sensory, affective/motivational, cognitive.
- Pain impact on ADL, relationships, finances.

Physical examination

The examination should cover the following aspects:

- Pain behavior – interpersonal communication.
- Observe function, both implicit and explicit.
- Hypersensitivity – allodynia, tenderness, reactivity.
- Mechanical signs.
- Autonomic features.
- Evidence of neurologic deficit – not just sensory but motor and reflexive alterations.

Disease severity classification

- There is no "pain-meter" – at least not yet!
- The quantification of pain is a necessary step in its clinical study and treatment, and can work within a context.
- Intra-observer consistency is best with acute or short-term comparisons, such as analgesic dosing trials.
- Pain intensity rating scales:
  - Numerical (0–10)
  - Verbal (no pain–worst possible)
  - Visual analog (horizontal line), faces: advantage: quick and simple to use; disadvantage: views only one dimension of pain.
- Pain questionnaires – able to capture multidimensionality of pain, but cumbersome:
  - McGill Pain Questionnaire
  - Descriptor differential scale

Laboratory diagnosis

List of diagnostic tests

- Blood tests – inflammatory markers, CPK, rheumatologic, glycohemoglobin.
- CSF – pleocytosis, substance P, protein, immune synthesis.
- CT or MRI – spine, bone, viscera, plexus.
- Nuclear bone scan.
- EMG/NCS.
- fMRI or brain PET – currently research only.

Potential pitfalls/common errors made regarding diagnosis of disease

- Pain must be considered as "real" even in the absence of an objective standard "pain meter."
- Chronic pain often lacks indicators of acute reaction.
- Pain may be denied as well as exaggerated, as a social communication and personal belief.
- Placebo response is not an indicator of pain fabrication. It is normal though variable.
- Analgesic tolerance is not a sign of addiction.
- A very small percentage of patients with access to opioids will develop issues of abuse.
- The most common error in treatment of pain is undertreatment.

Section 4: Treatment

Treatment rationale

- Ask about pain.
- Look for specific treatments for the underlying condition.
- Utilize medications according to the "analgesic ladder" (see below).
- Titrate to effect.
- Reassess regularly.
- Adjust for tolerance.
- Anticipate and treat side effects.
- Employ multiple modalities.

The analgesic ladder begins with NSAIDs, then adds low-potency opioids, then higher potency, then titrate dose and frequency. Adjuvants such as tricyclic antidepressants (TCA) or anticonvulsants should be considered at all rungs.

When to hospitalize

- Uncontrollable pain – unable to manage with present options due to reduced efficacy, limited routes of administration, or serious side effects.
- When escalating pain indicates dangerous disease progression.

Managing the hospitalized patient

- Assess pain at onset and on a frequent basis – the fifth vital sign.
- Begin regular medication dosing, depending on previous analgesic exposure and estimation of severity and feasible route of administration.
- Decide on standing or p.r.n. regimen, based on nursing response times and pattern of use.
- Consider PCA for appropriate candidates.
- Treat underlying condition.
- Access to all modalities – may involve consultation from Acute Pain team.
- Monitor and treat side effects – confusion, respiratory depression, constipation.

Table of treatment

Conservative treatment	
• Rest • Physical therapies • OTC analgesics	Minor trauma, musculoskeletal disorders, self-limited mild pain of any type; also to maintain function in any chronic disorder

Medical – analgesic ladder	Significant post-traumatic or postoperative
• NSAIDs • Add weak opioids – codeine, hydrocodone, tramadol • Add stronger opioids – morphine, hydromorphone, oxycodone, methadone • Add adjuvants/specifics – TCAs, SNRIs (serotonin norepinephrine reuptake inhibitors), anticonvulsants, steroids, muscle relaxants	pain; cancer pain; use in chronic non-malignant pains must be proportionate
Mildly invasive • Nerve blocks: local anesthetic injections, steroid injections, neurolysis	Mononeuropathies, radiculopathies, spinal mechanical pains, nerve invasion, regional pain disorders, central pains
Surgical • Nerve section, tractotomy, ablation, spinal cord stimulator, DBS	
Radiological • Focused RT	Trigeminal neuralgia, local tumor invasion
Psychological • Includes cognitive, behavioral, etc. therapies	Coping strategies for acute and chronic pain, psychotherapy for support Cognitive therapies for reinterpretation, behavioral therapies to improve performance
Complementary • Acupuncture, massage, chiropractic	Any patient who is inclined to pursue in preference to other therapies
Palliative	End of life

Prevention/management of complications

- Opioids: sedation may be counteracted by stimulants; constipation is best treated before it occurs; confusion must be suspected before it becomes florid; respiratory depression needs monitoring of respiratory rate and trends.
- NSAIDs at sustained doses require renal and GI monitoring; never give with steroids.
- Adjuvant anticonvulsants may add to CNS burden of confusion and falls.
- Opioid abuse/misuse: some patients are prone to utilize opioids in a manner that evokes misgivings in the treating physician. Either they report inadequate effect from doses we feel should work, or they request increments of drug at a rapid rate, or they seem to get "high" while they deny relief. Other patients left to their own initiative report erratic or inappropriate choices in self-dosing. The major portion of these may be corrected by education, while in others poor choices expose character flaws or habitual miscommunication in relationship to their support systems, such as family and physician. The last problematic group must be considered abusers. In these cases, explicit criteria for treatment must be worked out in anticipation of the inevitable conflicts between responsible care and the patient's demands.

Management/treatment algorithm

Pain disorder	Treatment
Traumatic	Depends on correct analysis of injuries; NSAIDs depend on bleeding; opioids IV with monitoring of vitals
Postoperative	PCA is gold standard, but be careful in neurologic patients; local and topical may be synergistic; frequent reassessment

Pain disorder	Treatment
Spinal	Initial immobilization, then mobilize; muscle relaxants and opioids (gabapentin is popular for presumed neuropathic component, but may be relaxant); epidural steroid injection
Visceral	Opioids are most effective, and reduce smooth muscle activity, which may not always be favorable
Arthritic	Anti-inflammatories are the core; specific therapies may be the effective solution
Soft tissue	If inflammatory, treat for such; if repetitive strain, alter mechanics; chronic non-inflammatory soft tissue pain is often refractory but pregabalin and several SNRIs have demonstrated benefit
Orofacial	Find specific mechanism; temporomandibular dysfunction may respond to prosthetics and medications that relax the muscles of mastication; neuralgias require anticonvulsants such as oxcarbazepine
Cancer	This demands a multifaceted approach, but there is little room for concerns about long-term consequences; opioids may need repeated escalation
Neuropathic	Less responsive to opioids; variably responsive to anticonvulsants such as gabapentin or pregabalin and antidepressants such as TCAs or SNRIs; consider nerve blocks or topical anesthetic or capsaicin
Radiculopathic	Combined spinal and neuropathic approaches; reducing sensitization of the nervi nervorum in the root may be a mechanism of epidural steroid injections (ESI)
Myelopathic	If compressive, the treatment is to relieve pressure; if inflammatory, try a neuropathic regimen
Central	There is no treatment with more than modest rates of success; again try neuropathic meds
Sympathetically mediated	Blocks of the sympathetic nerves to the affected region should be done as soon as the syndrome is recognized; neuropathic meds should be added. There is urgency to treat before irreversible changes occur

Section 5: Special populations

Pregnancy

- Opioid use early in pregnancy is associated with heart defects and spina bifida, but short-term use later in pregnancy appears safe (class B: specifically morphine, oxycodone, hydromorphone, fentanyl, and methadone).
- However, the newborn may suffer opioid abstinence.
- Breastfeeding mothers should avoid opioids, as ultra-rapid CYP2D6 metabolizers pass active metabolites of codeine, oxycodone, and hydrocodone.
- Aspirin is associated with fetal or newborn hemorrhage.
- NSAIDs may cause patent ductus arteriosus from third trimester exposure (class D).
- Acetaminophen is the analgesic of choice in pregnancy, and this plus ibuprofen are acceptable in breastfeeding.

Children

- Children in pain may not feel it is their right to complain, so always ask and offer.
- There is ample evidence to support the use of the analgesic ladder in children, with dose adjustments by weight, but fewer studies exist on the use of adjuvants.
- Young children can estimate pain severity using the Faces scale.

Elderly

- Pain is often undertreated in the elderly, either because of fear of medication side effects or the reduced physiologic expression of acute distress.
- Chronic pain declines somewhat in prevalence after mid-life, but the intensity does not.
- Multimodality treatment, including physical and psychological therapies, should be encouraged.
- Opioids must be adjusted for reduced metabolism and tolerance of side effects, but remain an essential ingredient for pain of any severity.

Others

- Patients with a known past or present history of substance abuse represent a notorious problem for the treating physician. Given the lack of any truly objective markers for pain, the clinician is always plagued with the suspicion that the patient is merely using this complaint as a ticket for satisfying a pleasurable habit, or acquiring a valuable commodity at the expense of a system guided by professional compassion.
- Perhaps more common is the patient's inappropriate attempts to treat a complex form of life distress as though it were opioid-responsive. In either case the physician–patient relationship is strained by lack of essential agreement as to the means.
- Treatment in the acute setting must be guided by the clinician's instincts, remembering that opioid-tolerant patients may look like drug seekers. In longer term treatment there are many techniques such as contracts and spot checks that support clinicians in their attempts to provide appropriate care.

Section 6: Prognosis

BOTTOM LINE/CLINICAL PEARLS
- Acute pain can generally be managed successfully by recognizing and attending to it.
- Most pain resolves with the subsidence of the acute condition.
- Chronic pain evolves out of the unsuccessful treatment of acute pain.

Natural history of untreated disease

- Painful conditions that persist risk becoming refractory, so that even when the underlying illness is addressed the pain does not abate.
- Experimental models demonstrate long-term neuronal plasticity in the form of altered gene expression and protein phosphorylation, even irreversible cell loss or formation of new synapses.
- Prolonged loss of function induced by pain may become permanent.

Prognosis for treated patients

- Acute pain treatment has a high rate of success overall.
- Chronic pain is refractory to resolution, and the rate of successful management depends on the criteria used.
- Restoration of function is a measurable goal for the clinician, while the elusive dimensions of meaning and autonomy remain central to the patient.

Follow-up tests and monitoring

- Pains tend to recur with their inciting conditions (e.g. low back pain), and there are pain-prone patients for whom pain complicates their unconnected maladies.

- Knowledge of individual pain histories is the best preparation for new instances.
- Chronic pain is a condition like diabetes or hypertension that requires frequent surveillance.

Section 7: Reading list

Key reading sources for this chapter can be found online at www.mountsinaiexpertguides.com

Suggested websites

American Pain Society: americanpainsociety.org

International Association for the Study of Pain: www.iasp-pain.org

National Institute of Neurological Disorders and Stroke Chronic Pain Information Page: www.ninds.nih.gov/disorders/chronic_pain

Section 8: Guidelines
National society guidelines

Title	Source	Weblink
IASP Guidelines	International Association for the Study of Pain (IASP)	http://www.iasp-pain.org/guidelines
Clinical Practice Guidelines	American Pain Society	http://americanpainsociety.org/education/guidelines/overview

Additional material for this chapter can be found online at:
www.mountsinaiexpertguides.com

This includes a case study, multiple choice questions,
and a reading list.

CHAPTER 38

Migraine and Other Headache Disorders

Mark W. Green

Icahn School of Medicine at Mount Sinai, New York, NY, USA

OVERALL BOTTOM LINE
- Ninety-four percent of recurring headaches that present to a primary care practitioner in the office are migraines.
- Tension-type headache is the most common variety of headache. However, it is never disabling and typically responds to simple OTC medications. Most patients who seek care for their headache do not have tension-type headaches.
- "Sinus headache" is overdiagnosed and most who have the diagnosis of "sinus headache" have migraines.
- Migraineurs often have a "spectrum" of headaches, including tension-type headaches and "mixed headaches." Their symptoms respond to migraine treatment and are likely all variations of migraine.

Section 1: Background
Definition of disease
- Migraine is a condition with recurring attacks of headache, lasting 4–72 hours, often pulsatile, moderately severe, unilateral, and worse with activity; not all features have to be present.
- Twenty percent of migraineurs have aura; usually visual or sensory symptoms precede the headache, but they can occur at any point within the migraine attack.

Disease classification
- Migraine without aura
- Migraine with aura
- Acephalgic migraine (migraines without headache).

Incidence/prevalence
- Eighteen percent of women, 6% of males (12% of the general population) experience at least one migraine attack yearly.

Economic impact
In the USA the associated direct medical costs of migraine headache are estimated to total approximately US$1 billion per year, but indirect costs such as loss of workplace productivity are likely to be much higher.

Mount Sinai Expert Guides: Neurology, First Edition. Edited by Stuart C. Sealfon, Rajeev Motiwala, and Charles B. Stacy.
© 2016 John Wiley & Sons, Ltd. Published 2016 by John Wiley & Sons, Ltd.
Companion website: www.mountsinaiexpertguides.com

Etiology

- The cause of migraine is not established.
- Since migraine is a phenotype, it is expected that migraine will have a variety of causes.
- Genetic factors are important but there are environmental triggers.
- Those who experience migraine possess a lower threshold for the development of headaches.
- The triggers of migraine are mundane; and migraineurs experience attacks in situations that would not ordinarily trigger an attack in others, such as stress or relaxation following stress, drops in estrogen levels, small amounts of alcohol, missing meals, and so forth.

Pathology/pathogenesis

The pathogenesis of migraine is uncertain. It might be due to "cortical spreading depression," a wave traversing the cortex at 3 mm/minute, activating trigeminal nociceptors in the cortex and ultimately activating the thalamus and cerebral cortex. Migraine involves meningeal inflammation as well as vasodilatation. This explains why symptoms of migraine are similar to those of meningitis, with pulsatile headaches, photophobia and phonophobia, nausea, and neck pain.

Predictive/risk factors

Disease: risk factor	Odds ratio compared to general population
Migraine with aura: stroke	8.4
Epilepsy: migraine	3.5
Migraine: depression	2.2
Migraine: bipolar	2.9
Migraine: Raynaud's	5.4

Section 2: Prevention and screening

> **BOTTOM LINE/CLINICAL PEARLS**
> - The number, severity, and duration of attacks at baseline predict progression.
> - It remains to be determined whether aggressive management of attacks, including preventive and acute therapy, is disease modifying.

Screening

The diagnosis of migraine is clinical, and usually based upon an individual and family history. Children who are carsick or have recurring vomiting or abdominal pain, particularly if they have a migrainous parent, are likely to develop migraine.

Primary prevention

- No known interventions affect the likelihood of developing migraine.

Secondary prevention

- Attacks can be minimized by reducing triggers including maintaining a regular sleep and meal schedule, a modest amount of caffeine ingested at the same time daily to reduce the likelihood of developing caffeine withdrawal headache, avoiding dehydration and excessive overheating, and the management of stress. Many other triggers cannot be ordinarily modified such as hormonal changes and weather.

- "Migraine diets" are sometimes useful in reducing attack frequency, but not with sufficient frequency to be routinely recommended.

Section 3: Diagnosis

BOTTOM LINE/CLINICAL PEARLS
- Although tension-type headache is more common, it is mild and easily self-treated.
- Therefore migraine is by far the most common headache seen in those who seek medical care for recurring disabling head pain.

Box 38.1 gives the criteria of the International Headache Society for the diagnosis of migraine. In practice, migraineurs may experience a variety of different types of headache attacks, which, for therapeutic purposes, should be considered variations along the spectrum of migraine.

BOX 38.1 INTERNATIONAL HEADACHE SOCIETY CRITERIA FOR THE DIAGNOSIS OF MIGRAINE

Migraine without aura: 80% of attacks (must satisfy all criteria)
- A. At least five attacks
- B. Headache attacks lasting 4–72 hours
- C. Headache with at least two of the following:
  - Unilateral location
  - Pulsating quality
  - Moderate to severe pain
  - Aggravation by or causing avoidance of physical activity
- D. During headache at least one of the following:
  - Nausea and/or vomiting
  - Photophobia and phonophobia
- E. Not attributed to another disorder

Migraine with aura (20% of attacks):
- At least two attacks fulfilling criteria B–D above
- Aura consists of one of the following; no motor weakness:
  - Fully reversible visual symptoms including positive and or negative features.
  - Fully reversible sensory symptoms including positive and or negative features.
  - Fully reversible dysphasic speech disturbance.
- At least two of the following:
  - Homonymous visual symptoms and/or unilateral sensory symptoms.
  - At least one aura symptom develops gradually over 5 minutes and/or different symptoms occur in succession over >5 minutes.
  - Headache fulfills criteria for migraine without aura.
  - Not attributed to another disease.

Hemiplegic migraine is considered to be a separate entity, according to current classification, rather than a subtype of migraine with aura.

Differential diagnosis

Differential diagnosis	Features
Tension-type headaches	Never severe or disabling, no significant photophobia, phonophobia, or nausea. Rarely present to physician as a significant complaint unless frequent. Most common headache type
"Sinus headache"	Not recognized as a diagnosis by the International Headache Society. No evidence that chronic sinusitis causes headache (some exceptions), and acute sinusitis is associated with purulent drainage, fever, and significant pathologic changes on sinus studies
Cluster headache	More common in males. Clusters of attacks vary in length, most commonly 4–6 weeks. During this time, one or more attacks/day lasting 30–120 minutes. Pain unilateral, often retro-orbital and temporal. Boring and knife-like in quality. Associated with ipsilateral lacrimation and rhinorrhea. Very severe. Sufferers rock and pace, as opposed to migraineurs, who prefer to remain still. In contrast with migraine, cluster headaches typically wake the patient

Typical presentation

Migraines usually present with recurring headaches, with or without auras. Attacks can be disabling but often migraineurs have a spectrum of attacks that mimic tension-type headaches and headaches with symptoms suggesting sinus disease. These are all considered to be variations in migraines rather than separate syndromes.

Clinical diagnosis

History
- Are these recurring? Attacks are typically recurrent, and five or more attacks are needed in order to make the diagnosis. The frequency of attacks is highly variable.
- How long do they last? In adults, attacks typically last 4–72 hours.
- What triggers attacks? Most attacks are spontaneous, but some may be triggered by stress, relaxation following stress, missing meals and a variety of foods and drinks, including alcohol. Oversleeping or undersleeping are common triggers. Estrogen withdrawal, often in association with ovulation and menstruation, can be a powerful trigger.
- If these triggers frequently bring on headache attacks, the diagnosis is highly likely to be migraine.
- How disabling are the attacks? Many migraines are disabling, and worsening with activity is the feature with the highest sensitivity. They are commonly associated with phonophobia and photophobia.

Physical examination
- Examination is typically normal although tenderness over the occipital grooves, supraorbital notches, and superficial temporal arteries can be found.

Useful clinical decision rules
- Migraine auras last less than 60 minutes. TIAs and strokes often cause headaches. It is important to distinguish these conditions when there is a focal neurologic complaint and concomitant head pain.

Disease severity classification

In clinical trials, headaches are rated 0–3:

0 no headache

1 mild; does not interfere with activity

2 moderate; impairs activity but does not require bedrest

3 requires bedrest

The 0–10 scale is not recommended as patients generally fail to understand the scale and may overrate their attacks. The 0–3 scale is more reflective of the disability suffered.

Laboratory diagnosis

List of diagnostic tests

- There are no blood tests for migraine.
- MRI scans commonly show small white matter lesions, but their significance is unknown and these reports may alarm patients.
- Electroencephalograms are not routinely recommended. While sometimes abnormal, they do not provide useful information other than rare cases where the headache is associated with epilepsy ("migralepsy").
- Imaging is appropriate:
  - When there is a significant change in the character and frequency of attacks, since those with migraine who develop a secondary headache often manifest this as a change in a pre-existing headache type.
  - If the neurologic examination is abnormal.
  - If the onset is apoplectic reaching full intensity instantly.

Potential pitfalls/common errors made regarding diagnosis of disease

- As migraineurs often experience a "spectrum of headaches," many attacks are often misdiagnosed as "sinus" or "tension" headaches, particularly in situations where stress and weather changes are triggers.
- Chronic sinusitis is not typically associated with headache.
- The triggers do not define separate subtypes. An attack triggered by stress, another triggered by alcohol, and a third by estrogen changes are not separate diagnoses.

Section 4: Treatment

Treatment rationale

Acute therapies are used to abort individual attacks. The most effective self-administered acute treatments are triptans and dihydroergotamine. Attacks may vary in their severity, and it is preferable not to over-treat each attack with these "migraine-specific" medications. However, if treatment is delayed, these agents will be less effective than if administered early in the attack. Therefore it is important to evaluate the natural history of each patient's attacks:

- Are all attacks severe? If not, can the patient distinguish early in the attacks which are likely to become disabling? If they can, treating these attacks with the "migraine-specific" agents, and others with less expensive medications, like NSAIDs, is appropriate. The frequency of attacks that are treated acutely is also a factor.
- The presence of nausea and vomiting is also considered. If early in the attack, nausea will impede absorption of oral medications, therefore non-oral routes of administration are appropriate.

- If a patient is experiencing more than six attacks monthly, preventive agents should be considered. The intent is to reduce the number of attacks (typically by 50%) and make the others more easily treated. These agents take several weeks at an adequate dose to become effective.

When to hospitalize
- Status migrainosus.
- Hypotension or severe dehydration, especially in pregnancy.
- Medication overuse headache, if not controllable as an outpatient.
  - Withdrawal of acute agents might be unsafe or not tolerated (commonly occurring with butalbital or opioid overuse).

Managing the hospitalized patient
- Intractable attack:
  - Intravenous dihydroergotamine, pretreating with intravenous antiemetics.
- Corticosteroids.
- NSAIDS, diphenhydramine can be useful.
- Parenteral hydration if severe vomiting and anorexia are present.
- Detoxify from overused acute drug, if relevant.

Treatment approach by headache type
Cluster headache
- Acute therapy:
  - sumatriptan subcutaneously 2–6 mg;
  - oxygen 10 L/min using a non-rebreathing mask.
- Bridge therapy (before preventive agents become effective):
  - prednisone;
  - occipital and supraorbital nerve blocks.
- Preventive therapy:
  - verapamil 80–720 mg (below may be added to verapamil);
  - topiramate;
  - divalproex;
  - lithium carbonate;
  - gabapentin;
  - melatonin 9 mg at night.

Migraine
- Acute therapy:
  - NSAIDs may be tried first.
  - If ineffective, triptans or dihydroergotamine.
  - NSAIDs can be added to triptans or dihydroergotamine.

  If six or more attacks/month, or if acute medications ineffective, preventive therapy is indicated.

Tension-type headaches
- Since, by definition, these are mild and easily self-treated, OTC agents are first line. If disabling, consider alternative diagnosis. Disabling "tension" headaches are usually part of the spectrum of migraines.
- If more than 2–3 times weekly, preventive agents, mirtazapine, or amitriptyline should be started as preventive therapy.
- Avoid narcotics and muscle relaxants. OnabotulinumtoxinA is not effective in the treatment of tension-type headaches.

Specific treatments

Behavioral treatments with documented efficacy in clinical trials • Relaxation training • Thermal biofeedback training • Electromyographic biofeedback therapy • Cognitive/behavioral therapy (CBT)	
Drugs for acute migraine	
Group 1 Fast-onset, short half-life triptans: • Almotriptan • Eletriptan • Rizatriptan • Sumatriptan • Zolmitriptan	6.25 mg and 12.5 mg tablets 20 mg and 40 mg tablets 5 mg and 10 mg tablets 5 mg and 10 mg orally dissolving wafers. These preparations are not sublingual and are not faster acting, nor do they improve efficacy when nausea and vomiting are present 25 mg, 50 mg, and 100 mg tablets 5 mg and 20 mg intranasal Single dose vial, 6 mg/0.5 mL for subcutaneous injection, 4 or 6 mg is usually administered 4 mg and 6 mg cartridges for autoinjector 6 mg needle-free single-use devices for subcutaneous injection Fixed-dose combination tablet of 85 mg sumatriptan with 500 mg naproxen sodium 2.5 mg and 5 mg tablets 2.5 mg and 5 mg orally dissolving wafers 5 mg intranasal
Group 2 Slower-onset, long half-life triptans • Frovatriptan • Naratriptan	 2.5 mg tablet 1 mg and 2.5 mg tablets
Other drugs • Dihydroergotamine • Non-steroidal anti-inflammatory drugs (NSAIDs)	 1 mg, s.c., i.m., i.v., intranasal Ibuprofen Ketorolac (i.v., p.o., intranasal) Diclofenac (tablets, powder)

Prevention/management of complications
- Acute agents should be administered early in an attack.
- Awakenings with migraine are difficult to manage but most likely to respond to injectable sumatriptan.
- If nauseated at the time of treatment, consider non-oral preparations, such as triptans or dihydroergotamine nasal sprays or injections.
- Vasoactive medications such as ergots and triptans are contraindicated in those with cardiovascular and cerebrovascular disease.
- Preventive agents are to be strongly considered if attacks occur at a frequency of six attacks per month or greater.
- Preventive agents may be used when the frequency of attacks is less if the episodes are disabling despite aggressive acute therapies.

Evidence-based prevention guidelines

Level A: Established efficacy (at least two class 1 trials)

- Divalproex sodium
- Topiramate
- Propranolol
- Metoprolol
- Timolol
- *Petasites* (butterbur)
- Frovatriptan (menstrually related migraine)

Level B: Probably effective (one class 1 or two class 2 studies)

- Beta-adrenergic blockers:
  - Atenolol
  - Nadolol
- Antidepressants:
  - Venlafaxine
- Amitriptyline
- Triptans for menstrually related migraine (used preventively in this setting):
  - Naratriptan
  - Zolmitriptan
- Herbals or natural:
  - Feverfew, riboflavin, magnesium

Level C: Possibly effective (one class 2 study)

- ACE inhibitors:
  - Lisinopril
- Angiotensin receptor blocker (ARB):
  - Candesartan
- Alpha-agonists:
  - Clonidine
  - Guanfacine
- AEDs:
  - Carbamazepine
- Beta-blockers:
  - Nebivolol
  - Pindolol
- Antihistamines:
  - Cyproheptadine
- Herbals
- CoQ10

Note: Botox (onabotulinumtoxinA) is FDA approved for migraine with 15 or more attacks/month and failure of conventional therapy, but as of January 2014 it had not yet received American Academy of Neurology evidence-based guideline assignment.

- Most preventive agents, with the exception of topiramate, can induce weight gain.
- Preventive agents should be initiated with a low dose and gradually increased to a therapeutic dose. A positive response is commonly not seen for 6 weeks, and side effects are minimized by slowly raising the dose.
- Medication overuse headache causing transformation of episodic attacks into the chronic form: all acute antimigraine medications can induce this problem, but triptans and NSAIDs are less likely than opioids and butalbital-containing preparations.

- Abrupt or gradual withdrawal of the offending agent. Some agents can be discontinued abruptly, like a triptan. Opioids and barbiturates in particular must be slowly tapered off.
- Education to avoid medication overuse headache in the future.

CLINICAL PEARLS

- Tension-type headaches are the most common type of headache. As they are not disabling, and are also easily treatable with OTC medications, these rarely present to physicians (if they appear to be disabling, question the diagnosis).
- Migraines often occur as part of a spectrum of headaches; with migraines, "mixed headaches," and tension headaches being components of the same disorder.
- Treatment of chronic tension-type headache is exceedingly difficult. Mirtazapine or amitriptyline are the most rational therapies. These headaches do not respond to muscle relaxants or onabotulinumtoxinA.
- Cluster headaches consist of severe recurring attacks. They are not a variant of migraine and treatment is very different.
- Prevention of cluster headaches is with verapamil (80–720 mg) used with topiramate, valproate, or lithium carbonate.
- Bridge therapy is with corticosteroids. Treatment should continue for at least 3 weeks after no attacks have been experienced, and then the agents are slowly reduced.
- Consider the diagnosis of hemicrania continua in all with side-locked, continuous head pain.
- A course of indomethacin (indometacin) is appropriate for all suspects to both treat and support the diagnosis: usually 75–150 mg daily.

Section 5: Special populations
Pregnancy
- Migraine commonly improves during the second and third trimesters of pregnancy.
- The safety of acute and preventive agents in pregnancy is unknown.
- Non-medication methods are first tried in pregnancy (biofeedback, occipital nerve blocks, aggressive trigger management); caffeine and acetaminophen used occasionally appear safe if not overused.

Children
- Children with migraine can present with recurring abdominal pain and attacks of vomiting.
- Migraine attacks in childhood have a more rapid onset compared to adults, but a shorter duration.
- Sleep commonly terminates attacks in children, and should be encouraged.
- Three triptans, rizatriptan, almotriptan, and Treximet® are FDA approved for use in children.
- Amitriptyline, topiramate, and propranolol are the most commonly employed preventive agents in the pediatric population.

Elderly
- Migraine commonly recedes in the elderly.
- The use of vasoconstricting agents (particularly ergots and triptans) in the elderly requires an evaluation to exclude significant vascular disease.
- NSAIDs are more likely to cause serious GI and renal toxicity in the elderly.
- Elderly patients commonly reject agents that can cause tremor, like divalproex.

Others

- Those with comorbid hypertension and migraine might benefit from the use of an appropriate beta-blocker or possibly verapamil, lisinopril, or candesartan.
- Those with comorbid depression might do best with venlafaxine or a tricyclic antidepressant. SSRIs and bupropion commonly increase migraines. Beta-blockers can increase depression in these individuals.
- Those with comorbid bipolar disease, if using an antidepressant that also improves migraine, need to be closely followed to assure it is not triggering mania. Divalproex can be used in the management of both migraine and bipolar disease.
- Those with comorbid migraine and insomnia might benefit from the nighttime administration of amitriptyline, although the architecture of their sleep on this agent differs from normal sleep architecture. Trazodone and nefazodone, often used to induce sleep, commonly worsen migraine.

Section 6: Prognosis

> **BOTTOM LINE/CLINICAL PEARLS**
> - Migraine prevalence peaks in the early 40s for both men and women.
> - Cluster headache prognosis is unpredictable; patients may develop prolonged remissions or it can continue into advanced age.
> - Tension-type headaches can persist throughout life, or spontaneously resolve.

Natural history of untreated disease

- Whether aggressive preventive and acute therapy is disease-modifying remains unknown.

Prognosis for treated patients

- Most acute medications can work in 70% of attacks if treatment is commenced early in the attack.
- Preventive agents typically reduce migraine attacks by 50%. Polytherapy and aggressive management of triggers are often necessary to improve this number. Those on preventive therapies often experience attacks, which are more amenable to acute therapies.
- When preventive agents are used successfully for 6–12 months, these agents can often be reduced or discontinued.

Follow-up tests and monitoring

- Monitor, via diaries, the number, duration, and intensity of attacks, their triggers, and the treatments employed.

Section 7: Reading list

Key reading sources for this chapter can be found online at www.mountsinaiexpertguides.com

Suggested websites

American Academy of Neurology headache guidelines: https://www.aan.com/Guidelines/Home/ByTopic?topicId=16

American Headache Society: http://www.americanheadachesociety.org/
International Headache Society: http://www.ihs-headache.org/
National Headache Foundation: http://www.headaches.org/

Additional material for this chapter can be found online at:
www.mountsinaiexpertguides.com

This includes advice for patients, a case study, multiple choice
questions, and a reading list.

CHAPTER 39

Sleep Disorders

Steven H. Feinsilver
Icahn School of Medicine at Mount Sinai, New York, NY, USA

OVERALL BOTTOM LINE
- Excessive daytime sleepiness is a distinct symptom warranting diagnostic evaluation.
- Assuming an adequate amount of sleep, the complaint of daytime sleepiness is most likely related to medical illness.
- The most common illness to cause daytime sleepiness is sleep-disordered breathing, followed by narcolepsy, which is the most common neurologic disease to cause sleepiness.
- Psychiatric etiologies (especially depression) are less common causes of sleepiness.
- Both obstructive sleep apnea and narcolepsy are underdiagnosed.

Section 1: Background

Definition of disease

Sleep-disordered breathing is defined by the presence of at least 10-second periods of cessation of breathing (apnea) or a reduction in airflow accompanied by an arousal or oxygen desaturation (hypopnea) occurring during sleep. Most sleep-disordered breathing is caused by upper airway obstruction (obstructive sleep apnea, OSA).

Narcolepsy can be viewed as a failure of normal sleep organization leading to symptoms that generally include daytime somnolence and may also include cataplexy, sleep paralysis, and hypnagogic hallucinations.

Disease classification

Obstructive sleep apnea is often classified on the basis of the number of apneas or hypopneas per hour (Apnea Hypopnea Index, AHI), with cutoffs of 5, 15, and 30 indicating mild, moderate, or severe.

Incidence/prevalence

One estimate is that one of every five adults has at least mild OSA, and one in 15 has at least moderate OSA, although not all will have symptoms, and the significance of OSA without symptoms is unclear.

The prevalence of narcolepsy with cataplexy is estimated at 25–50 per 100,000 of the general population; if cataplexy is not required for the diagnosis the prevalence is much higher.

Mount Sinai Expert Guides: Neurology, First Edition. Edited by Stuart C. Sealfon, Rajeev Motiwala, and Charles B. Stacy.
© 2016 John Wiley & Sons, Ltd. Published 2016 by John Wiley & Sons, Ltd.
Companion website: www.mountsinaiexpertguides.com

Economic impact

The economic impact of excessive daytime sleepiness is estimated in the hundreds of billions of dollars in its effect on work performance, absenteeism, and accidents. Perhaps more importantly, treatment of obstructive sleep apnea is highly cost-effective, with an extremely low estimated incremental cost-effectiveness ratio of less than US$4000 per quality-adjusted life year gained.

Etiology

- OSA is caused by a narrowed or excessively collapsible upper airway. The defect can be worsened by obesity or the use of alcohol and other sedatives.
- Narcolepsy with cataplexy is caused by a deficiency of the hypothalamic neuropeptide hypocretin (also known as orexin). The etiology of narcolepsy without cataplexy is less clear.

Pathology/pathogenesis

In sleep-disordered breathing, repetitive respiratory events are terminated by arousals or awakenings. This may lead to sleep fragmentation causing daytime sleepiness and frequent cycles of hypoxia and reoxygenation with cardiovascular consequences.

Narcolepsy with cataplexy is caused by destruction of hypocretin cells in the hypothalamus. Although rarely familial, there is a genetic predisposition with the strong association with HLA-DQB1*0602 suggesting an autoimmune basis.

Predictive/risk factors

Disease: risk factor	Odds ratio
OSA: male gender	2–3
OSA: obesity	6 for 10% increase in weight
OSA: family history	2–4 for first-degree relative with OSA
Narcolepsy: family history	10–40 for first-degree relative (but still low, <2% prevalence)

Section 2: Prevention and screening

> **BOTTOM LINE/CLINICAL PEARLS**
> - OSA may be prevented or improved by weight loss and avoidance of sedating medications, in particular alcohol.
> - No interventions are known to decrease the risk of disease onset or progression for narcolepsy.

Screening

Screening for sleep apnea is inherently problematic, as it is a common disease that generally presents with daytime sleepiness (vague) and snoring (common). The majority of patients with OSA remain undiagnosed. Questionnaires such as "STOP-Bang" (Table 39.1) or the Berlin questionnaire are simple, but have limited specificity or sensitivity. Home sleep studies are most useful in patients with a high pretest probability of disease, and are not suitable for screening low-risk populations.

No screening methods exist for diagnosing narcolepsy, also a frequently underdiagnosed disease for which a good sleep history is critical.

Table 39.1 The STOP-Bang Questionnaire.

Snoring (loud enough to be heard through closed doors?)	Yes = 1
Tired (do you often feel tired or sleepy during daytime?)	Yes = 1
Observed (has anyone observed apnea during your sleep?)	Yes = 1
P (blood pressure requiring treatment?)	Yes = 1
BMI	>35 = 1
Age	>50 = 1
Neck circumference	>40 cm = 1
Gender	Male = 1

Higher score increases the probability of sleep apnea: e.g. a score of 7 or 8 indicates a 60% probability of moderate or severe apnea.
Source: Chung F, Yegneswaran B, Liao P, et al. STOP questionnaire: a tool to screen patients for sleep apnea. Anesthesiology 2008;108:812–21.

Section 3: Diagnosis
See Algorithm 39.1.

> **BOTTOM LINE/CLINICAL PEARLS**
> - A history of daytime sleepiness and snoring should lead to high suspicion for sleep-disordered breathing.
> - A history of sleepiness dating back to adolescence should lead to consideration of narcolepsy even in the absence of ancillary symptoms (however, erratic sleep patterns in adolescence are common and usually not pathological).

Differential diagnosis

Differential diagnosis	Features
Depression	Both hypersomnolence and insomnia may be seen. Psychiatric evaluation, response to medications may be helpful
Insomnia	Most patients with insomnia will not complain of daytime sleepiness despite subjective complaints of inadequate sleep
Chronic fatigue syndrome	May be history of recent viral illness; complaint more of fatigue than difficulty staying awake
Periodic limb movement disorder	Often accompanied by "restless legs" during wakefulness; may disrupt sleep and lead to daytime sleepiness

Typical presentation
The typical OSA patient is an overweight middle-aged male who may complain of difficulty staying awake and may have a bed partner who observes severe snoring or even apnea. The average patient has at least a few years of symptoms before coming to medical attention.

Narcolepsy patients may have a history of somnolence beginning about the time of puberty, perhaps difficulties concentrating in school, although the diagnosis is typically made when patients are in their twenties or later. In addition to sleepiness, ancillary symptoms of *cataplexy* (an abrupt decrease in motor tone without loss of consciousness, typically lasting 30–120 seconds, brought on by strong emotions), *sleep paralysis* (paralysis on falling asleep or awakening, often with hallucinations), and *hallucinations* on falling asleep or awakening (hypnagogic or hypnopompic hallucinations) may be reported.

Clinical diagnosis

History
- A sleep history should include: typical bedtime and rise time, sleep latency (time to fall asleep), number of awakenings, observed snoring or apnea, morning headache, and daytime sleepiness. Observations from a bed partner may be necessary, particularly about snoring or apnea, and any unusual behavior during sleep.
- Inquiry should be made regarding ancillary symptoms of narcolepsy (cataplexy, sleep paralysis, hallucinations).
- Daytime sleepiness is best assessed by asking how likely it is that the patient would become drowsy or fall asleep under specific circumstances (e.g. the Epworth Questionnaire), as distinct from just feeling fatigued.
- Patients need to be asked about presence of respiratory, cardiac, or psychiatric disease and medication use. Social history must include use of alcohol, caffeine, tobacco, and recreational drugs.

Physical examination
Patients complaining of daytime sleepiness should have a standard medical examination with particular attention to the upper airway (including crowding of the oropharynx, position of the mandible, enlargement of tonsils, nasal patency), neurologic examination, mood and affect. See also Chapter 10: Sleep Disorders, Somnolence, and Fatigue.

Laboratory diagnosis

List of diagnostic tests
- *Overnight polysomnography* remains the gold standard for diagnosis of sleep disorders. Patients come to the Sleep Center a few hours before their usual bedtime and spend the sleep period in a quiet, private, controlled environment where EEG, respiration, limb movements, motor tone, EKG, oximetry, and video images are continuously monitored and recorded. Monitoring airflow from nose and mouth as well as chest and abdominal movements allows for the differentiation between obstructive and central respiratory events. Most patients are able to sleep reasonably close to their usual sleep in the home setting, and the Sleep Center polysomnogram allows for a standardized and controlled environment.
- *Unattended polysomnograms* ("home studies") are simpler than full polysomnography, generally involving only respiratory measurements of airflow, oximetry, and chest movement. EEG recording during sleep at home is not generally practical. Thus, sleep itself is generally not measured and the environment is not standardized. Although this can be diagnostic when sleep-disordered breathing is severe, it is less useful in milder cases.
- *Multiple sleep latency testing* (MSLT) is generally done in the daytime following overnight polysomnography. Beginning 2 hours after awakening, the patient is given 20-minute opportunities to nap at 2-hour intervals throughout the day while EEG, motor tone, and

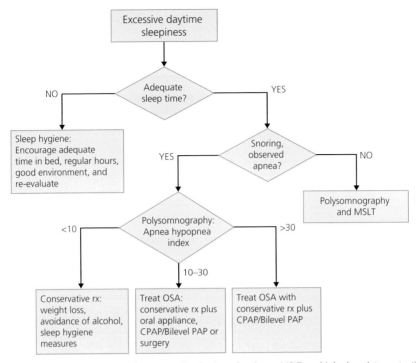

Algorithm 39.1 Diagnostic approach to excessive daytime sleepiness. MSLT, multiple sleep latency testing.

EKG are recorded in a dark room. The time until sleep occurs on each nap is recorded as sleep latency, given as 20 min if no sleep occurred. The average of five naps is the mean sleep latency. Mean latencies of less than 8 min are considered indicative of abnormal daytime sleepiness. Additionally, the presence of REM sleep on naps is not common, and the finding of two or more naps with REM may be consistent with narcolepsy, although this is neither completely sensitive nor specific.

- *Maintenance of wakefulness testing* is less commonly done. In this test, 40-minute periods are spent in darkness with EEG and muscle tone recorded while the patient is instructed to stay awake. Since this tests the ability to stay awake rather than the ability to nap, it might be expected to be a better surrogate for sleepiness than the MSLT, but this remains unproven.

- *CSF hypocretin levels* can be measured and may confirm the diagnosis of narcolepsy with cataplexy. This has good specificity and sensitivity, but because it requires lumbar puncture, it is not typically performed.

Potential pitfalls/common errors made regarding diagnosis of disease

- Somnolence cannot be assessed without an accurate sleep history, which may be difficult to obtain.
- Sleep may vary from night to night, and a single night's polysomnogram may not be representative.

Section 4: Treatment
Treatment rationale
Obstructive sleep apnea
- Nocturnal use of continuous positive airway pressure (CPAP machine) is the most reliably effective treatment for OSA. Pressure is applied to the oropharynx using a nasal or oronasal mask to keep the upper airway patent during sleep. Most patients will find this tolerable, and daytime sleepiness improves within several nights of treatment.
- One alternative includes the use of an oral appliance that is designed to advance the mandible to improve airway patency.
- Another option is surgery such as tonsillectomy, uvulopalatopharyngoplasty (UPPP), resection of the base of the tongue, or deviated nasal septum repair. Although surgery on the upper airway often improves snoring and eliminates the need for nightly interventions, it is less reliably effective for treating apnea. In one review UPPP successfully eliminated OSA less than 50% of the time.
- Tracheotomy is curative, but rarely performed for OSA.
- Surgical advancement of the mandible can be very effective but is more invasive.
- Weight loss is often helpful, and patients should be advised to limit use of alcohol or any sedatives.
- Despite optimal treatment, some patients will remain significantly sleepy and treatment with a wakefulness-promoting agent such as modafinil may be appropriate (see below).

Central sleep apnea
- Central sleep apnea is treated by addressing the underlying cause when possible (e.g. congestive heart failure, obesity), but may also be treated with CPAP or bilevel PAP, a form of non-invasive nocturnal ventilation.

Narcolepsy
Treatment of narcolepsy has been traditionally divided into treatments for excessive daytime somnolence, usually the primary symptom, and treatments for the ancillary symptoms of cataplexy, sleep paralysis, and hallucinations.
- The most common first-line treatment for sleepiness is modafinil, a wakefulness-promoting agent that is thought to be more specific for its action on the anterior hypothalamus than stimulants such as methylphenidate or amphetamines, which may needed for more severe sleepiness.
- Cataplexy is thought to represent the intrusion of REM sleep into wakefulness, with resulting loss of motor tone as normally seen with REM. Originally the most common treatments for cataplexy were antidepressants, particularly fluoxetine and venlafaxine.
- Sodium oxybate was originally used to treat cataplexy, but has also shown efficacy in improving daytime sleepiness. This is a very sedating drug taken at bedtime. It may take a few months to see maximal improvement in sleepiness.

When to hospitalize
In some cases OSA may complicate COPD or CHF with resultant hypoxia or CO_2 retention. Ensuing respiratory failure may require hospitalization.

Table of treatment

Conservative treatment • Sleep hygiene	All patients with sleep disorders should be instructed in sleep hygiene including regular hours, limiting non-sleep activities in bed, and allowing adequate sleep time Patients with OSA are helped by weight reduction and limiting alcohol and other sedatives
Medications • Modafinil	For treatment of sleepiness in narcolepsy or residual sleepiness in OSA on CPAP: 100–600 mg/day
• Armodafinil	Similar to modafinil, longer duration of action, lower dosing: 50–250 mg/day
• Methylphenidate	Less specific stimulant in narcolepsy Rx: 10–60 mg/day
• Dextroamphetamine	Similar to methylphenidate: 5–60 mg/day
• Sodium oxybate	Improves both sleepiness and ancillary symptoms in narcolepsy: 6–9 g/day
Surgery • Uvulopalatoplasty	More successful for snoring than for OSA, consider in mild disease
• Mandibular advancement surgery, tracheotomy	Success rate excellent, but more invasive
Dental appliance • Oral mandibular advancement device	Variably successful, probably best for mild OSA
Psychological • Cognitive behavioral therapy and desensitization techniques	Cognitive behavioral therapy useful for insomnia Desensitization techniques may help CPAP acceptance

Prevention/management of complications

- CPAP treatment for OSA is remarkably safe. Main complaints relate to tolerance and fit of facemask and oral dryness (improved with use of humidification).
- Modafinil is well tolerated except for occasional headaches. Tolerance and withdrawal are not reported.
- Stimulant medications can cause irritability, elevation of blood pressure, and tachyphylaxis. Dosage should be closely monitored.

> **CLINICAL PEARLS**
> - CPAP is almost always successful in treating OSA, and most patients can adapt to this.
> - Results of surgery for OSA remain disappointing.
> - Patients with narcolepsy may need treatment for sleepiness and for ancillary symptoms; sodium oxybate may treat both.

Section 5: Special populations

Pregnancy

- OSA may be treated in pregnancy with CPAP.
- Treatment of narcolepsy in pregnancy is problematic: modafinil, dextroamphetamine, and methylphenidate are all category C in pregnancy; sodium oxybate is category B.

Children

- In children with OSA, upper airway abnormalities such as enlarged tonsils constitute the major etiology, and surgery is more likely to be successful compared to adults. CPAP has been used successfully, even for very young children.
- Children with narcolepsy may be treated with methylphenidate or other stimulants. Treatment with modafinil has been recommended by some experts, but safety has not been established by the FDA in those younger than 16. Sodium oxybate is not recommended in children.

Section 6: Prognosis

> **BOTTOM LINE/CLINICAL PEARLS**
> - Successful treatment of OSA with CPAP leads to sustained improvement in daytime sleepiness and appears to decrease cardiovascular risk.
> - Narcolepsy is a lifelong although not progressive disease and, once controlled by medications, treatment is lifelong for most patients.

Natural history of untreated disease

- Untreated sleep apnea leads to complications of daytime sleepiness (e.g. accidents) as well as cardiovascular complications (hypertension, coronary disease, and stroke).
- Many patients with narcolepsy will remain undiagnosed (and untreated) for decades leading to disability mostly from sleepiness but also from ancillary symptoms.

Section 7: Reading list

Key reading sources for this chapter can be found online at www.mountsinaiexpertguides.com

Suggested websites

American Academy of Sleep Medicine: www.aasmnet.org
American Sleep Apnea Association: www.sleepapnea.org
Narcolepsy Network: www.narcolepsynetwork.org

Section 8: Guidelines

Title	Source	Weblink
Practice parameters for the use of continuous and bilevel positive airway pressure devices to treat adult patients with sleep-related breathing disorders	American Academy of Sleep Medicine (AASM), 2006	http://www.ncbi.nlm.nih.gov/pubmed/16553024
Practice parameters for the surgical modifications of the upper airway for obstructive sleep apnea in adults	AASM, 2010	http://www.ncbi.nlm.nih.gov/pubmed/21061864
Practice parameters for the treatment of narcolepsy and other hypersomnias of central origin	AASM, 2007	http://www.ncbi.nlm.nih.gov/pmc/articles/PMC2276123/
Clinical guideline for the evaluation, management and long-term care of obstructive sleep apnea in adults. Obstructive Sleep Apnea Task Force of the American Academy of Sleep Medicine	AASM, 2009	http://www.aasmnet.org/practiceparameters.aspx?cid=102

Section 9: Evidence for therapies

Type of evidence	Title and comment	Weblink
Systematic review	Surgical modifications of the upper airway for obstructive sleep apnea in adults: a systematic review and meta-analysis **Comment**: Surgical maxillomandibular advancement successful; data on other surgery (e.g. UPPP) less consistent	http://www.ncbi.nlm.nih.gov/pubmed/21061863
Systematic review	Continuous positive airways pressure for obstructive sleep apnoea in adults **Comment**: CPAP is effective in improving sleepiness, quality of life, and blood pressure	http://www.ncbi.nlm.nih.gov/pubmed/16437429
Systematic review	Sodium oxybate for narcolepsy with cataplexy: systematic review and meta-analysis **Comment**: Narcolepsy patients on sodium oxybate had improvement in cataplexy and sleepiness	http://www.ncbi.nlm.nih.gov/pubmed/22893778

Additional material for this chapter can be found online at: www.mountsinaiexpertguides.com

This includes advice for patients, a case study, multiple choice questions, and a reading list.

CHAPTER 40

Neurocritical Care

Errol L. Gordon
Icahn School of Medicine at Mount Sinai, New York, NY, USA

OVERALL BOTTOM LINE
- Improved outcomes in the care of critically ill neurologic patients can be achieved through specialized units and expertise in neurocritical care.
- Knowledge of the principles of brain and spinal pathophysiology is essential to render care to such patients.
- Management of intracranial pressure (ICP) is a central component of the care of the neurocritical patient and is the main focus of this chapter. See Chapter 4: Delirium and Coma, for the approach to diagnosis of patients with coma.

Section 1: Background
Definition
Neurocritical care is the comprehensive and multisystem care of critically ill neurologic patients. It therefore crosses the borders of several medical and surgical specialties, with a focus on life-threatening neurologic illnesses.

Disease classification
Common disorders leading to neurointensive care include:
- Ischemic strokes such as malignant MCA syndrome or vertebrobasilar infarction.
- Intracerebral hemorrhage.
- Subarachnoid hemorrhage, most commonly from ruptured cerebral aneurysm.
- Spinal cord injuries.
- Traumatic brain injury.
- Status epilepticus.
- Complications of brain tumors.
- Nervous system infections.
- Respiratory disorders of neurologic origin including myasthenia and acute inflammatory demyelinating polyneuropathy (AIDP).
- Post-neurosurgical complications or monitoring.
- Anoxic encephalopathy.

Mount Sinai Expert Guides: Neurology, First Edition. Edited by Stuart C. Sealfon, Rajeev Motiwala, and Charles B. Stacy.
© 2016 John Wiley & Sons, Ltd. Published 2016 by John Wiley & Sons, Ltd.
Companion website: www.mountsinaiexpertguides.com

Neurointensive care issues in the management of subarachnoid hemorrhage, intracerebral hemorrhage, and malignant MCA syndrome are found later in this chapter. Management of other disorders is discussed in relevant chapters elsewhere in this volume.

Pathophysiology of intracranial hypertension

Understanding the physiology of increased intracranial pressure is a key to neurocritical care.

- Increased ICP (intracranial pressure) can result from:
  - intracranial mass lesions;
  - edema;
  - CSF hypersecretion;
  - increased intracranial blood volume;
  - cerebral vasodilatation.
- Monroe–Kellie doctrine: given that the cranial vault has a fixed volume (~1500 cm³), an increase in the volume of one component must be accompanied by a corresponding decrease in the volume of another.
- The three components are:
  - brain parenchyma 70–80%;
  - blood in arteries and veins 10%;
  - CSF 10%.
- Mechanisms to compensate for an increase in the volume of one component include:
  - Shifting CSF into the spinal subarachnoid space.
  - Moving blood out of the dural sinuses.
    - About two-thirds of the blood in the cranial vault is contained in the venous system.
  - All told the cranial vault can displace 15–70 cm³ of volume using this mechanism before ICP begins to rise.

CNS compliance

- CNS compliance is the ability of the intracranial vault to accommodate changes in volume related to the change in pressure.
- As compensation fails, compliance falls sharply and ICP rises.
- It is not possible to calculate these values accurately.
- At steady state, the typical ICP = 8–10 mmHg.
- The typical compliant ICP waveform (Figure 40.1) contains three peaks of decreasing size:
  - P1, or the percussion wave, is the first peak, which is thought to be related to the arterial input, with the pressure wave being transmitted via the choroid plexus and brain parenchyma.
  - P2, or the tidal wave, is the second peak and represents the retrograde venous pulsation.
  - P3, or the dicrotic wave, is the third peak; it follows the dicrotic notch and represents venous drainage.
  - As the intracranial vault becomes less complaint, P2 and P3 will tend to increase in amplitude (Figure 40.2).
  - A-waves, or plateau waves (Figure 40.3), represent rapid rises in ICP from normal pressure to levels around 50 mmHg for 5 to 20 minutes followed by spontaneous resolution.
  - B-waves (Figure 40.4) occur when ICP rises quickly to around 30 mmHg lasting for 1 to 2 minutes.

- C-waves (Figure 40.5) are rhythmic elevations of ICP with peaks less than both A and B waves, and lasting only for 5 to 6 minutes at a time.
- These abnormal A, B, and C CNS waveform patterns indicate poor CNS compliance.

Cerebral autoregulation

- The critical element for brain health is the continuous maintenance of an adequate cerebral blood flow (CBF), normally about 15% of the total cardiac output, and approximately 750 cm³/min or 50 cm³/min/100 g of brain tissue.
- CBF depends on cerebral perfusion pressure (CPP), the difference in pressure between the arterial system and the intracranial vault:
  - CPP = MAP − ICP, where MAP is mean arterial pressure.
- In a non-hypertensive patient, CBF is unaffected by changes in MAP over a range of 60 to 160 mmHg, or by CPP over a range of 50 to 150 mmHg (Figure 40.6). Within these ranges, the cerebral arterioles change resistance to keep CBF unaffected by changes in CPP.
- Outside of this range, due to low blood pressure or increased ICP, autoregulation cannot achieve adequate CBF. Ischemia occurs at a CBF below approximately 20 cm³/min/100 g brain.
  Cerebral autoregulation may be impaired in acute brain injury, and CBF dysregulates within a CPP range that would otherwise be compensated. This may lead to a direct relationship between CBF and cerebral perfusion pressure CPP (Figure 40.7).
- Chronic hypertension will cause autoregulation to be maintained over higher MAP and CPP values.
- Hypercapnia or hypoxia lowers the upper limits of autoregulation because of vasodilatation.
  CBF and ICP can vary unexpectedly in a number of conditions observed in neurocritical care.
- Causes of decreased CBF and increased ICP:
  - increased intrathoracic and intra-abdominal pressure
  - hypotension
  - hypovolemia
- Causes of increased CBF and increased ICP:
  - hypoventilation
  - hyperthermia
  - hypoxia
  - pain
  - seizures
- Causes of decreased CBF and decreased ICP:
  - hyperventilation
  - hypothermia
- Relationship between CBF and ventilation and oxygenation:
  - Severe hypoxia (pO_2 < 50 mmHg) increases CBF.
  - CBF doubles at a pO_2 of 30 mmHg.
  - pCO_2 of 80 mmHg causes maximum cerebral vasodilation.
  - pCO_2 of 20 mmHg causes maximum cerebral vasoconstriction.

Intracranial pressure monitors

Several different approaches are utilized. These are:
- External ventricular catheter (EVD):
  - Most accurate way to measure ICP.
  - Requires catheter to pass through the brain parenchyma.

- Most technically difficult monitor to place.
- Intraventricular catheter also allows treatment of elevated ICP when due to hydrocephalus and infusion of therapeutic agents.
- Highest complication rate of all the devices.
- Intraparenchymal monitor:
  - Second most accurate way to measure ICP.
  - 1 to 2 mmHg/day drift in accuracy.
  - Lower complication and infection risk than EVDs.
- Subarachnoid monitor:
  - Older type of monitor in which device connects the subarachnoid space with a pressure transducer.
  - Typically secured with a bolting device.
- Subdural monitor:
  - Monitors are placed just under the dura.
  - Less accurate than both the intraventricular and subdural catheters.
- Epidural monitor:
  - Monitor that is placed superficial to the dura.
  - Considered to be the least accurate way of measuring ICP.

Cerebral herniation

In addition to the effects of increased intracranial pressure decreasing cerebral perfusion, an increase in volume can cause displacement of the brain and compression of vital areas. Depending on the location of the increase, several well-characterized herniation syndromes can be differentiated.

- Herniation represents an absolute neurocritical emergency, requiring prompt recognition and treatment.
- Types of herniation:
  - Subfalcine herniation: herniation of the cingulate gyrus underneath the falx cerebri.
  - Uncal herniation: herniation of the temporal horn inferiorly through the tentorium.
  - Tonsillar herniation: herniation of the cerebellar tonsils through the foramen magnum.
  - Upward herniation: herniation of the cerebellum through the tentorium.
- Patients with high risk for herniation, such as patients with hemispheric mass lesions showing midline displacement or cerebellar mass lesions, need close monitoring to detect early signs of herniation.
- Signs of cerebral herniation include:
  - Decreasing level of consciousness or responsiveness.
  - Unilateral or bilateral blown pupil (dilated, unreactive pupil) or oculomotor paresis.
  - Changes in respiratory pattern, such as development of Cheyne–Stokes respiration.
  - Posturing:
    - Decorticate posturing consists of extension of the lower extremities with flexion in the arms at the wrist and elbow.
    - Decerebrate posturing consists of extension of the lower extremities with extension and internal rotation of the upper extremities.
  - Flaccid paralysis.

Section 2: Prevention and screening

Not applicable for this topic.

Section 3: Diagnosis
Not applicable for this topic.

Section 4: Treatment
Treatment of elevated ICP and cerebral herniation

Conservative measures and prevention	Maintain quiet environment Elevate head of bed >35 degrees Avoid internal jugular compression by keeping the head in a neutral position Reduce activities that increase intrathoracic and intra-abdominal pressure
Hyperventilation	Used to achieve rapid, but short-lived reduction in ICP through vasoconstriction due to hypocapnia, usually with incipient herniation Secure airway and hyperventilate by hand with an Ambu bag Attempt should be made to reverse the clinical sign suggesting herniation (i.e. reversal of a blown pupil) The ICP lowering effect of hyperventilation does not persist Persistent pCO_2 of <17 mmHg may cause severe vasoconstriction and cerebral ischemia and infarction
Osmotherapy	Increases the tonicity of the blood Draws fluid from the extracellular space and cells into the bloodstream, essentially desiccating the brain Ideal osmotic agents would stay inside the bloodstream and not enter the extracellular space Requires an intact blood–brain barrier in order to exclude the movement of any solute but not impede the free flow of water Osmotherapies work on the intact parts of the brain Typical agents are mannitol and hypertonic saline
	Mannitol • Non-metabolizable sugar in humans • Reflection coefficient of 0.9 (90% of mannitol stays in blood) • 1–1.5 g/kg in emergencies • May be given scheduled in the order of 0.25–0.50 g/kg every 4–6 hours • Mannitol is excreted by the kidneys • Caution should be used in patients with renal failure • In patients with intact renal function, mannitol acts as a diuretic • In patients with renal failure mannitol acts as a volume expander, which could potentiate fluid overload Other complications: • Dehydration and hypotension • Hyperosmotic prerenal failure • Electrolyte disturbances (i.e. hypokalemia) Monitoring of mannitol should be done by monitoring the osmolar gap: osmolar gap = (measured osm – calculated osm) Mannitol should not be given if the osmolar gap is 20 or greater **Hypertonic saline** Sodium chloride solution that has a tonicity that is greater than the tonicity of the human body Available concentrations: 2%, 3%, 7%, and 23% Typically 2% and 3% are used for used for infusions 7% and 23% are used as bolus therapy

	Hypertonic saline is used to treat: • Cerebral edema • Midline shift • Intracranial hypertension • Hyponatremia • Cerebral herniation Some intensivists prefer to maintain sodium concentration in normal physiologic ranges and give bolus therapy only for emergent situations like spikes in ICPs and cerebral herniations Some intensivists prefer to keep sodium in at-risk individuals at a higher than physiologic range. This is attempting to reduce episodes of ICP spikes and possibly prevent herniation syndromes Complications of hypertonic saline: • Fluid overload • Pulmonary edema • Central pontine myelinolysis • Renal failure Na levels of 160 Meg/L are associated with worse outcomes In cerebral herniation syndromes bolus therapy is preferred: • 23% saline may be utilized in this manner • Typical dose is 30 cm^3 bolus infusion over 10 minutes • Transient hypotension is seen anecdotally with rapid administration of 23% saline Administration of any hypertonic saline solution greater than 2% concentration should be done through a central line
Hypothermia	Second- or third-line treatment for refractory elevated ICP. Used after failure of conservative measures and osmotherapy Moderate hypothermia reduces ICP by the reduction of the cerebral metabolic rate and the resultant reduction of cerebral blood flow Also reduces the release of excitatory neurotransmitter and blocks the inflammatory cascade Complications of hypothermia: • bradycardia and other cardiac arrhythmias • rebound intracranial hypertension • increased risk of sepsis and coagulopathy
Surgical intervention	Intracranial hypertension may become medically refractory to treatment. In these situations surgical intervention such as hemicraniectomy may be considered

Neurocritical treatment of aneurysmal subarachnoid hemorrhage (SAH)

• First phase of neurocritical treatment, prior to securing the aneurysm, may involve:
  • Resuscitation.
  • Dealing with potential concomitant medical complications related to aneurysm rupture.
  • Minimizing the risk of rupture or re-rupture.
  • Systolic blood pressure is maintained below 160 mmHg.
  • Intubation, if necessary, should be performed using a rapid sequence technique.
  • Immediate reversal of any coagulopathy. Most commonly, this is related to warfarin administration; fresh frozen plasma or prothrombin complex concentrate (PCC), and vitamin K should be administered. Protamine is used to counteract heparin.
  • Seizure prophylaxis (phenytoin or levetiracetam) to avoid seizure-induced re-rupture.
  • Placing an external ventricular drain can help relieve signs and symptoms of hydrocephalus, although overdrainage in a patient with an unsecured aneurysm may potentiate re-rupture.

Table 40.1 Modified Fischer score: CT grading for SAH

0	No SAH; no intraventricular blood
1	Thin diffuse or focal subarachnoid blood, no intraventricular blood
2	Thin diffuse or local subarachnoid blood with intraventricular blood
3	Thick focal or diffuse subarachnoid blood but no intraventricular blood
4	Thick local or diffuse subarachnoid blood with intraventricular blood

- The use of aminocaproic acid, an inhibitor of fibrinolysis, in order to prevent re-rupture, is controversial. Aminocaproic acid increases the risk of a venous thrombotic event.
  - Aminocaproic acid is contraindicated with a history of pulmonary embolism, in the presence of deep vein thrombosis, or with active ischemic changes on EKG.
  - Used prior to the vasospasm window (post bleed day numbers 4 to 21).
  - Loading dose of 4 g and then 1 g/h should be administered and stopped 3–6 hours prior to a catheter-based cerebral angiogram.
- Second phase of ICU care in a patient with an SAH occurs after securing the aneurysm either by clipping or coil embolization.
- Monitoring and treatment for delayed neurologic deterioration, including:
  - Seizures
  - Hydrocephalus
  - Cerebral vasospasm: risk of developing vasospasm is increased with history of hypertension, increased admission MAP, or elevated modified Fischer score (Table 40.1).
  - Angiographic evidence of vasospasm may not be associated with clinical symptoms or signs.
  - Clinical manifestations of cerebral vasospasm:
    - Headache
    - Focal neurologic deficits
    - Depressed mental status
    - Presence of new cerebral infarction
  - Studies for suspected vasospasm:
    - Transcranial Dopplers
    - CT angiography and perfusion studies
    - MR angiography and MR perfusion
  - Treatment of symptomatic cerebral vasospasm:
    - Triple "H" therapy (hypertension, hypervolemia, and hemodilution) is the mainstay of medical treatment.
    - Angioplasty of the affected cerebral vessel.
    - Intra-arterial administration of vasodilatory agent during catheter-based cerebral angiogram.

Cardiac complications of SAH
- Elevation in troponin – 35%
- Arrhythmias – 35%
- Abnormalities on ECHO – 25%
- "Neurogenic stress cardiomyopathy":
  - chest pain
  - dyspnea
  - hypoxia
  - cardiogenic shock
  - pulmonary edema
  - elevated cardiac markers

- occurs within hours of rupture
- may last 1 to 3 days.

- Seen in 20% of cases.
- Pulmonary edema (cardiogenic or neurogenic).
- Acute lung injury or ARDS (adult respiratory distress syndrome).
- Occur more often the higher the clinical grade.
- Associated with poor outcome.

Neurocritical treatment of other conditions
Intracerebral hemorrhage (ICH)
- Initial phases of treating patient with ICH driven by preventing further expansion of the hematoma.
- Most of the expansion occurs early.
- Reduce the blood pressure. Recent data suggest that a target of 140/90 is safe and may limit expansion.
- Any coagulopathy should be reversed if possible with the appropriate agent immediately. Patients who have been taking antiplatelet agents currently receive platelet transfusions and DDAVP, although the benefit is not established.
- Secondary neurologic deterioration may also occur from seizures or hydrocephalus in addition to hematoma expansion.
- Cerebellar ICH greater than 3 cm in diameter is a neurosurgical emergency requiring immediate evacuation. Deterioration can be sudden and prognosis for recovery is excellent in cases operated upon before stupor or coma develops.

Malignant MCA syndrome
- Large cerebral infarction involving a majority of the middle cerebral artery (MCA) territory on one side with the possible involvement of the anterior cerebral artery (ACA) territory may develop a malignant MCA syndrome.
- May rapidly develop uncal herniation.
- In younger patients, early hemicraniectomy (within 48 hours) improves survival and functional outcome.

Neuromuscular disease
- Patient with myasthenia gravis exacerbation and Guillain–Barré syndrome (GBS) may need ventilatory support.
- NIF (negative inspiratory force) <20 cm H_2O or VC (vital capacity) >15 mL/kg should be achieved before being extubated.

Traumatic brain injury (TBI)
- Spinal precautions should be maintained until CT imaging of the cervical spine can be obtained and the patient is found to have a stable c-spine.
- Patient with a GCS (Glasgow Coma Scale) <8 should be considered for an ICP monitor.
- Patient with significant contusions should usually have any coagulopathy corrected.
- Intubation if necessary should be performed using a rapid sequence technique in order to minimize spikes in ICP.

Section 5: Special populations
Not applicable for this topic.

Section 6: Prognosis

Prognosis is disease specific.

Section 7: Reading list

Key reading sources for this chapter can be found online at www.mountsinaiexpertguides.com

Suggested websites

Neurocritical Care Society: http://www.neurocriticalcare.org/
Neurocritical Care [journal]: http://link.springer.com/journal/12028

Section 8: Guidelines

Not applicable for this topic.

Section 9: Evidence for therapies

Not applicable for this topic.

Section 10: Images

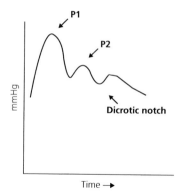

Figure 40.1 Normal intracranial pressure (ICP) waveform.

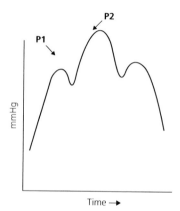

Figure 40.2 Non-compliant intracranial pressure (ICP) waveform.

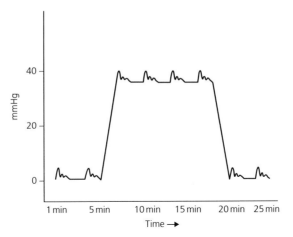

Figure 40.3 A-waves (plateau waves) typically last for 5 to 20 minutes followed by spontaneous resolution.

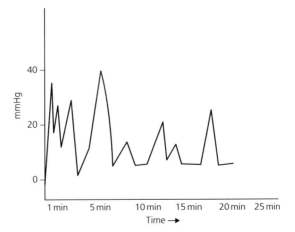

Figure 40.4 B-waves.

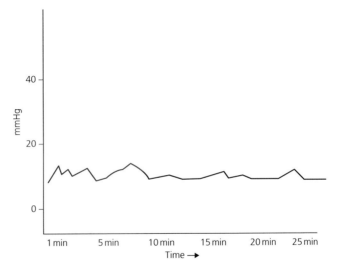

Figure 40.5 C-waves.

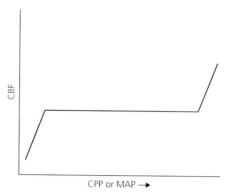

Figure 40.6 Cerebral autoregulation. CBF, cerebral blood flow; CPP, cerebral perfusion pressure; MAP, mean arterial pressure.

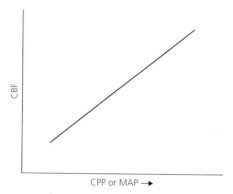

Figure 40.7 Cerebral autoregulation dysfunction. CBF, cerebral blood flow; CPP, cerebral perfusion pressure; MAP, mean arterial pressure.

Additional material for this chapter can be found online at:
www.mountsinaiexpertguides.com

This includes multiple choice questions and a reading list.

CHAPTER 41

Trauma

Jeremy M. Steinberger[1], Margaret Pain[1], and Jamie S. Ullman[2]
[1] Icahn School of Medicine at Mount Sinai, New York, NY, USA
[2] Hoftstra Northwell School of Medicine, Hempstead, NY, USA

OVERALL BOTTOM LINE
- Injury to the brain and brainstem is categorized as traumatic brain injury (TBI).
- Injury to the spinal cord and cauda equina is categorized as spinal cord injury (SCI).
- Injuries are divided into two categories: primary and secondary. Primary injury occurs at the time of the trauma; secondary injury occurs as an adverse result of the physiologic response after the initial impact.
- Diagnosis relies on correlating detailed neurologic findings with the mechanism of injury, and this can be supplemented by radiologic findings.
- Treatment for TBI is largely supportive; however, surgery is necessary when mass lesions, hydrocephalus, or edema cause significant displacement or compression of brain tissue.
- Treatment for SCI depends on the extent and mechanism of injury. The goals of treatment are stabilization of structural damage and relief of nervous system compression.

Section 1: Background
Definition of disease
Trauma is defined as injury caused by an external force.

Disease classification
Neurologic injury from trauma is divided according to the anatomic location of the injury and the mechanism of the injury.
- Traumatic brain injury involves the brain and brainstem.
- Brain injury associated with trauma stems from two causes: direct injury from the external force and secondary injury that develops as a reaction to the primary injury.
- Examples of primary brain injury are gunshot wounds that involve the brain, head injuries sustained during motor vehicle accidents, and injury to the head sustained during a fall. Examples of secondary injury include cell death related to persistent ischemia, reactive edema, intracranial hypertension, and venous infarction.
- Spinal cord injury involves the spinal cord and cauda equina. It is a clinical diagnosis based on a history of trauma with demonstrated physical deficits. It can also be divided into primary and secondary injury.

Mount Sinai Expert Guides: Neurology, First Edition. Edited by Stuart C. Sealfon, Rajeev Motiwala, and Charles B. Stacy.
© 2016 John Wiley & Sons, Ltd. Published 2016 by John Wiley & Sons, Ltd.
Companion website: www.mountsinaiexpertguides.com

Incidence/prevalence
- 1.7 million Americans suffer TBI each year – 1.4 million go to the Emergency Department, 275,000 are hospitalized, and 52,000 die.
- TBI-related deaths represent one-third of injury-related deaths.
- SCI: approximately 14,000 spinal cord injuries occur per year in North America.

Economic impact
- Direct medical costs and indirect costs (such as loss of productivity) of TBI totaled US$77 billion in the year 2000 alone.
- Some estimates for annual economic impact of spinal cord injury (including medical costs, household assistance and other support services) reach US$8 billion a year.

Etiology
- Major causes of TBI are falls (35.2%), motor vehicle accidents (17.3%), other collisions (16.5%), assault (10%), and unknown or other causes (21%).
- Leading causes of SCI across all demographics are motor vehicle accidents (32%), falls (25%), gunshot wounds (10%), and motorcycle crashes (7%). Falls were the leading cause in the elderly population, and motor vehicle accidents were the leading cause in individuals younger than 45.

Pathology
Traumatic brain injury (TBI)
Primary processes that contribute to TBI include:
- Skull fracture (displaced or non-displaced).
- Cerebral contusion – cerebral contusions are "bruising" of the brain. They are usually on the crest of the gyrus, often involved with clusters of small hemorrhages, and can be wedge-shaped with the apex toward the subcortical white matter. They tend to be progressive lesions and therefore require frequent monitoring. "Coup" contusions occur beneath the external point of impact. "Contrecoup" contusions occur opposite the point of impact. They are frequently associated with massive impact forces and can often be observed over the orbital surfaces, frontal poles, or temporal poles (Figure 41.1).
- Intracerebral hematoma – traumatic intracerebral hemorrhage may result from shearing forces, propagation of contusion, or direct extension of the external injury.
- Extra-axial hematoma (epidural, subdural) – epidural hemorrhages typically result from injury of the meningeal artery/vein complex or dural venous sinuses. Hemorrhage of these vessels leads to dissection of the dura away from the bone. They usually occur more frequently in younger patients and are often associated with skull fracture (Figure 41.2). In contrast, subdural hemorrhages tend to result from injury to the bridging veins. The blood accumulates in the space between the dura and arachnoid, causing mass effect (Figure 41.3).
- Subarachnoid hemorrhage and intraventricular hemorrhage – because of the extensive cortical vasculature, subarachnoid hemorrhage is a common finding in head trauma. Subarachnoid hemorrhage can lie over contusions, beneath areas of subdural hematomas, and can follow gunshot wounds or lacerations. Intraventricular hemorrhage can arise from diffuse axonal injury (DAI), adjacent contusion/laceration, or penetrating injury.
- Focal and diffuse axonal injury – DAI is a shearing injury to the axons and is usually sustained after a high-speed acceleration-deceleration injury. Areas at highest risk for DAI include the subcortical white matter, corpus callosum, deep gray matter, or periventricular white matter.
- Concussion – concussion is a reversible condition in which an impact to the brain, although not resulting in gross structural damage, results in biochemical disturbances ultimately leading to

mitochondrial dysfunction and impaired neuronal energy metabolism. The brain is particularly vulnerable to irreversible neuronal injury if a second concussion occurs prior to resolution of the initial metabolic derangements.

Secondary processes that contribute to TBI include:
- Edema
- Increased intracranial pressure
- Herniation syndromes
- Hydrocephalus
- Seizures
- Ischemic damage leading to neuronal membrane destruction.

Spinal cord injury (SCI)

Primary processes that contribute to SCI include:
- Primary processes affecting the vertebral column: fractures, dislocations, ligamentous injuries, disk herniation.
- Primary processes affecting the spinal cord: transection, shearing, cord or epidural hemorrhage, contusion, vascular disruption causing cord ischemia.
- Note that spinal cord injury can occur in the absence of radiologic changes, especially in children (spinal cord injury without radiologic abnormalities, SCIWORA).

Secondary processes that contribute to SCI include:
- Edema
- Mass effect causing impaired spinal cord perfusion and ischemia.

Risk factors
- Risk for TBI is highest among adolescents, young adults, and persons older than 75 years.
- Risk of TBI overall is two times greater in males than in females.
- For SCI, persons in their late teenage years and early twenties are at highest risk, while the pediatric population rates are lowest.
- SCI incidence is 3–4-fold higher in males than females.
- SCI risk is increased with underlying or pre-existing structural disease: for example, cervical spondylosis or stenosis, rheumatoid arthritis, tethered cord, osteoporosis, or spondylolisthesis.

Section 2: Prevention

> **CLINICAL PEARLS**
> - Using seatbelts, helmets, and other protective equipment can prevent or reduce devastating traumatic brain injury.
> - Maintaining adequate oxygenation and blood pressure can help to prevent secondary injury in brain and spinal cord injury.

Screening

Alcohol use screening is important to identify patients at risk for injury.

Prior history of trauma may indicate a patient's risk for injury (eg. falls due to gait imbalance). This risk is important to assess, especially in patients receiving anticoagulants or anti-platelet agents.

Primary prevention
- Primary prevention is the most effective way to avoid TBI and SCI.
- ThinkFirst is an example of a non-profit organization aimed at providing methods to children and teenagers to reduce their risk of injury. Guided by the mission of "leading injury prevention through education, research, and policy," ThinkFirst advocates wearing seat belts, avoiding drunk driving, and refraining from dangerous behaviors (e.g. diving into shallow pools) to lower the incidence, cost, and devastation of traumatic injury.

Secondary prevention
- Much of the neurologic devastation following traumatic brain injury does not occur at the moment of injury.
- In the aftermath of the injury, secondary insults can occur largely as a result of ischemia, which is most pronounced within the first 24 hours. In certain circumstances, these insults result in significant deterioration and can adversely affect outcome.
- Much research has been devoted toward the understanding of secondary injury and development of effective interventions to prevent it (see Treatment, below).

Section 3: Diagnosis

> **BOTTOM LINE/CLINICAL PEARLS**
> - High suspicion for TBI should be maintained in intoxicated obtunded patients with an otherwise unclear history.
> - Recognize the Cushing response: Clinical triad of hypertension, bradycardia, and slow, irregular breathing classically found in patients who have increased intracranial pressure. When CSF pressure is greater than the mean arterial pressure, blood supply to the brain, and importantly to the brainstem, is decreased, thus setting off the cascade that leads to the Cushing response, a paradoxical response caused by stimulation of both sympathetic and the parasympathetic responses. Reducing blood pressure during a Cushing response can result in devastating reduction in cerebral blood flow and brain ischemia. The primary treatment for the Cushing response is to reduce the intracranial pressure.
> - In SCI, monitor for bradycardia, hypotension, and cardiovascular instability. Acute cervical SCI may result in bradycardia, especially within the first 2 weeks after injury, due to reduced sympathetic tone. Intensive Care Unit monitoring and judicious use of vasopressors may be necessary to improve spinal cord perfusion to reduce ischemic damage.

Differential diagnosis
Traumatic brain injury (TBI)
There are two general situations in which traumatic brain injury and other acute neurologic conditions may be difficult to distinguish or the two may coexist. In the first instance, patients may have evident head trauma, such as a fall or motor vehicle accident, that is precipitated by a neurologic event such as a cerebrovascular accident or seizure. In this situation, careful attention to the history and workup is important in elucidating the etiology for signs and symptoms and guiding the appropriate interventions. In the second case, the history or signs of trauma may not be evident.

Differential diagnosis for TBI	Features
Cerebrovascular accident	Focal deficits, risk factors, characteristic CT or MRI
Acute encephalopathy or worsening of dementia	Possible evidence of infection or metabolic derangement, history of pre-existing impairment

(Continued)

Differential diagnosis for TBI	Features
Seizure	Witnessed convulsion, history of epilepsy, rapid fluctuations in neurologic status, drug or alcohol use, antiepileptics detected on blood tests
Brain tumor	History of systemic malignancy or progressive neurologic changes Contrast CT or MRI findings
Spontaneous subarachnoid hemorrhage	History of preceding headache, nuchal rigidity, CT and CTA may show lesion

Spinal cord injury (SCI)

Differential diagnosis for SCI	Features
Epidural or subdural infection, osteomyelitis, discitis	Back pain, fever, laboratory evidence of infection, diagnostic findings on MRI with contrast
Spontaneous epidural hematoma	History of coagulopathy or anticoagulant use, abnormal CT or MRI
Pathologic vertebral fracture	History of malignancy; pre-existing worsening back pain; CT shows characteristic fracture; contrast MRI best for identifying tumor; bone scan may identify other skeletal lesions; needle biopsy and pathologic diagnosis definitive
Epidural, intradural, or intramedullary neoplasm (benign or malignant, primary or metastatic)	Back pain, symptom progression, history of primary malignancy, contrast MRI may detect lesion

Typical presentation
- Typical presentation is a history of trauma but may not include explicit injury to the head or spine.
- In SCI, patients can present with either "complete" or "incomplete" injury. A "complete" injury involves loss of all sensory and motor function below the level of the lesion, while an "incomplete" injury consists of some sensory and motor sparing below the level of injury.
- A spinal "level" of injury refers to the lowest level that has normal sensory and motor function. For example, a patient with a "C4 level" has normal C4 function, but the caudal segments (C5 and below) have abnormal motor and/or sensory function.
- Quadriplegia is defined by the loss of movement of all four limbs; paraplegia involves the lower extremities.

Clinical diagnosis
History and examination
Efficiently obtaining adequate history from all emergency personnel, witnesses, and the patient is crucial, with special attention to a history of loss of consciousness, mechanism for injury, ethanol or drug abuse, witnessed seizure, known epilepsy, premorbid function, medication use (especially anticoagulation), and other symptoms listed below. Unwitnessed trauma in the obtunded patient presents as a diagnostic conundrum. Occasionally, it is unclear as to whether a syncopal episode or seizure preceded a fall resulting in TBI.
- Common TBI symptoms:
  - headache;
  - confusion, amnesia, irritability, somnolence or lethargy;

- nausea or vomiting;
- vertigo;
- tinnitus;
- gait instability.
- Common TBI signs:
  - Signs of trauma: lacerations, ecchymosis, "raccoon's eyes" (periorbital ecchymosis), "Battle's sign" (postauricular ecchymosis).
  - Loss of consciousness or reduced responsiveness.
  - Physical evidence of superficial or penetrating injury to the head.
  - Deficits in any cranial nerve: restricted extraocular movements, changes in pupil reactivity and pupil size.
  - Focal paresis.
  - Pathologic reflexes (e.g. Babinski sign).
  - Spontaneous posturing in an unconscious patient.
  - Abnormal respiratory pattern.
  - Hypertension with normal or slow heart rate (Cushing reflex, see below).
  - Seizure.
- Serial examinations should be performed to detect deterioration or improvement.
- Common SCI symptoms and signs:
  - Physical evidence of superficial or penetrating injury to the neck or back.
  - Midline posterior neck pain.
  - Weakness of individual muscle groups or extremities, especially at or below the suspected level of injury (quadriplegia, paraplegia).
  - Decreased sensation or paresthesias, especially with a defined sensory level.
  - Severe injury often causes initial spinal shock with acute loss of tone and deep tendon reflexes.
  - Increased or decreased deep tendon reflexes and pathologic reflexes (Babinski, Hoffmann sign).
  - Decreased anal sphincter tone.
  - Priapism.
  - Urinary retention.
  - Hypersensitivity or hyperalgesia in a dermatomal distribution.
  - Labile blood pressure.
- Diagnosis of SCI should be suspected in patients with a history of trauma and one or more of the following:
  - Midline posterior neck pain.
  - Weakness of individual muscle groups or extremities.
  - Decreased sensation or paresthesias, especially if associated with a spinal level.
  - Abnormal or absent deep tendon reflexes.
  - Decreased rectal tone.
  - Urinary retention.
  - Priapism.
  - Hypersensitivity or hyperalgesia in a dermatomal distribution.
  - Hypotension associated with normal or slow heart rate (neurogenic shock).

Disease severity classification

- GCS (Glasgow Coma Scale): This is the primary scoring system used in the management of TBI. The scale correlates physical examination findings with injury severity and likelihood of poor prognosis.

Table 41.1 The Glasgow Coma Scale.

	1	2	3	4	5	6
Eye	Does not open eyes	Opens eyes in response to painful stimuli	Opens eyes in response to voice	Opens eyes spontaneously	N/A	N/A
Verbal	Makes no sounds	Incomprehensible sounds	Utters inappropriate words	Confused, disoriented	Oriented, converses normally	N/A
Motor	Makes no movements	Extension to painful stimuli (decerebrate response)	Abnormal flexion to painful stimuli (decorticate response)	Flexion/ withdrawal to painful stimuli	Localizes painful stimuli	Obeys commands

GCS 3–8 denotes severe brain injury; GCS 9–12 moderate brain injury; GCS 13–15 mild brain injury.

- The examination is derived from three responses: eye, verbal, and motor, with scores ranging from 3 (worst prognosis) to 15 (best prognosis). The three values are recorded both separately and as a sum. See Table 41.1.
- ASIA (American Spinal Injury Association) Impairment Scale: The ASIA Scale is used to grade severity of SCI. ASIA A indicates complete injury and ASIA B–D partial injury.
  - ASIA A: no motor or sensory function below the level of injury and in the sacral segments S4–S5.
  - ASIA B: sensory but not motor function preserved below neurologic level.
  - ASIA C: motor function is preserved below the neurologic level and more than half of the key muscles below the level have a muscle strength grade less than 3.
  - ASIA D: motor function is preserved below the neurologic level, and at least half of the key muscles below the neurologic level have a muscle grade of 3 or more (antigravity function).
  - ASIA E: normal sensory and motor function.

Laboratory diagnosis

Laboratory workup rarely establishes the diagnosis of TBI or SCI but metabolic and hematologic abnormalities can worsen the severity of existing injuries. Hyponatremia can lead to increased brain swelling from an osmotic gradient and should be avoided.

Diagnostic tests

- Blood and urine toxicology, including blood alcohol level, serum chemistries, CPK, CBC, coagulation studies (may be desirable to include preoperative blood work).
- CT head is the diagnostic modality of choice for patients with TBI as it has high sensitivity for acute hemorrhage and short acquisition time. Imaging is critical for operative planning and so it should be obtained as soon as possible in the diagnostic workup.
- CT is also helpful in assessment of SCI. Because of varied presentation, the entire spinal column should be imaged if SCI is suspected. It is critical to obtain sagittal, coronal, and axial views. While CT is sensitive for bony abnormality of the spinal column, it lacks sensitivity for spinal cord and nerve root damage. MRI may be performed emergently if cord compression is suspected, as it will be able to demonstrate injury to the spinal cord itself as well as the surrounding soft tissue and ligamentous structures. If MRI is not available or is contraindicated, CT myelography may be performed to further assess for cord compression.

Potential pitfalls/common errors in diagnosis

- It is important to evaluate the entire spinal axis, especially the cervical spine, radiologically in patients with severe TBI as their neurologic examination will not reliably identify all spinal injuries.
- CT is the preferred method, and the entire thoracic and lumbosacral spine can be visualized on a routine chest, abdomen, and pelvis CT when obtained to evaluate other systemic injuries.

Section 4: Treatment

Treatment rationale for TBI

- The first objective in TBI is always airway and hemodynamic stabilization.
- TBI management typically focuses on control of intracranial pressure (ICP) and determination of the need for procedural intervention for hemorrhage or hydrocephalus.
- Patients may decompensate precipitously, especially in the presence of expanding supra- or infratentorial hemorrhages and hydrocephalus.
- Elevated ICP may be suspected based on the examination. There are both medical and procedural options for treating elevated ICP, and the rationale for treatment depends on patient factors as well as the severity of the pressure or examination findings.
- ICP monitoring may be necessary for obtunded or comatose patients. There are several options for ICP monitors (see Chapter 40); however, ventriculostomy is typically the treatment of choice as it can be used for diagnostic as well as therapeutic purposes. Subdural and epidural monitors are less accurate. The Brain Trauma Foundation recommends ICP monitors be placed for all patients with GCS of 8 or less and to maintain ICP values of less than 20 cmH$_2$O.
- The cerebral perfusion pressure (CPP) defines the adequacy of arterial blood supply to the brain. It is defined as the calculated difference between mean arterial pressure and intracranial pressure. The target should be 60–70 mmHg.
- Methods to decrease ICP include increasing sedation and analgesia, CSF drainage, head of the bed elevation, mild hyperventilation, and hyperosmolar therapy with mannitol or hypertonic saline. If these methods fail to reduce ICP, decompressive craniectomy, induced hypothermia, or high-dose barbiturates may be necessary to decrease the brain's metabolic needs and to improve perfusion.
- Some 4–25% of patients will suffer an "early" seizure after TBI within 7 days of injury. For this reason, TBI guidelines recommend administering an antiepileptic agent (e.g. phenytoin, levetiracetam, valproic acid) for the first 7 days post-injury. Long-term prophylactic therapy has not been shown to reduce the incidence of late-onset post-traumatic seizures.
- Surgery can be performed to evacuate blood collections that have significant mass effect or that are causing midline shift or herniation. The period of greatest risk for swelling is within the first 48 to 72 hours following injury. Decompressive operations include burr hole placement to evacuate chronic or subacute blood, craniotomy (bone removal, hematoma evacuation, and replacement of bone), or hemicraniectomy (removal of bone to allow hematoma evacuation and brain expansion).
- Severe TBI patients (GCS 3–8) should be intubated for airway protection. C-spine clearance down to the C7–T1 junction is essential in all TBI patients due to the relatively high incidence of associated cervical spine injury (4–8%). This association is particularly high in patients with GCS less than 9.

Treatment rationale for SCI

- The first objective in SCI is always airway and hemodynamic stabilization.
- "Spine precautions" should be instituted for patients with suspected spinal cord injury to avoid further injury. These precautions should be maintained until history, physical, and imaging studies indicate low likelihood of SCI.

- Systolic blood pressure less than 90 mmHg should be avoided in order to prevent further injury to the spinal cord. Maintaining mean arterial pressure greater than 85 mmHg for 7 days is recommended.
- There has been significant controversy regarding the administration of steroids to patients with SCI to prevent or decelerate the swelling and inflammatory response after injury. As per recent practice guidelines, steroids are not recommended for the initial treatment of SCI due to the risk of complications, although they have been used in selected patients.
- Early surgical spinal canal decompression should be performed with any deteriorating spinal cord injury. For neural compression, spinal instability, and presence of a neurologic deficit, surgery should be considered. A reduction (closed or open) should be done for patients with bilateral cervical facet dislocation.
- As in TBI, post-injury rehabilitation is an important part of recovery and should be instituted as soon as the patient's medical status has stabilized.

Prevention/management of complications

- Prevention of venous thromboembolism is important after brain and spinal injury. Pneumatic compression boots and chemoprophylaxis can reduce the incidence. Caution should be taken, however, when considering anticoagulants in TBI patients with intracranial hemorrhage that has not yet stabilized on imaging.
- Early cranioplasty can potentially reduce complications after decompressive craniectomy, such as hydrocephalus and the "syndrome of the trephined" (headache, focal deficits).
- Early operative stabilization after spinal cord and spinal column injury can potentially reduce the incidence of pneumonia and venous thromboembolism through early mobilization.

CLINICAL PEARLS
- Appropriate initial resuscitation attending to airway and circulation is necessary in all TBI and SCI patients; hypotension and hypoxia need to be avoided.
- Early decompression of large mass lesions in the brain is essential to prevent cerebral herniation and relieve intracranial hypertension in acute TBI.
- Surgical decompression of compressive spinal cord lesions is essential in maximizing recovery potential after acute SCI.
- Treatment of TBI and SCI is a multidisciplinary, cooperative team effort involving surgeons, intensivists, neurologists, medical consultants, rehabilitation medicine, and other ancillary providers such as speech pathology and respiratory therapy.

Section 5: Special populations
Pregnancy

- Trauma is the leading cause of maternal death in the USA. Approximately 6% of trauma cases involve pregnant women.
- The treatment of a pregnant patient with TBI/SCI should be similar to all patients with traumatic injury. The primary survey should begin with the standard ABCs of stabilization.
- One important rule to apply is that the mother should be stabilized first, and the fetus secondarily.
- Pregnancy can be confirmed by examination of the uterus, ultrasound, or serum hCG testing.

Children

- As discussed earlier, TBI is one of the leading causes of acquired disability and death in infants and children.

- Blood loss must be monitored closely in children as they are more likely to suffer hemodynamic side effects from large amounts of blood loss.

Elderly
- Elderly persons are at increased risk both for nervous system injury from trauma and for poor functional recovery following injury.
- Special attention should be given to the role of age in prognosis as severity of injury tends to be higher in the elderly.
- Because of potentially important indications for the prescription of anticoagulants, reversal of these agents for prevention of trauma-related hemorrhage should be done thoughtfully in consultation with others.

Others
- Sports participants and athletes merit special mention. Guidelines have been established for standardized assessment and management of concussion and acute spinal symptoms in an attempt to reduce the risk of more severe acute injury, repetitive brain injury, and permanent spinal cord injury. This currently is an active area of research.

Section 6: Prognosis

BOTTOM LINE/CLINICAL PEARLS
- Poor prognosis:
  - Age >60 years.
  - Low Glasgow Coma score.
  - Absent pupillary reflex.
  - Major extracranial injury.
  - CT head with: compression of basal cisterns, subarachnoid hemorrhage, midline shift, intracranial hemorrhage.
- Better prognosis:
  - Age <40 years.
  - Minimal medical comorbidities.
  - No prior history of TBI.
  - Rehabilitation services available.

Natural history of untreated disease
Untreated large intracranial mass lesions in acute TBI can lead to unnecessary morbidity and mortality. Untreated SCI with compressive lesions and skeletal instability can lead to painful spinal deformity, infection, thromboembolic events, respiratory complications and failure, and death. Care must be taken to weigh all factors relating to a particular patient's care, including presence of other life-threatening injuries, comorbidities, and other circumstances that would preclude intervention. Families should be apprised of the risk and benefits of treatment.

Prognosis for treated patients
The overall mortality for severe TBI has decreased from 50% in the 1970s to 25% currently, largely due to improvements in prehospital, emergency department, and intensive care with attention to proper resuscitation and medical/surgical management.

Recovery from brain and spinal cord injury is both variable and multimodal. Depending on the patient, a collaborative approach amongst physical and occupational therapists, neuropsychologists, and medical doctors may be necessary in determining the long-term plan for TBI and SCI patients, who often require significant rehabilitation after the immediate injury.

Follow-up tests and monitoring

Follow-up evaluation and imaging is important in many TBI and SCI patients. For many patients, return to work, play, or daily activities will need to be assessed through evaluation of post-injury symptoms and disability.

Section 7: Reading list

Key reading sources for this chapter can be found online at www.mountsinaiexpertguides.com

Suggested websites

American Spinal Injury Association: www.asia-spinalinjury.org/
Brain Trauma Foundation: www.braintrauma.org/
Centers for Disease Control and Prevention: Traumatic Brain Injury: www.cdc.gov/traumatic braininjury
ThinkFirst: National Injury Prevention Foundation: www.thinkfirst.org/

Section 8: Guidelines

Title	Source	Weblink
Guidelines for the Management of Severe Traumatic Brain Injury	Brain Trauma Foundation; American Association of Neurological Surgeons (AANS); Congress of Neurological Surgeons (CNS); Joint Section on Neurotrauma and Critical Care (2007)	https://www.braintrauma.org/pdf/protected/Guidelines_Management_2007w_bookmarks.pdf
Guidelines for the Management of Acute Cervical Spine and Spinal Cord Injuries	Joint Section on Disorders of the Spine and Peripheral Nerves of the American Association of Neurological Surgeons and the Congress of Neurological Surgeons (2013)	http://journals.lww.com/neurosurgery/toc/2013/03002
Guidelines for the acute medical management of severe traumatic brain injury in infants, children, and adolescents – second edition	Kochanek PM, Carney N, Adelson PD, et al. (2012)	https://www.braintrauma.org/pdf/guidelines_pediatric2.pdf

Section 9: Evidence for therapies

See above Guidelines (Section 9) for information on the evidence to support management of TBI and SCI.

Section 10: Images

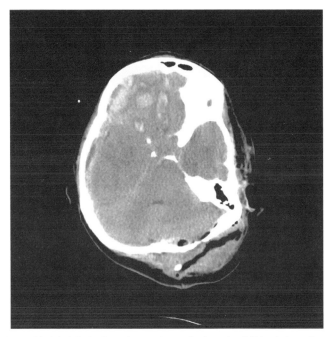

Figure 41.1 Patient with right inferior frontal contusion and subarachnoid blood along the tentorium. There is a right fronto-temporal subdural hematoma. This patient underwent left occipital craniotomy for epidural hematoma evacuation.

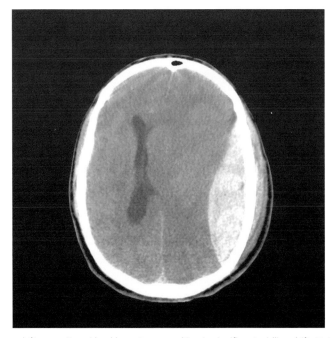

Figure 41.2 Large left convexity epidural hematoma resulting in significant midline shift. Note the convex lens shape that is typical of epidural hematomas, which are limited by the sutures where the dura is most adherent to the skull.

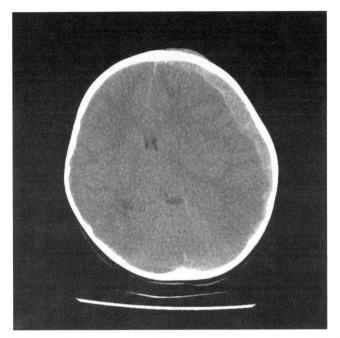

Figure 41.3 Child with acute left fronto-parietal subdural hematoma with significant midline shift. Note the concave, crescent shape of this type of hematoma, which does not respect suture lines.

Additional material for this chapter can be found online at:
www.mountsinaiexpertguides.com

This includes a case study, multiple choice questions, and a reading list.

CHAPTER 42

Postoperative Neurosurgical Patients

Justin Mascitelli, Asha Iyer, and Joshua Bederson
Icahn School of Medicine at Mount Sinai, New York, NY, USA

OVERALL BOTTOM LINE
- A basic understanding of potential surgical complications and treatments is important for any provider caring for neurosurgical patients.
- Prevention of postoperative complications is crucial.
- Adherence to certain postoperative protocols allows for timely screening and treatment of potential postoperative conditions.
- Good communication among services and providers is essential.

Section 1: Background

- Of the many postoperative complications that can occur, the most common include hematoma, seizure, and infection.
- These can manifest in different fashions depending on the type of surgery and the individual patient characteristics.
- This chapter will review specific salient postoperative considerations for a variety of common neurosurgical procedures, including coiling and clipping for aneurysmal subarachnoid hemorrhage (SAH), posterior fossa surgery, brain tumor surgery, shunting, spine surgery, and carotid revascularization surgery.

Section 2: Prevention and screening

BOTTOM LINE/CLINICAL PEARLS
- There are a few basic protocols to prevent and screen for postoperative complications (Table 42.1).
- The majority of patients undergoing cranial surgery, and a smaller subset of patients undergoing spine surgery, should be monitored in a specialized intensive care unit (ICU) setting for the first postoperative day.
- In the ICU, vital signs can be continuously monitored and kept within a normal range (except for specific scenarios when blood pressure should be either increased or lowered).
- A tailored postoperative neurologic assessment of the patient can elucidate complications and permit intervention. For example, a comprehensive bedside visual system examination (including red desaturation, acuity, and visual fields by confrontation with special attention to

---

Mount Sinai Expert Guides: Neurology, First Edition. Edited by Stuart C. Sealfon, Rajeev Motiwala, and Charles B. Stacy.
© 2016 John Wiley & Sons, Ltd. Published 2016 by John Wiley & Sons, Ltd.
Companion website: www.mountsinaiexpertguides.com

the bitemporal fields) is mandatory for all patients who have undergone surgery in the sellar or suprasellar region.
* Patients who have had SAH or surgery in the sellar or suprasellar region should have fluid status closely monitored to screen for both hypo- and hypernatremia.
* Standard postoperative laboratory studies include serum basic metabolic panel (BMP), complete blood count (CBC), coagulopathy panel (PT/PTT), and anticonvulsant level (if applicable) to identify common abnormalities, such as hyponatremia or surgical anemia, that can be readily identified and corrected.
* Postoperative imaging is determined on a case-by-case basis. Any change in neurologic status should prompt a stat CT head.

Table 42.1 Specific preventive measures for the postoperative neurologic patient.

Condition	Preventive measure
Early seizures	• Prophylaxis with antiepileptic drug (AED; typically phenytoin or levetiracetam) for 7 days after insult (SAH, TBI, surgery, etc.)
Late seizures	• Prophylaxis not recommended
Post-SAH vasospasm	• Nimodipine for 21 days associated with improved outcomes
	• Daily transcranial Doppler (TCD) to screen for vasospasm
Infection	• Perioperative antibiotics for 24 hours following surgery
	• Daily wound care
	• Early mobilization for spine surgery patients
Cerebral edema	• High-dose perioperative dexamethasone followed by appropriate taper
	• Induced hypernatremia
	• Avoid hypotonic fluids; cautiously administer isotonic fluids; consider prophylactic hypertonic fluid therapy if edema is expected
Embolic stroke after CEA/ CAS	• Aspirin alone for carotid endarterectomy (CEA)
	• Aspirin + clopidogrel for carotid artery stenting (CAS)
Post-CEA hyperperfusion syndrome	• Strict BP control
	• SBP < 140 mmHg in normotensive patients
	• SBP < 160 mmHg in hypertensive patients
Deep vein thrombosis/ pulmonary embolism	• Subcutaneous heparin or enoxaparin should be initiated as early as postoperative day 2 (although exceptions exist)
	• Early mobilization
	• Sequential compression devices

Section 3: Diagnosis

BOTTOM LINE/CLINICAL PEARLS
* The diagnosis of certain postoperative complications is based on a combination of clinical, laboratory, and radiographic data.
* A complication is usually (but not always) heralded by a change in the neurologic examination.

Differential diagnosis of change in mental status in postoperative patients

Differential diagnosis	Features
Mass effect (hematoma, edema, abscess, instrumentation)	• Symptoms of increased intracranial pressure (ICP) • Focal neurologic deficit; normal vital signs (unless elevated ICP Cushing's triad (see below)) • Normal laboratory values (unless infectious) • Abnormal CT/MRI
Seizure	• Witnessed convulsive activity • Altered level of consciousness; focal neurologic deficit • Subtherapeutic anticonvulsant levels • Possibly normal CT, MRI
Vasospasm	• Possibly headache • Focal neurologic deficit; hypertensive • Normal laboratory values • Increased velocity on transcranial Doppler (TCD); infarction on CT and MRI; small caliber vessels on CTA, MRA, and conventional digital subtraction angiography (DSA)
Shunt malfunction	• Symptoms of increased ICP • Cushing's triad; febrile (if infectious cause) • Normal laboratory values (unless infectious) • Hydrocephalus on CT; shunt discontinuity on shunt series

Typical presentation

A postoperative complication often presents as a change in neurologic examination. The patient will be noted to have a new deficit, be obtunded, or may have a seizure. After a thorough history and neurologic examination, focused laboratory tests and imaging should be obtained immediately. It is typical to begin with a non-contrast CT head, but other imaging studies may be more appropriate if guided by clues in the history and examination. For example, a SAH patient may have a sudden change in the neurologic examination associated with hypertension and elevated TCD velocities. When there is a high suspicion for vasospasm, it may be more appropriate to move directly to CT angiogram (CTA) or digital subtraction angiogram (DSA).

Clinical diagnosis

History and physical examination

These will depend on the specific complication and location in the neural axis. Specific scenarios require different laboratory or imaging studies (see Diagnostic tests, below).

Laboratory diagnosis

Diagnostic tests

Condition	Study
Hematoma	CT head (better for brain hematoma) MRI (better for spine hematoma)
Infection	CBC, erythrocyte sedimentation rate (ESR), C-reactive protein (CRP) Contrast enhanced CT or MRI Lumbar puncture (LP)

(Continued)

Condition	Study
Edema	MRI
Hydrocephalus	CT head
Seizure	AED level EEG or continuous monitoring CT head to rule out new mass or bleed
Vasospasm	TCD, CTA, MRA, or DSA
Hyponatremia	Serum electrolytes Urine electrolytes/osmolarity
Diabetes insipidus	Serum electrolytes Urine electrolytes/osmolarity
Addisonian crisis	Cortisol, ACTH, electrolytes
Shunt malfunction	Shunt series CT head Shunt tap/lumbar puncture
Post CEA/CAS deficit	CT head MRI DSA

Section 4: Treatment of specific postoperative complications
Aneurysmal subarachnoid hemorrhage
The primary treatment for aneurysmal SAH is clipping or coiling of the aneurysm. There are a number of conditions that can commonly arise in the weeks following this primary treatment such as seizures, hydrocephalus, hyponatremia, and vasospasm (Table 42.2).

Posterior fossa surgery
- Posterior fossa surgery is associated with many of the most rapidly progressive and dangerous complications that neurosurgeons and neurologists encounter.
- Problems such as postoperative hematoma, brain edema, and infarction can quickly lead to acute hydrocephalus and brainstem compression.
- As patients can rapidly deteriorate from any of these complications, vigilance is of utmost importance.
- A subtle change in vital signs may be the earliest symptom to herald an ominous posterior fossa complication. The pattern often follows the Cushing's triad, with bradycardia, hypertension, and abnormal respirations. Progression is marked by changes in mental status and level of consciousness, brainstem and long-track findings, coma, and death. All of these changes can occur within minutes.
- If any of these changes occur, it is paramount that the neurosurgeon is immediately notified.

Management
- Intubate the patient for airway protection and hyperventilation.
- Initiate immediate empirical measures for ICP control, including head-of-bed elevation, hyperosmolar therapy with mannitol or hypertonic saline (either 3% NaCl at a high rate or a one-time bolus of 23.5% NaCl), and hyperventilation.
- Obtain stat head CT.
- If the CT scan reveals hydrocephalus, place an external ventricular drain (EVD) as soon as possible. If an EVD has already been placed, increase cerebrospinal fluid (CSF) drainage until ICP

Table 42.2 Treatments for specific complications following primary treatment of aneurysmal subarachnoid hemorrhage (SAH).

Complication	Treatment
Seizure	• All patients should continue on either phenytoin or levetiracetam for at least 7 days for early seizure prophylaxis and only continue beyond 7 days if a seizure occurs • Seizures should be treated with a bolus of the current AED or addition of a second AED
Hydrocephalus	• Patients with depressed mental status or radiographic evidence of hydrocephalus should undergo external ventricular drainage (EVD) with ICP monitoring • Medical strategies to maintain ICP <20 cmH$_2$O include but are not limited to: head-of-bed elevation, hyperosmolar therapy, sedation, paralysis, and cautious hyperventilation
Hyponatremia	• Fluid status and sodium homeostasis should be monitored • Patients with SAH can experience both the syndrome of inappropriate ADH secretion (SIADH) or cerebral salt wasting (CSW) • The cause of hyponatremia should be immediately determined • Hyponatremia can be treated with hypertonic saline and fludrocortisone, and occasionally by fluid restriction for true hypervolemic SIADH
Vasospasm	• Once the aneurysm has been secured, blood pressure may be liberalized • SAH patients should be monitored with daily TCD to screen for vasospasm • If there are any elevations of TCD velocities or, more importantly, changes in neurologic examination, hypervolemic, hypertensive, hemodilution therapy (triple-H therapy) should be initiated and DSA considered • If vasospasm is identified on DSA, intra-arterial verapamil and angioplasty are therapeutic options

is less than 20 cmH$_2$O. However, one must also avoid over-drainage, which can cause upward transtentorial herniation.
- If the CT scan reveals brainstem compression, the patient should be taken back to the operating room immediately. It is important to note that EVD drainage should not be performed without surgical decompression for patients with brainstem compression.
- Once the patient has been stabilized, ICP has been controlled, and hydrocephalus or brainstem compression has been treated, the source of the complication should be rapidly elucidated. Postoperative vasogenic brain edema can be treated with high-dose dexamethasone. A postoperative hematoma should usually be removed surgically. If antiplatelet or anticoagulant use was known or suspected, further appropriate reversal should be initiated.
- Infarction is another possible complication of posterior fossa surgery. While arterial infarction presents immediately, postoperative venous infarction typically presents 24 to 48 hours after surgery (Figure 42.1). This is especially relevant following posterior fossa surgery given the multiple venous sinuses and potential for injury or obstruction. If swelling is significant enough to cause changes in the neurologic examination, hydrocephalus, or brainstem compression, immediate return to the operating room for suboccipital decompression should be strongly considered.

Brain tumor surgery
- A variety of different scenarios and complications can arise following brain tumor surgery depending on the tumor type and location.
- Postoperative hemorrhage and edema are possible after resection of any brain tumor. This is especially true for glioblastoma multiforme (GBM), which when partially resected has a propensity for hemorrhage and swelling, a.k.a. "wounded glioma" (Figure 42.2).
- Given the proximity of the pituitary gland to sellar and suprasellar tumors, diabetes insipidus can begin within the first few hours after surgery in that region.

Table 42.3 Treatment of specific complications following surgery for a brain tumor.

Condition	Management
Edema	• Steroids • Discontinue hypotonic and isotonic fluids • Administer hyperosmolar therapy (hypertonic saline or mannitol)
Hematoma	• Surgical evacuation • Reversal of coagulopathy or thrombocytopenia (if applicable)
Seizure	• AED
Diabetes insipidus	• Match urinary losses with IV fluids or oral intake • Desmopressin (ddAVP)
Addisonian crisis	• Fluid resuscitation • IV hydrocortisone • Vasopressors (if necessary)

Table 42.4 Treatment by type of shunt complication.

Type	Features
Mechanical	Proximal obstruction: • Surgical revision of the ventricular catheter • If the patient is experiencing an ICP crisis, an external ventricular drain (EVD) should be placed immediately, followed by surgical revision of the shunt Distal obstruction: • Similarly, a distal obstruction requires surgical revision • If ICP is a concern, temporary measures include withdrawing large quantities of CSF via tapping the reservoir or complete externalization of the shunt at the clavicle
Infection	• Empiric broad-spectrum antibiotics should be initiated after CSF is obtained and narrowed once a species and sensitivity identified • It is important to determine if the patient is shunt dependent either clinically or radiographically • If the patient is shunt dependent, then the shunt should be externalized while the infection is treated to allow for continued CSF drainage • If the patient is not shunt dependent, then the shunt can be completely removed while the infection is treated and then replaced at a future date • Often, shunt infection may cause shunt obstruction, and both the infection and the obstruction need to be addressed

Caution: After MR scanning, shunts with adjustable valves should be checked and reprogrammed.

- Patients with Cushing's disease manifest a dramatic and rapid reduction in cortisol following successful removal of an ACTH-secreting microadenoma. Some neurosurgeons prefer to withhold postoperative steroids in order to detect the cortisol decrease that accompanies successful resection of an ACTH-secreting tumor. Those patients who are not given postoperative steroids can develop a condition similar to an Addisonian crisis with dangerously low blood pressure.
- Treatment of specific complications is summarized in Table 42.3.

Shunting

- While ventricular shunting can prevent the life-threatening progression of hydrocephalus and increased intracranial pressure, complications in both the acute and long-term care of shunt patients require immediate recognition and treatment (Table 42.4).
- Mechanical shunt complications underlie more than half of all shunt failures.

Table 42.5 Treatment of specific complications following spine surgery.

Condition	Treatment
Surgical anemia	• IV fluids for acute volume restoration • Blood transfusions if symptomatic
Hematoma	• Surgical evacuation if symptomatic
Infection	• Empiric broad-spectrum antibiotics • Image-guided aspiration/culture • Specific antibiotics once organisms identified • Surgical washout; removal of foreign material (hardware can usually be left in place during initial management, but may need removal if infection persists)
Spinal cord injury	• High-dose methylprednisolone (controversial) • Blood pressure elevation
Instrumentation misplacement	• Surgical revision if symptomatic
CSF leak	• Bed rest • Lumbar drain • Blood patch • Surgical revision

Spine surgery

- The mainstays of postoperative management of patients after spine surgery include pain control, wound care, and early mobilization with physical therapy (Table 42.5).

Carotid revascularization

- Carotid stenosis can be surgically treated with either carotid endarterectomy (CEA) or carotid artery stenting (CAS).
- Postoperative complications following CEA include arteriotomy dehiscence with neck hematoma formation, stroke, TIA, seizures, cerebral hyperperfusion syndrome, and cranial nerve injury. See Table 42.6.

CLINICAL PEARLS

- The treatment of neurosurgical postoperative complications should be rapid.
- Subarachnoid hemorrhage patients can have many reasons for postoperative neurologic decline, including hydrocephalus, seizure, and vasospasm. It is important to determine the diagnosis because the treatments vary.
- Patients who develop bleeding or swelling after posterior fossa surgery are at risk for rapid decline and there should be a low threshold to bring a patient back to operating room if new symptoms of mass effect develop.
- Patients with Cushing's disease are at risk for Addisonian crisis after successful surgery and should be treated immediately with intravenous steroids.

Section 5: Special populations
Pregnancy

- Neurosurgery on pregnant patients is feasible in both the second and third trimesters.
- It is important that the obstetrician is closely involved to perform both pre- and postoperative prenatal ultrasound to assess the fetus.
- Teratogenic medications, X-ray, and CT should be avoided whenever possible in pregnant patients.

Table 42.6 Management of complications following early post-carotid endarterectomy (CEA) and post-carotid artery stenting (CAS).

Condition	Management
Early post-carotid endarterectomy	
Transient focal deficit	• CT head to rule out hemorrhage • Angiogram to assess for occlusion • Return to OR if occlusion seen
Fixed deficit	• Immediate return to OR (without obtaining further imaging)
Disruption of arteriotomy	• This potentially fatal complication can be recognized by a rapidly expanding neck mass and respiratory distress • Open wound, evacuate clot, attempt to clamp artery • Intubate • Return to OR
Early post-carotid artery stenting	
Groin hematoma	• Manual pressure
Hypotension	• Hold antihypertensives except beta-blockers
New focal deficit	• IV bolus of glycoprotein IIb/IIIa inhibitor
Arterial occlusion	• Angiogram • Clot retrieval
ICH	• Reduce blood pressure • Discontinue and reverse antiplatelet medications • Consider surgical evacuation for large symptomatic ICH
Reperfusion syndrome	• Reduce blood pressure • Treatment based on manifestation (seizure, deficit, headache, hemorrhage)

Children

- While adults undergoing cranial surgery rarely lose enough blood to require transfusion, this is not true for pediatric patients (especially those in the first few years of life).
- This is an important consideration, for example, in young children undergoing craniosynostosis surgery, who may need multiple pre- and postoperative transfusions.

Elderly

- It is common that elderly patients experience altered mental status in the days to weeks after surgery.
- In elderly patients, metabolic causes of altered mental status are common and should be addressed.

Section 6: Prognosis

BOTTOM LINE/CLINICAL PEARLS
- While the goal is always to avoid postoperative complications, some will occur despite optimal preventive measures and operative technique.
- Consistent screening, rapid diagnosis, and prompt treatment can help minimize long-term sequelae from neurosurgical complications.

Section 7: Reading list

Key reading sources for this chapter can be found online at www.mountsinaiexpertguides.com

Section 8: Guidelines

Title	Source	Weblink
Guidelines for the management of aneurysmal subarachnoid hemorrhage: a statement for healthcare professionals from a special writing group of the Stroke Council, American Heart Association	American Heart Association (AHA), 2009	http://stroke.ahajournals.org/content/40/3/994.extract
Guidelines for the management of spontaneous intracerebral hemorrhage	American Heart Association/American Stroke Association, 2015	http://stroke.ahajournals.org/content/early/2015/05/28/STR.0000000000000069
Decompressive craniectomy for space occupying hemispheric and cerebellar ischemic strokes: Swiss recommendations	Swiss Working Group of Cerebrovascular Diseases with the Swiss Society of Neurosurgery and the Swiss Society of Intensive Care Medicine, 2009	http://www.ncbi.nlm.nih.gov/pubmed/19659825
Practice parameter: anticonvulsant prophylaxis in patients with newly diagnosed brain tumors	American Academy of Neurology, 2000	http://www.ncbi.nlm.nih.gov/pubmed/10822423
The role of steroids in the management of brain metastases: a systematic review and evidence-based clinical practice guideline	Ryken TC, McDermott M, Robinson PD, et al., 2010	http://www.ncbi.nlm.nih.gov/pubmed/19957014
Pharmacological therapy for acute spinal cord injury	Hurlbert RJ, Hadley MN, Walters BC, et al., 2013	http://www.ncbi.nlm.nih.gov/pubmed/23417182

Section 9: Evidence for therapies

Type of evidence	Title and comment	Weblink
Class IIb, Level B	Guidelines for the management of aneurysmal subarachnoid hemorrhage: a statement for healthcare professionals from a special writing group of the Stroke Council, American Heart Association, 2009 **Comment**: The administration of prophylactic anticonvulsants may be considered in the immediate post-hemorrhagic period	http://www.ncbi.nlm.nih.gov/pubmed/19164800
Class III, Level B	Bederson, 2009 **Comment**: The routine long-term use of anticonvulsants is not recommended	http://www.ncbi.nlm.nih.gov/pubmed/19164800
Class IIa, Level B	Bederson, 2009 **Comment**: Ventriculostomy can be beneficial in patients with ventriculomegaly and diminished level of consciousness after acute SAH	http://www.ncbi.nlm.nih.gov/pubmed/19164800

Type of evidence	Title and comment	Weblink
Class IIa, Level B	Bederson, 2009 **Comment**: The use of fludrocortisone acetate and hypertonic saline is reasonable for correcting hyponatremia	http://www.ncbi.nlm.nih.gov/pubmed/19164800
Class I, Level A	Bederson, 2009 **Comment**: Oral nimodipine is indicated to reduce poor outcome related to aneurysmal SAH	http://www.ncbi.nlm.nih.gov/pubmed/19164800
Class IIa, Level B	Bederson, 2009 **Comment**: One approach to symptomatic cerebral vasospasm is volume expansion, induction of hypertension, and hemodilution (triple-H therapy)	http://www.ncbi.nlm.nih.gov/pubmed/19164800
Class IIb, Level B	Bederson, 2009 **Comment**: Cerebral angioplasty and/or selective intra-arterial vasodilator therapy may be considered after, together with, or in the place of triple-H therapy, depending on the clinical scenario	
Class I, Level B	Guidelines for the management of spontaneous intracerebral hemorrhage: a guideline for healthcare professionals from the American Heart Association/American Stroke Association, 2010 **Comment**: Patients with cerebellar hemorrhage who are deteriorating neurologically or who have brainstem compression and/or hydrocephalus from ventricular obstruction should undergo surgical removal of the hemorrhage as soon as possible. Initial treatment of these patients with ventricular drainage alone rather than surgical evacuation is not recommended	http://www.ncbi.nlm.nih.gov/pubmed/20651276
Class III, Level C	Decompressive craniectomy for space-occupying hemispheric and cerebellar ischemic strokes: Swiss recommendations **Comment**: Indications for decompressive craniectomy include neurologic signs of brainstem compression, mass effect on imaging, and exclusion of other causes of impaired consciousness	http://www.ncbi.nlm.nih.gov/pubmed/?term=michel+2009+decompressive
Level II, Guideline	Practice parameter: anticonvulsant prophylaxis in patients with newly diagnosed brain tumors. Report of the Quality Standards Subcommittee of the American Academy of Neurology, 2000 **Comment**: In patients with brain tumors undergoing craniotomy, prophylactic AEDs may be used, and if there has been no seizure, it is appropriate to taper off AEDs starting 1 week postop	http://www.ncbi.nlm.nih.gov/pubmed/10822423
Level III	The role of steroids in the management of brain metastases: a systematic review and evidence-based clinical practice guideline, 2010 **Comment**: Corticosteroids are recommended to provide temporary symptomatic relief of CNS symptoms related to increased intracranial pressure and edema secondary to brain metastases	http://www.ncbi.nlm.nih.gov/pubmed/?term=ryken+2010+steroid

(Continued)

Type of evidence	Title and comment	Weblink
Class I	Pharmacological therapy for acute spinal cord injury, 2013 **Comment**: A variety of Class III medical evidence has been published supporting the neuroprotective effect of methylprednisolone (MP) in SCI	http://www.ncbi.nlm.nih.gov/pubmed/23417182
Class I	Hurlbert, 2013 **Comment**: Both consistent and compelling Class I, II, and III medical evidence exists suggesting that high-dose MP administration is associated with a variety of complications including infection, respiratory compromise, GI hemorrhage, and death	http://www.ncbi.nlm.nih.gov/pubmed/23417182

Section 10: Images

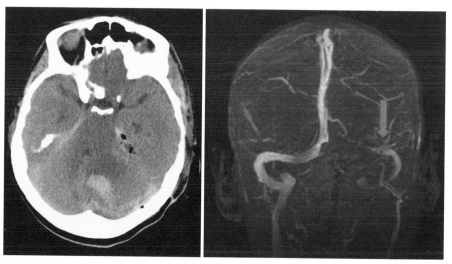

Figure 42.1 A middle-aged man who deteriorated on postoperative day 2 after resection of a left-sided cerebellopontine angle meningioma. CT head (left) revealed cerebellar hemorrhage, fourth ventricular compression, hydrocephalus, and brainstem compression. MRV (right) revealed a disruption of the left transverse sinus that likely led to a venous infarction of the left cerebellum.

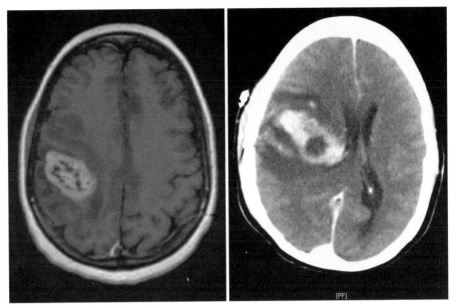

Figure 42.2 An elderly man who underwent a right-sided craniotomy for a partial resection of a glioblastoma multiforme (GBM; left). The patient presented 5 days after surgery with worsening left-sided hemiparesis and mental status, and was found to have worsening edema and hemorrhage within the residual tumor (right).

Additional material for this chapter can be found online at: www.mountsinaiexpertguides.com

This includes a case study (including multiple choice questions) and a reading list.

Index

Page numbers in **italics** denote figures, those in **bold** denote tables.

Mount Sinai Expert Guides: Neurology, First Edition. Edited by Stuart C. Sealfon, Rajeev Motiwala, and Charles B. Stacy.
© 2016 John Wiley & Sons, Ltd. Published 2016 by John Wiley & Sons, Ltd.
Companion website: www.mountsinaiexpertguides.com